Low Back Pain:
A Symptom-Based Approach
to Diagnosis and Treatment

Low Back Pain: A Symptom-Based Approach to Diagnosis and Treatment

Karen S. Rucker, M.D.

Professor and Chair (Retired) of Physical Medicine and Rehabilitation,
Virginia Commonwealth University School of Medicine, Richmond

Andrew J. Cole, M.D.

Assistant Clinical Professor, Department of Rehabilitation Medicine, University of
Washington, Seattle; Medical Director, The Spine Center at Overlake Hospital and
Medical Center, Bellevue, Washington; Private Practice, Northwest Spine and
Sports Physicians, Bellevue

Stuart M. Weinstein, M.D.

Clinical Associate Professor, Department of Rehabilitation Medicine, University of
Washington, Seattle; Private Practice, Puget Sound Sports and Spine Physicians, Seattle

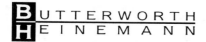

Boston   Oxford   Auckland   Johannesburg   Melbourne   New Delhi

Every effort has been made to ensure that the drug dosage schedules within this text are accurate and conform to standards accepted at time of publication. However, as treatment recommendations vary in the light of continuing research and clinical experience, the reader is advised to verify drug dosage schedules herein with information found on product information sheets. This is especially true in cases of new or infrequently used drugs.

 Recognizing the importance of preserving what has been written, Butterworth–Heinemann prints its books on acid-free paper whenever possible.

 Butterworth–Heinemann supports the efforts of American Forests and the Global ReLeaf program in its campaign for the betterment of trees, forests, and our environment.

Library of Congress Cataloging-in-Publication Data
Low back pain : a symptom-based approach to diagnosis and treatment / [edited by]
Karen S. Rucker, Andrew J. Cole, Stuart M. Weinstein.
    p. ; cm.
  Includes bibliographical references and index.
  ISBN 0-7506-9485-8
  1. Backache. I. Rucker, Karen S. II. Cole, Andrew J., 1958– III. Weinstein, Stuart M.
  [DNLM: 1. Low Back Pain—diagnosis. 2. Low Back Pain—therapy. WE 755 L9125 2001]
  RD771.B217 L6845 2001
  617.5'64—dc21

                                                                        00-036007

British Library Cataloguing-in-Publication Data
A catalogue record for this book is available from the British Library.

The publisher offers special discounts on bulk orders of this book.
For information, please contact:

Manager of Special Sales
Butterworth–Heinemann
225 Wildwood Avenue
Woburn, MA 01801-2041
Tel: 781-904-2500
Fax: 781-904-2620

For information on all Butterworth–Heinemann publications available,
contact our World Wide Web home page at: http://www.bh.com

10 9 8 7 6 5 4 3 2 1

Printed in the United States of America

Contents

Contributing Authors

Venu Akuthota, M.D.
Clinical Instructor of Physical Medicine and Rehabilitation, Northwestern University Medical School, Chicago; Attending Physiatrist, Center for Spine, Sports, and Occupational Rehabilitation, The Rehabilitation Institute of Chicago

Paul A. Anderson, M.D.
Clinical Associate Professor of Orthopaedic Surgery, University of Washington, Seattle

Steven J. Anderson, M.D.
Clinical Professor of Pediatrics, University of Washington and Children's Hospital and Regional Medical Center, Seattle

Mark R. Bookhout, M.S., P.T.
Adjunct Associate Professor of Physical Medicine and Rehabilitation, College of Osteopathic Medicine, Michigan State University, East Lansing; President, Physical Therapy Orthopaedic Specialists, Inc., Minneapolis

Marla M. Bookhout, M.S., P.T.
Guest Lecturer, Department of Physical Therapy, University of Minnesota and College of St. Catherine's, Minneapolis; Physical Therapist, Physical Therapy Orthopaedic Specialists, Inc., Minneapolis

Susan J. Dreyer, M.D.
Assistant Professor of Orthopaedics and Physical Medicine and Rehabilitation, Emory University and Emory Spine Center, Atlanta

Paul Dreyfuss, M.D.
Clinical Associate Professor of Rehabilitation Medicine, University of Texas Health Science Center, San Antonio; ETMC Neurological Institute, Spine Specialists, Tyler, Texas

Michael Giovanniello, M.D.
Attending Physician, Physical Medicine and Rehabilitation, The Ohio State University Medical Center, Columbus

R. Norman Harden, M.D.
Associate Professor of Physical Medicine and Rehabilitation, Northwestern University, Chicago; Director, Center for Pain Studies, Rehabilitation Institute of Chicago

Ernest W. Johnson, M.D.
Professor of Physical Medicine and Rehabilitation, The Ohio State University, Columbus

A. John Kuta, M.D.
Staff Neuroradiologist, Radiology Associates of Richmond, Inc., Henrico Doctors' Hospital, Richmond, Virginia

Fred J. Laine, M.D.
Associate Professor of Radiology and Otolaryngology, Department of Diagnostic Radiology, Virginia Commonwealth University School of Medicine, Richmond

William S. Pease, M.D.
Associate Professor and Chairperson of Physical Medicine and Rehabilitation, The Ohio State University, Columbus; Medical Director of Dodd Hall Rehabilitation Center, The Ohio State University Medical Center, Columbus

Robert H. Perkins, M.D.
Resident in Physical Medicine and Rehabilitation, The Ohio State University Medical Center, Columbus

Hubert L. Rosomoff, M.D., D.Med.Sc., F.A.A.P.M.
Professor and Chairman Emeritus of Neurological Surgery, University of Miami School of Medicine, Miami; Medical Director and Vice Chairman of Florida Pain Management Commission, Comprehensive Pain and Rehabilitation Center at South Shore Hospital and Medical Center, Miami Beach

Renee Steele Rosomoff, B.S.N., M.B.A, C.R.C., C.D.M.S., C.R.R.N.
Adjunct Associate Professor of Neurological Surgery and Anesthesiology, University of Miami School of Medicine and School of Nursing, Miami; Programs Director, Comprehensive Pain and Rehabilitation Center at South Shore Hospital and Medical Center, Miami Beach

Karen S. Rucker, M.D.
Professor and Chair (Retired) of Physical Medicine and Rehabilitation, Virginia Commonwealth University School of Medicine, Richmond

Steven H. Sanders, Ph.D.
Clinical Professor of Physical Medicine and Rehabilitation, University of Tennessee College of Medicine, Chattanooga; Director of Center for Pain Rehabilitation, Siskin Hospital for Physical Rehabilitation, Chattanooga

Aloysia L. Schwabe, M.D.
Fellow in Physical Medicine and Rehabilitation, Baylor College of Medicine, Houston

David J. Tauben, M.D.
Clinical Associate Professor of Medicine, University of Washington School of Medicine, Seattle; Active and Consulting Staff, Swedish Hospital Medical Center and Providence Hospital Medical Center, Seattle

Robert G. Viere, M.D.
Clinical Assistant Professor of Orthopaedic Surgery, University of Texas Southwestern Medical Center, Dallas; Staff Physician, Baylor Spine Center, Baylor University Medical Center, Dallas

Michael D. West, Ph.D.
Assistant Professor, Rehabilitation Research and Training Center on Supported Employment, Virginia Commonwealth University, Richmond

Stuart E. Willick, M.D.
Assistant Professor of Physical Medicine and Rehabilitation, University of Utah, Salt Lake City

Preface

From the start, the concept of this book has been to present a unique approach to a common problem: low back pain. The plan was twofold: first, to re-emphasize the clinical assessment, namely symptoms and signs, as the foundation of the diagnostic process and functional rehabilitation plan, and second, to assemble a group of authors whose cumulative clinical experience would exemplify the art, as well as the science, of medicine.

The journey from the initial idea to this final product has taken a great deal of time and effort but has been very gratifying. Many thanks are due to those who demonstrated patience and perseverance. Special thanks to Karen Oberheim, Senior Medical Editor, who inherited this project in its early stages from a previous publishing house and rekindled the fire. And thanks to all the authors who at the time had to respond to a rather demanding editorial pen; Thank you for both your flexibility when necessary and your steadfastness when appropriate.

Many expert clinicians have contributed to this book, and the reader will greatly benefit from their pearls and wisdom. However, this is not a cookbook or a step-by-step guide; rather, this book should serve as a stepping stone to enhance one's practical understanding and management of patients with low back pain. So read, learn, and criticize, but most of all, enjoy!

K.S.R.
A.J.C.
S.M.W.

PART I

Low Back Pain:
A Symptom-Based Approach

Chapter 1
Adolescent Lumbar Spine Disorders

Steven J. Anderson

When compared to adults, back pain in adolescents is less frequent, has different causes, different treatments, and different outcomes. As a result, any comfort that comes from familiarity and practice in dealing with adult back pain is not sufficient to deal with adolescent back pain.

Low back pain in the adolescent patient should always raise suspicion for the possibility of serious underlying medical pathology. Even when serious or life-threatening conditions are ruled out, a careful clinical evaluation usually reveals a specific physical or mechanical cause for back pain.

This chapter discusses the various ways in which problems originating in the lumbar spine may present clinically. By learning to identify and follow the trail of back-related complaints, progress toward an accurate diagnosis can be made. Identifying the pathway to back pain can also help plan treatment that not only relieves symptoms but also disrupts the cycle of continued pain.

Back pain in adolescents can present suddenly or gradually, with acute or repetitive trauma, and in previously healthy or ill individuals. Back pain may be constant or associated only with specific activities. Back pain can be confined to the back or can radiate to the extremities. Some problems originating in the spine may present with no back pain, and some spine problems may present with pain that occurs in areas other than the back. Back pain in young people can be due to conditions unique to skeletal immaturity or can be due to conditions in which skeletal immaturity is not a factor. Back pain can be amplified with psychological stresses, but is rarely due to psychological factors alone. A given symptom complex may be due to more than one underlying etiology, and a specific spine problem may manifest as more than one symptom complex. The clinical value of any symptom, physical finding, or test result is largely dependent on how it fits into a larger clinical context.

By recognizing the presentations of common back problems, the clinician can better determine when rare or exceptional cases require further consideration. Early recognition of unusual cases permits a more selective allocation of diagnostic resources and use of subspecialty consultants. By recognizing symptom patterns, related findings from physical examination and radiologic evaluation can be interpreted and integrated in an appropriate clinical context.

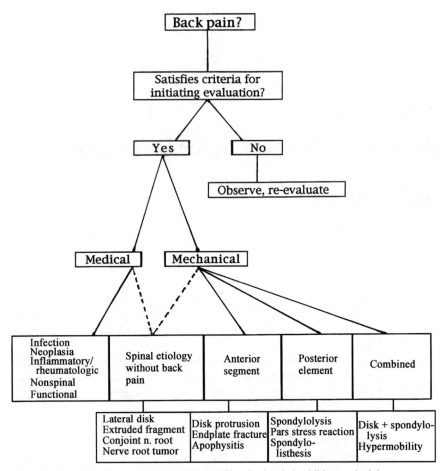

Figure 1.1 Algorithm for categorizing etiology of low back pain in children and adolescents.

BACK PAIN BREAKDOWN

An algorithm for evaluating and categorizing the various causes of back pain in young people is shown in Figure 1.1. Once it has been determined that an evaluation is indicated, the first question in this analysis is whether the back pain is medical or mechanical. Medical causes of back pain include infections, neoplastic processes, inflammatory conditions, or back pain originating from nonspinal conditions. Although medical causes are rare, they represent a disproportionate number of the more serious, or even life-threatening, causes of back pain. Mechanical back pain may be due to acute trauma, repetitive trauma, postural abnormalities, structural variations, biomechanical abnormalities, or a combination of these factors.

If back pain follows a mechanical pattern, the next question relates to the portion of the spine that is acting as a pain generator. Anterior segment pain usually stems from an injury or abnormality in the vertebral body, the vertebral end plate, or the intervertebral disk. Posterior element pain in young people usually stems from abnormalities in the facet joints or the pars interarticularis.

The following discussion shows how a symptom-based analysis can trace the etiology of back pain in the adolescent patient. The keys to differentiating medical versus mechanical and anterior segment versus posterior element back pain are emphasized. Particular attention is focused on symptoms that indicate serious underlying medical pathology, as well as the symptoms or symptom complexes that indicate common conditions. Symptoms that indicate a medical (rather than mechanical) etiology of back pain, or symptoms that deviate from known or common patterns, are good indicators that the standard clinical evaluation for back pain should be modified or expanded.

When to Initiate a Clinical Evaluation

Even before the question of medical versus mechanical back pain can be addressed, one must first determine who should be evaluated and when. Although back pain in young people should always be taken seriously, not every back pain complaint warrants a formal medical evaluation. On the other hand, there are some characteristics of a back pain complaint that should prompt an earlier investigation. More immediate evaluation is indicated when back pain develops after major physical trauma, when back pain is associated with spinal cord or neurologic dysfunction, or when back pain restricts activities of daily living. Back pain that occurs with fever, systemic illness, or is rapidly progressive also warrants earlier medical attention. If back pain is associated with a visible spinal deformity, there is little reason to delay the evaluation. Finally, a clinical evaluation is justified for any back pain that has persisted for more than 2 weeks or is unresponsive to standard home therapies (e.g., ice, heat, massage, or nonprescription analgesic or anti-inflammatory medications).

Medical Back Pain

Back pain may be due to medical conditions that directly involve the spine or nonspinal medical conditions in which back pain occurs secondarily. Inflammatory conditions, such as infectious and neoplastic conditions, may cause back pain by direct involvement of the musculoskeletal structures (bones, joints, muscles, intervertebral disks) or neurologic structures (spinal cord, nerve roots, meninges). Rheumatologic disorders may cause back pain due to direct inflammatory effects on the spine or associated structures such as the sacroiliac joints.

Back pain may accompany problems that originate outside of the musculoskeletal system. Problems in the kidney, ureters, liver, gallbladder, esophagus, intestines, and pancreas can all refer to the back. Similarly, abnormalities of the heart, great vessels (including thoracic and abdominal aorta), the lungs, and the pleura may cause back pain. Many excellent references discuss the diagnosis and management of medical conditions that cause back pain. The emphasis in this chapter is to correctly recognize a medical cause of back pain. Because the approach to medical back pain differs so greatly from the approach to structural and mechanical causes of back pain, an early distinction is critical for the evaluation process to follow the correct investigative pathway.

Characteristics of a medical cause of back pain include pain that follows or develops concurrently with an illness. The presence of constitutional symptoms, including fever, sweats, chills, malaise, weight loss, or anorexia, suggests underlying medical pathology, as does jaundice, iritis, skin rashes, mouth sores, chronic cough, or swollen, erythematous joints. Back pain in an adolescent with menstrual irregularities or weight gain should raise suspicion for intrauterine or ectopic pregnancy. Unlike mechanical back pain, medical back pain is more likely to be independent of posture, activity, or injury history. Back pain that cannot be relieved by rest or changes in position, occurs at night, or disrupts sleep is more likely to be medical in origin.

The evaluation of every patient with low back pain should include a medical review of systems that addresses the organ systems, abnormalities, and disease processes that can cause back pain. Positive findings should be correlated with back symptoms to establish if a temporal or a causal relationship exists. The purpose of this initial evaluation is to determine if sufficient evidence for a medical problem exists to warrant further medical investigation. A more detailed medical evaluation, with radiologic and laboratory studies, is usually required to reach a specific diagnosis. With effective historical screening, the number of young individuals requiring more extensive and more costly medical evaluations can be minimized.

Mechanical Back Pain

Mechanical back pain implies that the pain originates from the effects of acute or repetitive loading to structural elements of the spine. The loading may come from excessive loads to normal spinal structures or from normal loads to a spine with abnormal spinal structure. The loads transmitted to the spine can be influenced by factors such as posture, body mechanics, and trunk strength, as well as flexibility and strength in the muscles of the pelvic girdle and lower extremities. The effects of acute or repetitive loading can compromise the spine's capacity to handle subsequent demands and can lead to progressive breakdown. Because of the interdependence of bony and soft tissue elements of the spine, injury or compromise of one component of the spinal mechanism can have consequences that extend beyond the site of the original problem.

The choice to pursue an investigative pathway of mechanical back pain depends on first ruling out a medical pattern, and then identifying a pattern of symptoms that can be explained mechanically. In general, mechanical back pain occurs in otherwise healthy individuals who have a history of acute or repetitive trauma that can be related to their symptoms. A recent change or increase in activity—particularly activity that involves lifting, bending, twisting, or hyperextension—may accompany the onset of mechanical back pain. Injuries or dysfunction in the lower extremities may precede a mechanical back problem because changes in flexibility, strength, or gait may alter spinal mechanics or place additional demands on the spine.

Mechanical back pain is usually worse with specific positions or activities and can be relieved by other specific positions or activities. If a position of complete pain relief cannot be found, the symptoms of mechanical back pain should still follow a gradient whereby some positions are clearly better than others. This position-dependent symptom gradient is not seen as frequently with medical back pain.

Finally, the distribution of symptoms for mechanical back pain should follow a pattern consistent with known referral patterns for the structures most commonly injured. Pain coming from an injured disk, facet joint, or nerve root should follow a pattern compatible with injuries to the structure in question. If the timing and distribution of symptoms do not follow a pattern that can be attributed to any of the commonly injured structures, further inquiry into nonmechanical causes of back pain should take place.

Anterior Segment versus Posterior Element Pain

If a pattern of mechanical back pain has been identified, the next question relates to the structural origin of the pain. The functional unit of the spine is the three-joint complex. This complex includes the intervertebral disk joint and the paired facet joints. The vertebrae, vertebral end plates, and the intervertebral disks form an anterior column that functions primarily to support weight. The posterior elements of the spine include the pedicles, lamina, facet joints, pars interarticularis, transverse processes, and spinous processes. The posterior elements, in conjunction with the anterior segments, form a bony canal to protect the spinal cord and nerve roots. The facet joints function primarily to control spinal motion—particularly extension and rotation.

A simple paradigm for understanding mechanical back pain relates to how spinal function and demand are matched. Generally speaking, injury to the load-bearing anterior segments occurs if these structures are subjected to excessive load. Injury to the motion-controlling posterior elements (especially the facet joints and pars interarticularis in young people) occurs with exposure to excessive motion. The less obvious, but potentially more significant, scenario for injury occurs when a load-bearing structure (like an intervertebral disk) is subjected to excessive motion or when a motion-controlling structure (like a facet joint) is subjected to excessive loads. With either of these mismatches, a structure is being asked to perform a task that it was not designed to perform. Injury from mismatches of function and demand is not unusual.

Based on the pathomechanical forces involved and the location of the injured structure, mechanical back pain can be divided into an anterior segment or posterior element pattern. The conditions commonly seen in children and adolescents that follow an anterior segment pattern are intervertebral disk injuries, vertebral end plate fractures, and injuries to the vertebral ring apophysis. Common posterior element conditions include pars interarticularis defects (e.g., pars stress reaction, spondylolysis, spondylolisthesis) and lumbar facet joint injuries. Some conditions follow a mixed pattern in which there is a combination of anterior segment and posterior element symptomatology. Each of these patterns is discussed according to their characteristic symptoms.

Anterior Segment Pain. Anterior segment structures are most likely to be injured from trunk flexion or trunk flexion combined with rotation. Bending forward to lift a heavy weight, pulling against resistance, vertebral compression from a motor vehicle accident, or trunk flexion or rotation from sports activities, such as weight lifting, rowing, football, gymnastics, diving, tennis, and golf, are all common causes of anterior segment pain or injury. In younger or less skeletally mature individuals, the vertebral end plate or the ring apophysis may be more susceptible to injury than the intervertebral disk. As the bones mature, the disk is increasingly susceptible to injury as it becomes the weak link.

Low back pain from injury to anterior segment structures tends to be felt slightly lateral of midline and may extend into the buttock area. If there is nerve root involvement, symptoms may radiate further down the leg. Radicular complaints may be constant or intermittent, may extend distally or remain proximal, and may involve pain, numbness, tingling, burning, weakness, or any combination of these symptoms. The quality of back or leg pain is not usually specific to any given diagnosis. However, symptoms from muscle spasm frequently accompany anterior seg-

Table 1.1 Anterior Segment versus Posterior Element Pain Pattern

	Anterior Segment	Posterior Element
Stand	—	+
Walk	—	++
Run	—	+++
Sit	++	—
Bend forward	+++	—
Bend backward	—	+++
Twist	++	++
Lift	+++	—
Carry	++	—
Cough/sneeze/strain	++	—
Lie prone	—	++
Lie supine	++	—

+ = increases symptoms; ++ = significantly increases symptoms; +++ = maximally increases symptoms.

ment problems and may be the primary complaint. Muscle spasm can be associated with additional symptoms of cramping, stiffness, achiness, or fatigue. Muscle spasm is usually a response to an injury, not the primary cause. Nonetheless, muscle spasms or muscle strains are often misinterpreted as a diagnosis rather than a symptom.

The pain from an anterior segment problem tends to be more pronounced with postures or activities that cause loading to anterior segment structures (Table 1.1). For anterior segment problems, sitting is typically worse than standing; bending forward (trunk flexion) is worse than bending backward (trunk extension); lying supine is worse than lying prone. Tying a shoe or pulling on a sock can be painful, as can be sitting in a soft chair. Anterior segment pain tends to be worse with anything that increases intra-abdominal pressure such as coughing, sneezing, or straining. Changing positions can increase pain—particularly getting in or out of a car, getting out of a low chair, or even getting out of bed.

Anterior segment pain can usually be relieved by shifting the load to a nonpainful structure. With acutely injured disks, patients may literally shift to one side as they attempt to move away from the locus of pain. The acute onset of painful "scoliosis" or the patient's inability to reach an upright posture may be a compensation for an injured anterior segment structure. Idiopathic scoliosis is not typically a source of back pain, nor does the deformity from this condition develop acutely. A painful compensatory shift should not be confused with scoliosis, and a diagnosis of scoliosis should not be used to explain an acutely painful back.

A more subtle strategy to relieve a painful anterior segment structure is standing. Standing or extending the spine preferentially puts more load on the facet joints. Relief may also come from lying in a prone position, lying sideways, or lying supine with the knees and hips flexed. Traction or distraction forces may also help to reduce pain from anterior segment injury.

Patients with anterior segment back pain often report that their symptoms are paradoxically worse while sitting or resting and better when they are up and moving. Even some forms of strenuous exercise, such as running, may be relatively well tolerated by patients with anterior segment problems. Because muscle strength and endurance is critical for modulating stress on anterior segment structures, it is not unusual for patients to report that their back pain is worse when they are inactive or deconditioned and better when they exercise regularly.

The physical findings in a patient with an anterior segment injury are easily predicted from the symptoms. Patients may be found standing or lying down in the examination room and may have a visibly shifted posture when trying to stand upright. Range of motion tends to be painful and restricted going forward (trunk flexion) or when trying to correct a compensatory shift. Lumbar extension is often normal and may be associated with relief of pain. When there is pressure on a nerve root, dural tension signs may be present. Nerve root irritation may be accompanied by changes in sensation, strength, or deep tendon reflexes. Lower grades of radicular involvement may produce referred pain with a distinct lack of tenderness or other local findings at the site where the pain is perceived.

Palpation often has limited value in the physical examination for anterior segment injuries. The injured structures cannot be readily palpated, and the structures that are tender with palpation are usually not the source of the problem. Nonetheless, palpation can help rule out conditions in the differential diagnosis, including posterior element injuries, sacroiliac abnormalities, sacral or coccygeal abnormalities, and apophyseal avulsions along the iliac crest or ischium. When pain is referred, the absence of palpable swelling, tenderness, or spasm in the area of concern can help rule out a local injury. Tenderness over the sciatic notch or pyriformis may be an exception to this generalization. Tenderness or palpable spasm in these areas is commonly seen with disk injuries but usually does not indicate local muscle injury.

Radiographic studies can confirm the degree of skeletal maturation and help identify injuries to the vertebral body, including vertebral wedging and end plate irregularities. Disk space narrowing is rarely found in pediatric patients—even those with known disk injuries. Bone scans can help identify the presence of more subtle bony injuries or confirm if a given radiographic finding is an injury or an asymptomatic anatomic variation. Magnetic resonance imaging is most useful to confirm suspected soft tissue injuries such as an intervertebral disk protrusion.

Treatment for anterior segment problems is geared toward the relief of symptoms and the restoration of normal spinal function. Rest or traction, or both, can reduce injury-producing stresses on the affected structure. After acute pain has subsided, therapeutic exercise can help restore normal segmental motion, optimize flexibility in the hips and lower extremities, build trunk strength, and restore normal body mechanics. Bracing may be indicated for fractures or injuries associated with spinal deformity. Surgical consultation is warranted for patients with painful deformities; persistent or progressive neurologic deficits, or both; or pain refractory to conservative treatment. Rehabilitation of the spine should also include treatment of any predisposing conditions, including injuries or dysfunction in the lower extremities.

Posterior Element Pain.   Injuries to the posterior elements produce symptoms that are distinct from anterior segment problems. In young people, the facet joints and the pars interarticularis are the most commonly injured posterior element structures. Lumbar extension, or extension combined with rotation, can cause injury by producing excessive loads to structures designed primarily to control motion.

In patients with a hyperlordotic posture, the cumulative stresses of normal daily activity may be sufficient to produce posterior element pain. More commonly, physical activities or sports that require forceful or repetitive lumbar extension cause injury. Despite the amount of impact involved, running and jumping tend to be more stressful to the posterior elements than the anterior segments. Running with a long stride, running down hill, or running on hard surfaces with inadequate shock absorption can contribute to a posterior element injury. Extreme lumbar extension occurs by design with activities such as ballet, gymnastics, figure skating, and diving. Tennis, throwing sports, football, and soccer involve intermittent maximal extension and frequent submaximal stresses to the posterior elements. Some of these same sports can also cause anterior segment injury, but have this effect through mechanisms that are distinct from those that cause posterior element injury.

In the skeletally immature patient, the pars interarticularis is more susceptible to injury than the facet joint, although symptoms from injury to the two structures may be indistinguishable. A congenital pars defect, or spondylolysis, may become symptomatic from extension stresses. Similarly, an intact pars may develop a fatigue fracture or pars stress reaction from the same extension forces. If a pain from the pars interarticularis has been ruled out, injury to other posterior element structures can be considered. Facet joint pain may be seen in patients with segmental hypermobility. Anatomic variations such as facet tropism or a transitional vertebra may contribute to uneven facet loading and a greater likelihood of injury. Pedicle fractures and stress fractures produce a posterior element pain pattern, as do other pathologic processes in the pedicle such as an osteoid osteoma.

Pain from injury to a posterior element structure tends to be localized to the area of the affected structure and is less likely to radiate than anterior segment injuries. When radicular symptoms do occur with posterior element injuries, one should suspect spondylolisthesis or a bony abnormality creating stenosis in the neuroforamen. The quality of posterior element pain is nonspecific but may occasionally be characterized as sharp or pinching. Generalized muscle spasm may be reported, but a localized area of tightness may be more commonly noted.

Posterior element pain is usually worse with standing, walking, back extension, or lying in a prone position (see Table 1.1). Pain may be relieved by sitting, bending forward, or even slouching. Curling up in a knee-to-chest position can also provide relief. Activities of daily living are less likely to be adversely affected by a posterior element condition than an anterior segment problem. However, it may be more difficult to find aerobic activities or sports that can be tolerated with a posterior element injury because many of these activities involve repetitive stresses to the posterior elements.

The physical findings in a patient with a posterior element injury may reflect both the cause and the consequences of his or her problem. A hyperlordotic posture, tight hip flexors, and weak abdominal muscles combine to increase the demands and decrease protection to the posterior elements. The consequences of posterior element injury usually lead to restricted or painful lumbar extension with normal, pain-free lumbar flexion. A standing one-legged extension test is frequently positive on the side ipsilateral to a symptomatic spondylolysis. Because lumbar extension decreases tension on most back muscles, pain produced with active or passive extension can help convince the patient and the physician that the pain is not due to a strained muscle. The physical examination should also evaluate lower extremity flexibility because leg and hip flexibility determines pelvic position, as well as how much the hip and pelvis contribute to overall trunk flexion, extension, or rotation.

A neurologic examination to evaluate reflexes, sensation, and strength should be performed on any patient with pain, numbness, or weakness, or any combination of these symptoms, in their extremities. Referred pain or neurologic abnormalities are seen less frequently with posterior element problems than anterior segment problems.

The posterior elements are more accessible to palpation than the anterior segments. It is possible to assess alignment of the spinous processes, tenderness over the spinous processes or interspinous ligaments, and the presence of a step-off with spondylolisthesis. The laminae, pars interarticularis, facet joints, and transverse processes cannot be directly palpated, but the injured or abnormal spinal segment can usually be identified in a lean patient. Patients with posterior element injuries are less likely to have spasm or tenderness in the sciatic notch or along the pyriformis. Tenderness in the hip flexors is unlikely to be seen as a direct result of a posterior element injury but may be part of a separate injury that contributes to increased lordosis and increased loading on the posterior elements.

Plain radiographs of the lumbar spine are a useful component in the evaluation of posterior element pain in the adolescent. The 4-view spine series (anteroposterior, lateral, and obliques) can reveal spondylolytic defects, bony abnormalities of the spinous processes, transverse processes, facet joint, and pedicles. Because symptomatic pars defects are not always radiographically apparent, scintigraphy with a single photon emission computed tomography (SPECT) scan may add diagnostic sensitivity and specificity to the radiologic workup. A SPECT scan can also help determine if a visible defect in the pars interarticularis is acute and can help identify symptomatic abnormalities to the pars, the facets, the lamina, the pedicle, or the spinous and transverse processes. Computed tomography can help define complex bony abnormalities and can be used to monitor bony healing in spondylolysis.

Treatment for posterior element problems varies with the specific diagnosis as well as the pathomechanical factors in the injury. The unifying themes in treatment for all posterior element problems include correction of hyperlordotic postures and improvement of abdominal strength and trunk stability. Correction of hyperlordosis may require flexibility exercises for the hip flexors and lumbodorsal fascia as well as strengthening of the hamstrings, hip extensors, and the abdominals.

When posterior element pain is due to an acute bony injury or a pars lesion accompanied by a positive SPECT scan, a period of rest may be necessary before commencing therapeutic exercises. An antilordotic thoracolumbar sacral orthosis, such as a Boston overlap brace, can provide an added level of protection for a young person who needs to reduce stress on posterior element structures by forcing activity restrictions. Bracing is also used for problems of instability with conditions such as spondylolisthesis. Surgical consultation should be considered for instability uncontrolled with conservative measures or any spinal condition with persistent or progressive neurologic compromise.

Combined Anterior Segment and Posterior Element Pain

Because of interdependent anatomy in the three-joint complex, abnormalities affecting one component eventually have consequences for the others. For example, collapse or narrowing of a disk space transmits more load and, potentially, more motion to the facet joints. Conversely, hypermobility in facet joints may allow greater motion or shear stresses at the disk. Facet joint narrowing or subluxation may result in more loading on the disk. The time frame for significant progression of this degenerative cascade usually extends beyond adolescence. Nonetheless, over time, injuries may develop at secondary sites, and the pattern of symptoms may change or evolve accordingly. An anterior segment pain pattern may change to a posterior element pain pattern, or a mixed pattern may develop in which anterior segment and posterior element symptoms exist concurrently.

Patients with a mixed or combined anterior segment and posterior element pattern often have a history of a prior back condition in which the symptoms have evolved into a different pattern. This change may include pain that now occurs in a new area, pain that is brought on by activities that previously were not painful, or pain that can no longer be relieved by strategies that were previously effective. Some patients who have been diagnosed and treated earlier for spondylolysis may start experiencing back pain with sitting, bending, or lifting. Segmental hypermobility from a spondylolysis or spondylolisthesis may subject a disk to excessive motion. When disk degeneration develops in patients with spondylolysis, it is usually at the level of a pars defect.

Another scenario for combined pain patterns is the patient who has concurrent problems in the anterior segments and posterior elements. Adolescents with thoraco-lumbar Scheuermann's disease may have an anterior segment pattern with painful kyphosis, wedged vertebra, and irregular vertebral end plates. The kyphosis proximally in the spine is associated with a compensatory hyperlordosis distally. A facet joint injury or pars stress reaction can cause a posterior element pain pattern in the low back. Therapy for combined injuries is problematic because unloading one painful structure risks shifting the load to another painful structure.

Finally, a combined pattern may be seen in patients who participate in activities that create high demands on both anterior segment and posterior element structures. Ballet dancers, gymnasts, figure skaters, divers, and athletes who participate in football, track and field, and tennis all routinely challenge their spine's ability to withstand loads and control motion. Simultaneous injury to an anterior segment and posterior element structure is unusual, but sequential injuries leading to overlapping symptoms are not.

BACK PROBLEMS THAT DO NOT PRESENT WITH BACK PAIN

A number of problems that originate in the spine may present with symptoms only in an extremity. When a back problem manifests itself with extremity symptoms but no back pain, tracking down the source can be challenging. Extremity pain coming from the back but without back pain is most likely due to pathology in the neuroforamen or the lateral recess. Narrowing or stenosis in this area can result in nerve root compression and symptoms referred in the distribution of the nerve root. Narrowing can be a result of a lateral disk protrusion, an extruded disk fragment, a conjoint nerve root, spondylolisthesis, or tumors (e.g., neurofibroma, meningioma, Schwanomma) involving the nerve root or nerve sheath.

Neuroforaminal narrowing and resultant nerve root irritation may be due to a combination of structural changes and the effects of posture or position. For example, a conjoint nerve root may be asymptomatic until the patient further narrows the neuroforamen by standing or extending the lumbar spine. Similarly, neurologic symptoms from a spondylolisthesis may not occur unless the patient further stretches or compresses the nerve by an activity such as running. Narrowing a neuroforamen to a critical level with movement or activity is often referred to as *dynamic lateral stenosis*. Radicular pain associated with activities known to narrow the neuroforamen may help make a diagnosis of lateral stenosis by history alone.

A patient with fixed or dynamic lateral stenosis may present with symptoms along the course of the sciatic nerve or may only report symptoms distally. A calf strain with tightness or cramping in the calf, but no history of calf injury, may be due to compression of the first sacral (S1) nerve root. Chronic hamstring injuries, without a history of an obvious hamstring strain and without local signs of a hamstring injury (e.g., swelling, tenderness, weakness), may also signal a problem originating in the spine. What may be perceived as a quadriceps strain may be an abnormality affecting the L4 nerve root.

Pain in the posterior portion of the hip may be the most common spine problem mistaken for an extremity problem. Problems originating in the hip joint typically cause groin pain or anterior hip pain that radiates to the medial thigh or knee. Hip abnormalities are usually associated with restrictions of hip range of motion, particularly flexion and internal rotation. Patients may report difficulty walking up stairs, crossing their legs, putting on a shoe, or walking without a limp. Standing, walking, or any weightbearing activity usually worsens symptoms from a hip problem, whereas sitting usually relieves symptoms. Conversely, hip pain due to a spine problem usually occurs posteriorly in the buttocks region, does not limit hip joint range of motion, and does not typically become worse from weightbearing activity. Even if there is no complaint of back pain in this group of patients with posterior hip pain, activities that are known to stress the back may cause more pain than activities that stress the hip.

Correctly diagnosing the source of extremity symptoms originating in the spine, without back symptoms, requires an index of suspicion and familiarity with the clinical findings that support both local and referred origins of the problem. Muscle strains in the calf, hamstring, or buttock area that persist long enough to warrant medical evaluation are usually associated with a specific and memorable injury or event. Patients with muscle strains are expected to have a history of participation in activities in which involved muscles are forcibly stretched or muscles contract in an explosive manner while being stretched. Muscle symptoms that just appear in a sedentary individual are more typical for spine problems than muscle strains. If extremity symptoms are not supported by a good history for an extremity injury, a complete spinal history should be obtained. This should include a history of prior back problems, previous diagnostic studies, treatments for back-related conditions, and any residual impairments. If there is no past or present back complaint, the patient still should be queried as to whether the extremity symptoms are influenced by various stressors to the back. This includes the effects from standing, walking, running, arching, twisting, bending, sitting, lifting, coughing, sneezing, straining, or lying prone or supine.

In some cases, it may be difficult to separate a muscle injury from a spine condition. Tightness in the hamstring that is worse with stretching the hamstring may be due to a muscle injury or tension on the sciatic nerve. In such cases, the mechanism of injury, distribution and timing of symptoms, and the physical examination are crucial to make a clear distinction. Diagnostic studies, such as radiographs or magnetic resonance imaging scans of the spine, may also reveal a source for extremity symptoms in patients who do not complain about their backs.

Treatment for extremity pain originating in the spine depends on establishing a specific diagnosis. Often, a presumed muscle strain that is unresponsive to therapy for a muscle injury is a clue that the muscle symptoms are originating from a remote source. For lateral recess stenosis that has a dynamic component, exercise to prevent hyperlordosis and maintain an open neuroforamen can reduce symptoms. For more fixed lesions, surgical treatment should be considered.

SUMMARY

The symptoms of individual patients with low back pain may not match perfectly with the composite clinical descriptions provided in textbooks. Furthermore, symptom patterns alone are not sufficient to confirm a diagnosis. Despite these limitations, a symptom-based approach to low back pain in adolescents can narrow diagnostic possibilities, permit more selective use of diagnostic procedures and consultants, and can help in the planning and monitoring of rehabilitation. Familiarity with common symptom patterns and their related diagnoses can allow for earlier recognition of the conditions that are unusual or pose greater diagnostic challenges. The ability to diagnose by symptom analysis is not limited by the training of the practitioner or the medical resources available to the patient. A symptom-based approach can enhance the yield of clinical evaluations without enhancing the cost or need for subspecialty input.

RECOMMENDED READINGS

Anderson SJ. Assessment and management of the pediatric and adolescent patient with low back pain. Phys Med Rehabil Clin North Am 1991;3:157–185.

Anderson SJ. Children and Adolescents. In AJ Cole and SA Herring (eds), The Low Back Pain Handbook: A Practical Guide for the Primary Care Physician. Hanley & Belfus, Mosby, 1996, 323–344.

Anderson SJ. Evaluation and treatment of back pain in children and adolescents. J Back Musculoskel Rehabil 1991;1:49–65.

Burton AK, Clarke RD, McClune TD, Tillotson KM. The natural history of low back pain in adolescents. Spine 1996;21:2323–2328.

Duggleby T, Kumar S. Epidemiology of juvenile low back pain: a review. Disabil Rehabil 1997;19:505–512.

Emans JB. Diagnosing the cause of back pain in children and adolescents. J Musculoskel Med 1989;6:46–56.

Harvey J, Tanner S. Low back pain in young athletes: a practical approach. Sports Med 1991;12: 394–406.

Hollingworth P. Back pain in children. Br J Rheumatol 1996;35:1022–1028.

King HA. Back pain in children. Pediatr Clin North Am 1984;31:1083–1095.

Letts M, MacDonald P. Sports injuries to the pediatric spine. Spine: State of the Art Reviews 1990;4:49–83.

Micheli LJ, Wood R. Back pain in young athletes. Significant differences from adults in causes and patterns. Arch Pediatr Adolesc Med 1995;149:15–18.

Rosenblum BR, Rothman AS. Low back pain in children. Mt Sinai J Med 1991;58:115–120.

Salminen JJ, Erikintalo M, Laine M, Pentti J. Low back pain in the young. A prospective 3-year follow-up study of subjects with and without low back pain. Spine 1995;20:2101–2107.

Sherry DD. Musculoskeletal pain in children. Curr Opin Rheumatol 1997;9:465–470.

Sponseller PD. Back pain in children. Curr Opin Pediatr 1994;6:99–103.

Taimela S, Kujala UM, Salminen JJ, Viljanen T. The prevalence of low back pain among children and adolescents. A nationwide, cohort-based questionnaire survey in Finland. Spine 1997;22: 1132–1136.

White JI, Gardner JI, Takeda H. Back pain in the pediatric patient: assessment and differential diagnosis. Spine: State of the Art Reviews 1990;4:1–24.

Chapter 2

The Adult Spine: A Practical Approach to Low Back Pain

Venu Akuthota, Stuart E. Willick, and R. Norman Harden

EPIDEMIOLOGY

Low back pain (LBP) is epidemic in the United States. The annual incidence of back pain has been estimated to be 5%.[1] In fact, 90% of people have LBP at some point in their lives.[2] The 1 month prevalence of LBP is as high as 43% of the population.[3] Furthermore, LBP follows only the common cold as a presenting complaint to primary care physicians.[4]

The cost of LBP is staggering. In the late 1980s, direct and indirect medical costs of LBP were estimated to be $50 billion per year, an amount that grew substantially through the 1990s.[5] Of note, a small number (10–25%) of LBP patients accrue a large percentage (79–95%) of the total cost of total back injury claims.[5–7]

LBP is the leading cause of disability in people younger than age 45 years and the third leading cause of disability in people older than age 45 years. Disability can occur with vocational and avocational activities. Return to work is extremely poor if LBP lingers. The chance of returning to work is 50% if a patient is off work more than 6 months, 25% if off work more than 1 year, and approaches 0% if off work for 2 years or longer.[8] Back pain has also been identified as a frequent problem in many sporting activities, such as gymnastics, football, weight lifting, wrestling, rowing, swimming, golf, tennis, and baseball.[9,10]

The natural history of LBP appears to have been misinterpreted by many health care professionals and the lay public. Although 90% of LBP resolves within the first 6–12 weeks, the rate of recurrence is high.[8,11] In fact, between 70% to 90% of patients have additional episodes of LBP after their initial bout of pain.[11] Long-term studies show that one-third of patients continue to have persistent or intermittent LBP after their initial back pain episode.[12] Reasons for recidivism are multifold. One reason for a high rate of LBP recurrence may be the lack of multifidi muscle recovery after an acute LBP episode.[13] Additionally, patients who do not minimize risk factors may have continued episodes of LBP.

Table 2.1 Potential Pain Generators of the Lumbosacral Spine

Periosteum
Intervertebral disk—outer one-third of the annulus
Facet joint—capsule and ligaments
Sacroiliac joint—capsule and ligaments
Spinal nerve root—anterior dura
Ligaments
Muscles

ANATOMY

A full description of the anatomy of the lumbosacral spine is beyond the scope of this text. There are many excellent texts with a detailed review of the anatomy of the lumbar spine and pelvis.[14–16] Structures of the lumbar spine are conveniently divided into the anterior and posterior elements. The anterior elements consist of the vertebral bodies and the intervertebral disks (IVDs). The IVD has an outer cartilaginous annulus fibrosis, a central gelatinous nucleus pulposus, and sandwiching cartilaginous vertebral end plates. The anterior elements serve to distribute axial compressive loads. The posterior elements consist of the lamina, zygapophyseal joints (z-joints), transverse processes, and spinous processes. The anterior and posterior elements are joined by two pedicles, which are stout pillars of bone connecting the vertebral bodies to the laminae, forming the neural arch. The osseous and disk structures of the vertebral column have limited inherent stability. Static stability is provided by numerous ligaments, whereas dynamic control is provided by the short and long paravertebral musculature.

Any structure innervated by afferent nerve fibers has the potential to be a pain generator (Table 2.1). In addition to innervating the limb musculature, ventral rami of the spinal nerves innervate selected muscles around the spinal axis, including the psoas major and quadratus lumborum. Other paravertebral muscles are innervated by dorsal rami of the spinal nerves. The medial branches of the dorsal rami innervate the z-joints, multifidi, and interspinous ligaments. The sinuvertebral nerves innervate the outer one-third of the posterior annulus fibrosis, the posterior longitudinal ligament, and the ventral dura (Figure 2.1).[14]

The basic functional unit of the spine is the three-joint complex, consisting of the IVD and two z-joints. The degenerative cascade, coined by Kirkaldy-Willis, describes the changes of the three-joint complex with age.[17] The cascade starts with segmental dysfunction, or abnormally reduced motion, at the level of the facets or the IVD. Segmental dysfunction eventually progresses to relative segmental instability. Finally, age-related bony overgrowth leads to segmental stabilization and stenosis. Initial presentation of symptoms can occur anywhere along this continuum (Figure 2.2).[17]

MAKING THE DIAGNOSIS

Making a diagnosis in LBP can be challenging because of the widespread sensory innervation of spinal structures. Also, some terminology may be ambiguous, as the same diagnosis may mean something different to each health care professional.[18]

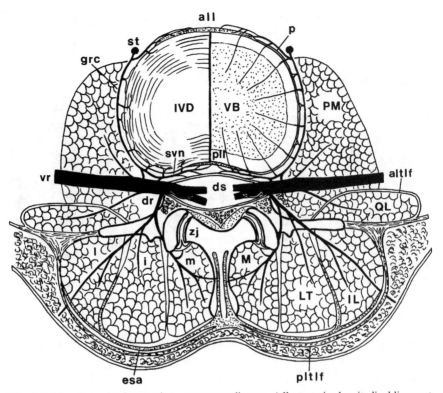

Figure 2.1 Lumbar spine innervation—transverse diagram. (all = anterior longitudinal ligament; altlf = anterior layer of thoracolumbar fascia; dr = dorsal ramus; ds = dorsal sac; esa = erector spinae aponeurosis; grc = gray ramus communicans; i = intermediate branch; IL = iliocostalis lumborum; l = lateral branch; LT = longissimus thoracis; m = medial branch; M = multifudus; pll = posterior longitudinal ligament; pltlf = posterior layer of thoracolumbar fascia; PM = psoas major; QL = quadratus lumborum; st = sympathetic trunk; svn = sinuvertebral nerve; vr = ventral ramus; zj = zygapophyseal joint.) (Reprinted with permission from N Bogduk. Clinical Anatomy of the Lumbar Spine and Sacrum [3rd ed]. New York: Churchill Livingstone, 1997;143.)

Diagnoses should be as specific and mechanistic as possible. Specific diagnoses yield more specific treatment plans and predictable outcomes, and naming a specific diagnosis may also reduce the patient's fear of the unknown and reassures the patient that the physician understands the problem.[18] However, a definitive diagnosis is not always possible, particularly during the initial presentation, and is not a requirement to institute reasonable and appropriate care. The authors propose that three parallel diagnostic axes be made with each patient with LBP. First, a functional descriptive diagnosis (similar to the Quebec Task Force Classification) should be given.[19] This should include the acuity of symptoms, provoking symptoms, and biomechanical deficits. Acute pain duration of symptoms is defined as pain lasting less than 6 weeks, subacute pain as from 6 to 12 weeks, and chronic pain as longer than 12 weeks. Biomechanical deficits include deficits in strength, endurance, range of motion, motor control, and neural mobility. Second, a working pathoanatomic diagnosis should be given if possible. In other words, the clinician should attempt to identify the pain generator. Third, a differential diagnosis should be listed. Nebulous terms, such as *lumbago* and *mechanical LBP*, should be avoided. Algorithms for specific diagnoses can sometimes be used as guidelines for

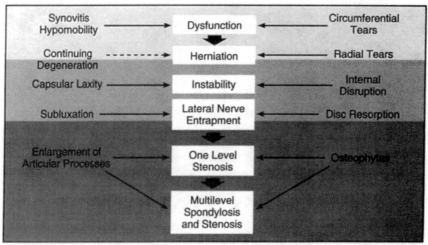

Figure 2.2 Degenerative cascade. (I.V. = intravenous.) (Reprinted with permission from WH Kirkaldy-Willis, CV Burton. Managing Low Back Pain [3rd ed]. New York: Churchill Livingstone, 1992;63.)

care; however, it is important to keep in mind that each patient needs and deserves an individualized plan of action.

History

Many etiologies of LBP can be identified through a thorough history. A systematic history identifies key facts without inadvertently omitting important questions. A systematic history of a specific pain complaint can be obtained using the OPQRST mnemonic.

Onset (sudden versus insidious)
Pain provocation/relief
Quality of pain
Referral—relief of pain
Severity—spatial pattern of pain
Time frame of pain

It is important to identify positions of both pain provocation and relief. The history should be useful in differentiating referred and radicular pain. Referred pain is perceived as a diffuse, achy, deep-set pain. Radicular pain, on the other hand, is perceived as a shooting pain that travels down the leg along a dermatomal band.[14] Prior history of LBP and previous successful and unsuccessful treatments should be discussed. Serious underlying medical conditions can be partially ruled out with questions concerning a history of cancer, immunosuppression, intravenous drug abuse, or infection. History should also elicit if the patient has had unexplained weight loss, no improvement with previous therapy, symptoms longer than 1 month, or pain with rest.[20] These so-called red-flag symptoms should be kept in mind while performing the history and review of symptoms (Table 2.2).

Table 2.2 Symptoms Requiring Further Investigation: The Yellow and the Red Flags

Sleep difficulty—inability to fall asleep or early morning awakening
Unusual pain qualities
  Pain worsened by walking
  No relief with bed rest
  Pain at rest
  Continuous pain
Significant past medical history of
  Cancer
  Immunosuppression
  Intravenous drug abuse
  Other infections
  Steroid usage
Unexplained weight loss
Fever
Cauda equina symptoms—bowel or bladder difficulty, bilateral lower extremity complaints,
    saddle anesthesia

History should also assess for cauda equina syndrome, as this constitutes a surgical emergency. Injury to the cauda equina presents with bowel or bladder difficulty (usually symptoms of urinary retention); bilateral lower limb pain and weakness; and saddle anesthesia.[20] If cauda equina syndrome is suspected, the patient should be sent for emergent imaging and surgical consultation.

Psychosocial, occupational, and functional histories are also important. The identification and subsequent treatment of psychosocial factors may help reduce disability in patients with LBP. In addition, a functional and work history should be done. A detailed description of the patient's job, including type of physical activity, description of work station, job satisfaction, amount of work missed because of pain, litigation, and workers' compensation status, can be crucial to developing a proper treatment plan. Family history should also be obtained because there may be a genetic factor in the development of lumbar herniated disks, disk degeneration, and other spinal conditions.[21,22] Much of the history can be obtained with a standardized questionnaire; however, there is no substitute for face-to-face history taking and the ability to interpret nonverbal communication.[18]

Physical Examination

The physical examination acts as an adjunct to a thorough history. After the differential diagnosis is established from the patient history, the examination can be used to confirm or refute particular diagnostic entities. The examination begins with observation. For example, a patient walking in with a lumbar shift has an acute disk herniation until proven otherwise.[23] A complete examination involves properly exposing the spine and lower limbs. The examination should also be serialized so that the patient does not need to change positions frequently.

The physical examination of spine patients extends beyond the standard orthopedic and neurologic examination so that subtle and specific abnormalities may be

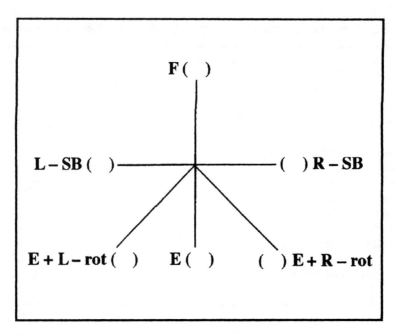

Figure 2.3 STAR diagram. (E = extension; F = flexion; L = left; L-SB = left side-bending; R = right; rot = rotation; R-SB = right side-bending.) (Reprinted with permission from MC Geraci, JT Alleva. Physical Examination of the Spine and Its Functional Kinetic Chain. In AJ Cole, SA Herring [eds], The Low Back Pain Handbook. Philadelphia: Hanley and Belfus, 1997;64.)

identified. In addition to the standard examination in which the motor strength, sensation, and reflexes are elicited, several items should be kept in mind. Lumbosacral spine range of motion should be tested in all cardinal planes (flexion, extension, side-bending, and extension-rotation) (Figure 2.3). Palpatory examination can be useful to identify bony landmarks, assess symmetry, and look for trigger points. However, many asymptomatic people have trigger points[18] and asymmetries. Trigger-point analysis is further complicated by poor interrater reliability[24] but may be improved by training and experience.[25] Sensory examination of the back and lower limbs is also important, but dermatomes are often variable. Table 2.3 lists tests to use for various lower limb dermatomes, myotomes, and muscle stretch reflexes.

Provocative maneuvers are integral to the spine examination. Adverse dynamic neural tension maneuvers (dural tension tests), such as the slump-sit, supine straight

Table 2.3 Dermatomes and Myotomes

Level	Dermatome Testing Site	Myotome—Key Muscles to Test	Muscle Stretch Reflexes
L4	Distal anterolateral thigh/ proximal medial lower leg	Knee extensors	Knee jerk
L5	First web space	Extensor hallucis longus	Medial hamstrings
S1	Lateral aspect of foot	Repeated toe raises	Achilles

leg raise, and femoral stretch tests, sensitize or stretch dura. Because the dura is irritated in cases of radicular pain, these tests can be invaluable in identifying a nerve root origin of pain. These dural tension maneuvers can gain sensitivity if additional components are applied. For instance, the slump-sit and the straight leg raise tests can be further sensitized by adding hip internal rotation or dorsiflexion, or both.[26] Furthermore, the supine straight leg raise, which is classically positive if pain occurs below 60 degrees, can gain sensitivity if higher degrees are used as a threshold. In addition, there are many provocative maneuvers to stress the sacroiliac joint (SIJ), but none has been validated by scientific studies.[27,28] Provocative tests for spinal stenosis, in which lumbar extension is held for 30 seconds, can be helpful.[29]

The following so-called Waddell's signs can be used to identify nonphysiologic pain behavior.[30]

- Superficial or nonanatomic tenderness
- Sham provocation of pain or discomfort
- Inconsistencies
- Regional weakness and sensory loss
- Overreaction

However, many practitioners use Waddell's signs inappropriately. Waddell's signs are used as signs of psychosocial distress and do not represent malingering. These signs should be used to determine if conclusions drawn from other portions of the examination are valid.[18] Waddell also showed that the presence of nonanatomic pain symptoms results in poor surgical outcome.[30]

Biomechanical assessment of the spine also adds valuable information. The examination should include not just the spine but also its functional kinetic chain. *Kinetic chain* refers to the joints, muscles, and fascia being systemically linked wherein a distal or proximal structure may influence the kinetically linked injured tissue.[31] The functional or biomechanical kinetic chain evaluation can identify poor postural habits, resultant muscle imbalances, hypomobile spinal segments, and functional limitations. A manual or osteopathic examination can be used to determine if lumbar spinal functional units are hypomobile. This type of examination has been validated in the cervical spine.[32] However, no single manual or osteopathic maneuver is pathognomic.[33] Instead, many manual practitioners advocate that a group of positive tests, rather than single tests, be used to determine dysfunctional levels. An assessment of muscle imbalances, such as tight and weak muscles linking the pelvis to the spine, identifies barriers to appropriate quality and quantity of motion. Abnormal muscle recruitment and gait patterns can also impair quality of motion. In conclusion, the biomechanical examination is an assessment of structure and function.

Putting It All Together

Because of the variable innervation of the lumbar spine and the autonomic contribution to the plexuses of the lumbar spine, localizing the pain generator based on the history and physical examination alone can be difficult. Additional diagnostics are often necessary to correlate history and physical findings.[34] Relying on a single positive finding on the physical examination to yield a definitive diagnosis is not ideal. Although each test alone does not have much power, a combination and analysis of all of the positive physical examination findings increases the sensitivity and specificity for a particular diagnosis.[35,36] The more precise the working diagnosis, the more directed functional rehabilitation becomes. Even in the absence of a definitive diagnosis, advancement of an early rehabilitation program based on history and physical examination evidence of pain provocation and relief is often possible and frequently successful. Correcting biomechanical deficits can be the missing therapeutic link in advancing a long-term solution to the problem of LBP.

DIAGNOSTIC SUBSETS OF REGIONAL LOW BACK PAIN

LBP and leg pain can occur due to multiple etiologies. Specific symptoms and signs taken together with available diagnostic tests can lead to an organized differential diagnosis. For the purposes of this chapter, diagnostic subsets have been divided according to their usual mode of presentation. We have broadly separated LBP presentation to flexion-based pain and extension-based pain. In general, flexion-based pain indicates pathology in the anterior column of the spine, and extension-based pain indicates pathology in the posterior column. It must be emphasized, however, that because each spinal segment is a three-joint complex, alterations in anterior column mechanics may affect the posterior column and vice versa. Specific symptoms and signs based on provocative testing, even with limited ancillary tests, can lead to a practical differential diagnosis. These schemes also lend themselves to reasonable initial treatment plans (Table 2.4).

Flexion-Based Pain

LBP exacerbated by flexion is common. Biomechanically, flexion of the lumbosacral spine is a combined motion involving sagittal rotation and anterior translation of each motion segment. Anterior translation is limited mainly by z-joint orientation and fibers of the annulus fibrous. Sagittal rotation is limited by fibers of the annulus fibrosis, z-joint capsule, ligaments, paravertebral muscles, and the thoracolumbar fascia. Pure

Table 2.4 Diagnostic Subsets of Low Back Pain and Leg Pain

Flexion-based pain
  Muscles
  Ligaments
  Intrinsic disk pain (diskitis, internal disk disruption, annular tears)
  Extrinsic disk pain (disk herniations)
  Vertebral bodies (compression fractures, osteoporosis)
Extension-based pain
  Spinal stenosis
  Spondylolysis
  Spondylolisthesis
  Baastrup's disease (kissing spines)
  Lamina impaction
Transitional pain
Pain associated with constitutional symptoms

---

flexion in a normal lumbar spine typically is not injurious. However, repetitive flexion can provoke pain, and flexion combined with torsion is potentially damaging.[14]

Muscles

Myofascial pain can occur with acute muscle strains and so-called muscle spasm. Muscle or myofascial pain can also be secondary to an underlying entity, such as an injured z-joint or disk. Muscle damage can occur because of unaccustomed eccentric activity, such as when the paraspinal muscles are contracting while being stretched, as with forceful lumbar flexion. Rarely, muscle injury occurs with concentric action, as with forceful lumbar extension. With disruption of muscle fibers, delayed-onset muscle soreness presents 24–48 hours after unaccustomed activity.[37] Patients often state that they have "muscle spasms." Rather, the patient is usually experiencing muscle guarding interpreted as a spasm. On physical examination, the patient has tenderness to palpation as well as pain with contraction or stretching of the muscle.[18] True trigger points have been defined as points of local tenderness with taut bands and referred pain to a remote site. Trigger points are thought to be plentiful in myofascial pain syndrome, a chronic pain condition. Persistent trigger points are often observed in the piriformis and quadratus lumborum muscles.

Ligaments

Ligament injury is also frequent with flexion activity and is also included in the myofascial axis. However, the "back or ligamentous strain" diagnosis is often used as a general term for any patient with LBP. "Which ligament is injured?" is a question requiring definition for diagnostic accuracy. The anterior longitudinal ligament and the posterior longitudinal ligament blend with the annulus fibrosis and therefore are considered with disk-related pain. The ligamentum flavum and supraspinous ligaments are not considered to be a major source of back pain due to their relative paucity of afferent nerve fibers. That leaves only the interspinous ligament and the iliolumbar ligaments as significant potential ligamentous sources of LBP. Injury to the iliolumbar ligament or overlying attachment of the lumbar intermuscular aponeurosis is often called *iliac crest syndrome* because tenderness is appreciated over the medial posterior iliac crest. Treatment has not been well defined for this syndrome, but may include anesthetic or steroid injection, or both, for temporary relief.[14]

Intervertebral Disks

Diskogenic pain is a common cause of flexion-based LBP. Formerly, the disk was not considered a potential pain generator, but now the disk is known to be innervated, particularly at the outer one-third of the annulus fibrosis.[14] The disk has been proven to cause pain by provocative studies such as diskography and outer annulus probing during conscious surgery.[14,38] Diskogenic pain can be divided into intrinsic disk pain (IDP) and extrinsic disk pain. IDP is further divided into a continuum of diagnoses: diskitis, internal disk disruption, and torsion injuries to the annulus fibrosis. According to Schwarzer's prevalence study, IDP constitutes close to 39% of chronic LBP.[34]

Diskitis is the prototypical IDP. Diskitis is usually an intensely painful infection diagnosed by magnetic resonance imaging (MRI) or bone scan. Intrinsic

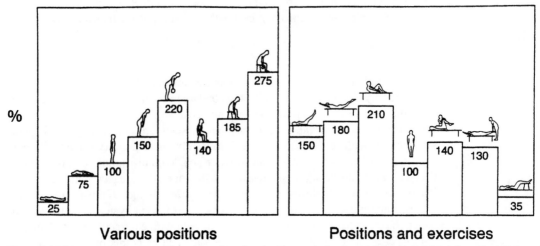

Various positions   **Positions and exercises**

Figure 2.4 Disk pressure changes with position. (Reprinted with permission from M Sinaki, B Mokri. Low Back Pain and Disorders of the Lumbar Spine. In RL Braddom [ed], Physical Medicine and Rehabilitation. Philadelphia: Saunders, 1996;817.)

disk disruption (IDD) has been defined as a condition in which the internal anatomy of the disk is changed but its external surface remains relatively normal. IDD remains a controversial diagnosis because it is difficult to prove IDD with objective testing. IDD is thought to become painful when inner annular tears extend to the innervated outer annulus. Nachemson's classic studies showed that the disk has its greatest pressure when patients are seated with their arms unsupported (Figure 2.4).[39] Patients often give a history of a flexion or rotation injury and complain of a sitting intolerance. Pain is usually confined to the low back and is described as deep-seated, diffuse, and achy. Pain may be increased with coughing and sneezing, as this may increase intradiskal pressure. Further diagnostics may be helpful in identifying IDP. Plain x-rays and MRI can reveal a degenerated disk but cannot directly identify if the disk is painful or asymptomatic. IDD is diagnosed with computed tomography (CT) following diskography demonstrating painful annular tears extending to the periphery of the disk. Diskography or disk stimulation may isolate a specific disk as a pain generator if adjacent disks do not reproduce pain on the same procedure.[14] High-intensity zones on T2-weighted MR images have also been correlated with painful annular tears, although some reports suggest high-intensity zones may be present in normal asymptomatic individuals.[40] At the end stage, internal disk disruption may lead to disk degeneration or frank disk herniation, or both. The term *degenerative disk disease* may be often used synonymously with IDP; however, this is confusing. Disk degeneration is part of the normal aging process and is not always symptomatic. Treatment options for IDP have not undergone randomized controlled trials. Similar treatment principles are used to treat IDP and disk herniations. Specifically, active exercise and physical therapy is used to unload the lumbar disks. The surgical option for IDP has traditionally been lumbar spinal fusion. Intradiskal electrical thermoplasty, an experimental treatment theoretically used to stimulate collagen growth to reconstitute annular tears, has been introduced in some centers, but further studies are necessary to evaluate long-term efficacy. In

contrast to IDD, extrinsic disk pain consists of diagnostic entities such as disk herniations. Extrinsic disk pain usually causes radicular pain and is discussed under
Radiculopathy.

Vertebral Bodies

Damage to the vertebral body can also cause flexion-based LBP. Although the vertebral body itself does not have extensive sensory nerve endings, the surrounding
periosteum is clearly pain sensitive. The vertebral body may be injured through
traumatic or atraumatic means, including infection (osteomyelitis), tumors, or metabolic disorders (Paget's disease, osteoporosis).[14] Most commonly, the bodies are
injured as a result of compression fractures. Although vertebral fractures may be
asymptomatic, they also have the capacity to cause disabling pain.[41] The pain is
described as a dull ache, worse with flexion of the spine; however, pain may also be
present even without spinal motion. Additional imaging tests, such as plain films,
CT scans or MRIs, may be helpful to identify fracture sites and associated soft tissue pathology. However, microfractures are often not evident even with the most
sophisticated images. Acute fractures can often be managed with relative immobilization for 2–3 weeks. Narcotic analgesics may be necessary for severe pain but
should be quickly switched to non-narcotic agents because of the risk of constipation and possible cognitive impairment in patients who are immobilized and perhaps disoriented by hospital stays. Calcitonin, either via nasal spray or injection,
may offer analgesia and deter further osteoporosis. Various back braces have also
been used for acute fractures but are generally not well tolerated.[41] Physical and
occupational therapy with the judicious use of modalities is appropriate during the
acute pain-relieving phase of rehabilitation. Therapy should progress to more functional goals as pain decreases and healing occurs.

   Osteoporotic patients may continue to have chronic pain and remain at risk for
further injury. The etiology of chronic pain in this context remains, for the most part,
uncertain. Most hypotheses state that the chronic spine pain is related to degenerative changes of the spine and dysfunctional paraspinal muscles. Treatment of chronic
pain should be directed to these possible etiologies. Therapy for osteoporosis should
emphasize postural correction either through back extensor strengthening or back
supports, or both. Back extensor strengthening reduces progressive kyphotic deformity. Precautions should include the avoidance of trunk flexion exercises, as they
may cause further vertebral body fractures. Abdominal strengthening should be done
isometrically for similar reasons. Deep breathing techniques and a low-impact aerobic exercise round out a well-balanced exercise program. Of course, comprehensive
medical treatment of osteoporosis should be initiated, if not already addressed.[41]

Extension-Based Pain

LBP provoked with extension of the lumbar spine usually indicates pain generation
from the posterior elements. Patients often complain that it hurts to lie on their
stomach or flat on their back (with their legs straight) because these positions can
increase lumbar lordosis, and they frequently find that the pain is worse with standing than with sitting. The specific diagnostic subsets usually associated with extension-based LBP include spinal stenosis, spondylolysis, facet-mediated pain,
Baastrup's disease, and lamina impaction.[42]

Spinal Stenosis

Central or lateral lumbar spinal stenosis occurs frequently in the older population. Although spinal stenosis may cause LBP, this condition is more commonly associated with pain and altered sensation in one or both legs. A further discussion of spinal stenosis can be found under the section Neurogenic Claudication.

Spondylolysis and Spondylolisthesis

Spondylolysis refers to a defect of the pars interarticularis, whereas *spondylolisthesis* refers to forward slippage of one vertebra on another. *Spondylosis* refers to degenerative disk narrowing and osteophyte formation (likely a normal part of aging). A pars defect can be acute or chronic. Spondylolysis can be particularly troublesome in adolescents and should be aggressively evaluated and treated in that age group. Spondylolisthesis is defined as a heterogenous group of disorders and involves forward displacement of one vertebra on another.[43] Each group is treated differently, thus it is important to distinguish between the different types. Wiltse and Rothman have proposed a convenient classification scheme for spondylolisthesis (Figure 2.5).[44]

Facet-Mediated Pain

Pain emanating from the lumbar z-joints (or facet joints) has been estimated to occur in 15% of patients with chronic LBP.[45] Anatomically, the lumbar facets are synovial, knuckle-sized joints innervated by two adjacent medial branches of the lumbar posterior rami. These joints act mainly to control motion, with the sagittally oriented facets limiting axial rotation and the coronally oriented facets limiting flexion and extension. The lumbar facets also provide 15% of the axial weightbearing of the spinal three-joint complex. This percentage rises in extension and falls in flexion.

Facet-mediated pain usually presents as localized paravertebral pain possibly provoked with extension or rotation, or both, of the lumbar spine.[46] (Theoretically, facet-mediated pain may also be provoked with forward bending because of stretching of sensitized nociceptors in the joint capsule.) Facet-mediated pain may also extend into the lower limb in a sclerotomal distribution. The causes of facet-mediated pain are uncertain but include degenerative and inflammatory arthropathies, meniscoid entrapment, microtrauma, and synovial cysts.[47] This uncertainty is compounded by several prospective trials demonstrating a lack of correlation between history and physical examination findings and significant pain relief with anesthetic facet blocks.[45,48,49] Thus, the history and physical examination cannot definitively distinguish facet-mediated pain from other sources of LBP. Imaging studies are also poor identifiers of facet-mediated pain. Facet degeneration is commonly seen in CT scans and plain films of asymptomatic individuals.[47,50] Thus, there remains no noninvasive gold standard for diagnosing facet-mediated pain. The current diagnostic gold standards are facet intra-articular anesthetic injections or two-level medial branch blocks, or both. These interventional tests can be used if conservative treatment is unsuccessful and if more specific treatment is contemplated.

An interdisciplinary treatment plan is used with facet-mediated pain, as with other LBP disorders. Specifically, an exercise program for facet pain should include a flexion-based lumbar dynamic stabilization program. The goal of any lumbar stabilization is to maximize motor control of all the muscles that influence spinal movement. The exercise program should be designed to unload the posterior ele-

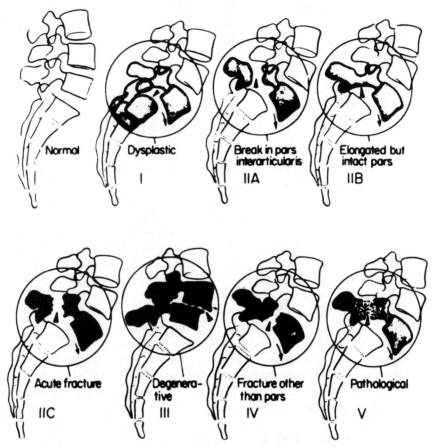

Figure 2.5 Classification of spondylolisthesis. (Reprinted with permission from LJ Grobler, LL Wiltse. Classification, and Nonoperative and Operative Treatment of Spondylolisthesis. In JW Frymoyer [ed], The Adult Spine: Principles and Practice. Philadelphia: Lippincott–Raven, 1997;1867.)

ments. Eliminating excess anterior pelvic tilt prevents compensatory lumbar spine extension. Manual therapy or manipulation appears to work best for acute facet pain and may be short lived.[47] There is considerable controversy about manipulation for chronic facet-mediated pain, but little compelling research. Facet corticosteroid injections may work to reduce pain; however, their efficacy has not been demonstrated by randomized controlled trials.[51,52] Radiofrequency neural ablation of the medial branches of the lumbar posterior rami may be an alternate option.

Baastrup's Disease (Kissing Spines) and Lamina Impaction

Baastrup's disease, or *kissing spines*, refers to pain resulting from the impaction of adjacent spinous processes. Impaction is due to lumbar extension or excessive lumbar lordosis. *Lamina impaction* refers to pain from the abutting of the inferior articular process of a lumbar vertebra onto the lamina below. The pain-generating structures appear to be the periosteum of the bony structures involved. Treatments that have been proposed include flexion-based lumbar stabilization, diagnostic injection of the interspinous ligament, medial branch blocks, and surgical excision of the lesion. Neither Baastrup's disease nor lamina impaction has been studied by proper clinical trials.[14]

Transitional Pain

Sacroiliac Joint

The SIJ has been implicated as a pain generator. Before 1934, the SIJ was thought to be a common source of pain, but once Mixter and Barr ushered in the dynasty of the disk in their seminal 1934 *New England Journal of Medicine* article, the SIJ as a source of pain fell out of favor.[53] Critics have argued that because there is such limited range of motion—only 4 degrees of movement and 1.6 mm of total translation—the SIJ was unlikely to be a pain source.[54] However, injection studies have confirmed the SIJ as a potential pain generator.[55,56] The surrounding ligaments likely also possess pain-generating capability. Furthermore, the SIJ has been a known and accepted source of pain in the seronegative spondyloarthropathies, such as ankylosing spondylitis (AS), and in third-trimester pregnant females, in whom the hormone relaxin causes ligamentous laxity and gapping of the SIJ.

Anatomically, the SIJ is an auricular or C-shaped diarthrodial synovial joint containing both hyaline and fibrocartilage that serves to transmit and dissipate upper trunk loads to the lower limbs during weightbearing. The SIJ is probably innervated from the anterior and posterior rami of L4–S4,[54] although Grob, in a cadaveric histologic study, demonstrated the innervation was exclusively from the posterior rami of S1–S4. A potential wide range of segmental innervation may account for the wide range of referred pain found with SIJ syndrome even distal to the knee.[57]

As with the diagnosis of facet-mediated pain, there is no completely validated method to diagnose a painful SIJ. The history and physical can often lead the clinician in the correct direction. Typically, the pain is worsened with transitional maneuvers, such as going from sit-to-stand positions, or sudden unexpected movement, such as stepping off an uneven surface. The pain may refer in a variable distribution, but the core referral zone is from the posterior superior iliac spine to the greater trochanter.[55,56] Patients often point to their posterior superior iliac spine as the site of maximal tenderness.[58] Physical examination includes assessment of muscle imbalances, quality of motion (Gillet's test), and provocative maneuvers (Patrick's, Gaenslen's, sacral thrust test). Imaging studies, such as plain films, CT scans, MRIs, and bone scans, rarely aid in diagnosis (except in cases in which infection, inflammation, metabolic, or traumatic conditions are considered).

The treatment of SIJ dysfunction is based on the etiology, and an integrated approach using osteopathic medicine, chiropractic, manual physical therapy, and medical management is best. Usually, a focused exercise program is started to correct muscle imbalances. Inhibited and weak muscles, such as the gluteus maximus, gluteus medius, and hip external rotators, are facilitated, whereas contracted and often-painful muscles, such as the iliopsoas, rectus femoris, and the hamstrings, are stretched. Manipulation or mobilization, medications, education, and sacroiliac belts all may have roles in the treatment of SIJ dysfunction. SIJ injections have diagnostic and treatment benefits. These injections should be performed under fluoroscopic guidance to confirm entry into the joint. Other modes of treatment, including SIJ fusion, SIJ denervation, prolotherapy, and acupuncture, have also been described with anecdotal success.

Instability

Instability is a biomechanical, rather than a clinical, term. Frymoyer defines segmental instability as a loss of spinal motion segment stiffness, such that force application to that motion segment produces greater displacement than would be seen in a normal structure, resulting in a painful condition, potential for progressive deformity, and neurologic structures placed at risk.[59] Some have proposed criteria wherein instability is diagnosed if two of three spinal columns are disrupted. However, this criterion is not applicable in chronic conditions such as spondylolisthesis. Rather, instability should be diagnosed on an individual basis taking into account history, examination, and radiographic findings. The etiologies for instability are multifold and are classified as

   I. Fractures, fracture dislocations
   II. Infection of the anterior elements
  III. Neoplasms
  IV. Spondylolisthesis
   V. Degenerative (primary or after surgery)

    Patients with spinal instability present with LBP with occasional referred pain into the leg and positionally related neurologic symptoms. Furthermore, patients often describe an "instability catch" when moving from a flexed to extended posture.[59] Radiographically, disk space narrowing, traction spurs, and spinal malalignment may be present. Traction spurs, as described by McNab, are bony adaptions to the tensile stresses of the outer annulus.[60] Traction spurs differ from claw osteophytes in that osteophytes are benign adaptions to compressive forces (Figure 2.6). On lumbar radiographs, if there is greater than 4 mm of translation from flexion to extension, or if there is greater than 11 degrees of wedging from flexion to extension, spinal instability can be inferred. The natural history of instability is favorable in that pain often improves with time, but bracing and surgical fusion are possible treatment options.

Low Back Pain with Constitutional Symptoms

Spinal Tumors

Spinal tumors represent a rare but important diagnosis in the evaluation of LBP (Table 2.5). Typically, patients younger than age 21 years tend to have benign lesions, whereas patients older than age 21 years tend to have malignant lesions.[61] Primary sites of spinal metastasis are the *p*rostate, *t*hyroid, *b*reast, *l*ung, and *k*idney (Mnemonic: *PT B*arnum *L*oves *K*ids). Metastases from extraspinal carcinomas account for the great majority of spinal tumors. Thus, the evaluation of spinal tumors should include a thorough search for an extraspinal source of cancer. Metastatic cancer most commonly occurs in the thoracic spine; however, metastatic tumors that are painful are most common in the lumbar spine.

    Tumors of the spine usually present as back pain. Pain associated with tumors is persistent, progressive, worse at night, and unrelieved by rest or position change.[62] Pain may be due to bony destruction (pathologic fracture), instability, or direct pres-

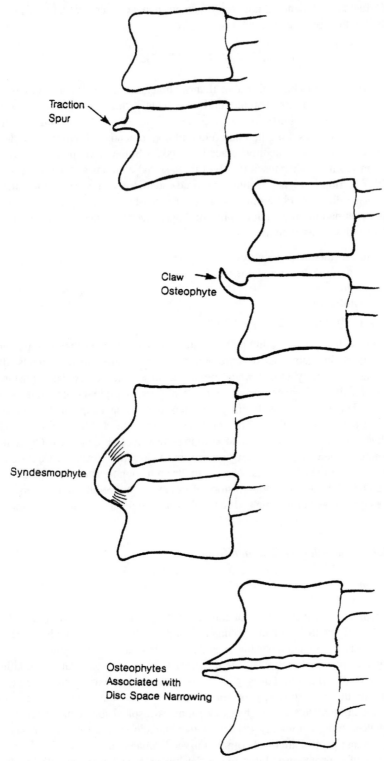

Figure 2.6 Traction spurs, osteophytes, and syndesmophytes. (Reprinted with permission from HJ Griffiths. Imaging of the Lumbar Spine. Gaithersburg, MD: Aspen, 1991;31.)

Table 2.5 Common Primary Spinal Tumors

Myeloma—osteolytic small "punched out" lesions
Chordoma—arises from notochord remnants
Lymphoma
Aneurysmal bone cyst—cystic cavity filled with blood, in young
Osteoid osteoma—smaller than 2 cm diameter
Osteoblastoma—larger than 2 cm
Eosinophilic granuloma—child with vertebral plana (vertebral body collapse)
Hemangioma
Intradural tumors—usually gliomas (ependymomas or astrocytomas)

---

sure on pain-generating structures. Constitutional symptoms such as weight loss and cachexia may be present. Physical examination often reveals localized tenderness, mass, decreased spinal motion, and an irritative scoliosis.[62] A complete neurologic assessment for cord or cauda equina compression should always be done.

Arthritides

Osteoarthritis of the spine (a term synonymous with degenerative joint disease, osteoarthrosis, or spondylosis) is a ubiquitous condition that typically represents age-related changes of the spine.[14] Seronegative spondyloarthropathies comprise the majority of rheumatic disorders affecting the spine. These seronegative spondyloarthropathies include AS, reactive arthritis or Reiter's syndrome, and arthritides associated with concomitant disease such as psoriasis and inflammatory bowel disease. All of these are associated with the HLA-B27 antigen. AS, specifically, is an inflammatory condition affecting mainly ligamentous insertions, particularly the annulus fibrosis of the IVD, the facet capsule, and peripheral skeletal insertion sites. AS usually presents in young adult white men with long-standing LBP or stiffness, or both. Reactive arthropathy (Reiter's syndrome) is triggered by genitourinary or gastrointestinal bacteria. Classically, Reiter's syndrome is a triad of urethritis, conjunctivitis, and arthritis. Psoriatic arthritis is another inflammatory arthropathy characterized by a seronegative rheumatoid factor status and involvement of the distal interphalangeal joints in patients with skin psoriasis. Finally, enteropathic arthropathies occur in some cases of inflammatory bowel disease, also without evidence of serum rheumatoid factor.

Polymyalgia rheumatica is a pain syndrome presenting with proximal shoulder or hip girdle pain and stiffness. Often, polymyalgia rheumatica occurs in elderly white women with laboratory values showing an increased sedimentation rate. Patients respond well to low-dose steroids. Polymyalgia rheumatica is associated with temporal arteritis, a cause of blindness, in 40–50% of patients.[37]

Paget's disease is a disorder of bone metabolism. Pagetic bone results in bone pain because of the weak structure of the affected bone. Back pain occurs in up to 40% of individuals with Paget's disease. Bone scans and plain films with evidence of lytic lesions confirm the diagnosis. Elevated alkaline phosphatase and urinary hydroxyproline are common. Along with achieving adequate pain control, Paget's disease is often successfully treated with biphosphonates or calcitonin.[37]

Infection

Spinal infection commonly occurs as epidural abscesses, vertebral osteomyelitis, or diskitis. Epidural abscesses typically occur in immunocompromised individuals, such as intravenous drug abusers. Abscesses can encroach on the spinal cord and nerve roots, thus treatment should be aggressive. Treatment is long-term antibiotics and possibly surgical débridement. Vertebral osteomyelitis is another dangerous condition that can be missed if not suspected. Patients often complain of constitutional symptoms and frequently have marked tenderness over the spinous process of the involved vertebrae. Treatment is similar to spinal abscesses. Disk space infection can often occur after an invasive procedure. This diagnosis should be considered in those patients with unsuccessful back surgery or persistent postdiskogram pain.[63]

Pseudospine Pain

Visceral sources of pain should also be considered with any patient presenting with back pain. A thorough and routine review of systems allows the clinician to cover the major organ systems that may refer to the back.

DIAGNOSTIC SUBSETS OF LEG PAIN WITH OR WITHOUT BACK PAIN

Definitions

Distinguishing between radicular and referred pain is critical to advancing proper treatment. *Radicular pain* is defined as pain that arises as a result of irritation of a spinal nerve or its roots.[14] Typically, radicular pain is described as shooting, band-like pain. On the other hand, *referred pain* is defined as pain perceived in a region innervated by nerves other than those associated with the primary pain generator. Typically, referred pain is a dull, achy, deep, vague discomfort. Also, a distinction can be made between radicular pain and radiculopathy. Radiculopathy implies that conduction is blocked in the axons of a spinal nerve or its roots, resulting in sensory or motor deficits, or both. Although there may be neurologic compromise, patients with radiculopathy do not necessarily have pain.[14] When neurologic compromise is evident, the distinction between radicular and referred pain is straightforward (Table 2.6). However, when neurologic compromise is not evident, as is often the case, the patient's description of pain and examination findings assist with this determination.

Leg Pain with Neurologic Signs and Symptoms

Radiculopathy

Radicular pain or radiculopathy can be due to a variety of mechanisms. Classically, radiculopathy has been attributed to mechanical compression of a nerve root. However, radiculopathy may result from a combination of factors, with compression often priming an inflammatory and ischemic cascade.[64] The location of a disk her-

Table 2.6 Distinguishing Referred and Radicular Pain

Characteristics	Referred Pain	Radicular Pain
Symptoms	Deep, boring, ill-defined, poorly localized	Sharp, well localized, electric-like
Radiation	Posterior joint, sacroiliac joint, and muscle syndromes may radiate to the posterolateral thigh, calf, and rarely to the foot	Follows the sciatic nerve distribution to the buttocks, posterior thigh, and calf to the foot; or femoral nerve distribution to the anterior thigh
Sensory alteration	Rare	Frequently follows a dermatomal distribution
Motor weakness	May have subjective weakness, but objective weakness or atrophy is rare	Frequent objective weakness and atrophy with prolonged duration of symptoms
Reflex deficit	Rare	Frequent
Nerve root tension signs	Absent; sciatic stretch testing may cause back pain or reveal hamstring tightness	Frequent sciatic notch tenderness and popliteal and peroneal nerve tenderness

niation determines which nerve root is affected. With posterolateral disk herniations, the traversing nerve root is usually affected. For example, with an L5–S1 posterolateral disk herniation, the S1 nerve root is typically injured. With large central disk herniations, traversing nerve roots, which can exit two levels or more below the level of herniation, may be affected. With lateral or far lateral disk herniations, the exiting nerve root can be affected. For example, with an L5–S1 lateral disk herniation, the exiting L5 nerve root is typically injured. Spinal stenosis is also a common cause of radiculopathy. Central spinal stenosis typically causes bilateral, multilevel radiculopathy. Conversely, foraminal stenosis usually causes unilateral, unilevel radiculopathy. Less commonly, space-occupying lesions, such as synovial cysts and tumors, can cause radiculopathy. Infectious agents, such as herpes zoster, and metabolic processes, such as diabetes mellitus, have also been implicated with radicular pain.

Cauda Equina Syndrome

When bilateral leg pain is associated with bowel or bladder dysfunction or saddle anesthesia, cauda equina syndrome must be considered. Injury to the cauda equina is typically due to a large central disk herniation. Other causes, such as epidural hematoma, epidural tumor, and fractures, should also be considered. To determine the exact cause, an urgent MRI or CT scan should be obtained. Surgical decompression should be accomplished as quickly as possible to optimize neurologic outcome. Of note, cauda equina syndrome may present acutely, in which case neurologic symptoms develop abruptly, or subacutely, in which case symptoms may take days to manifest. Urinary retention may be the most common symptom of cauda equina syndrome preoperatively.[65]

Other Neurologic Problems

Patients presenting with leg pain and neurologic compromise should also be investigated for neurologic injury other than nerve root compromise. Lesions anywhere along the lower motor neuron pathway can be mistaken for lumbar radiculopathy. Entrapment neuropathies of the lower limb can be confused with lumbar radiculopathies. For example, common peroneal nerve entrapment at the fibular head can be mistaken for an L5 radiculopathy. Lateral femoral cutaneous nerve palsy (meralgia paresthetica) presenting with discomfort in the anterolateral thigh could be mistaken for L3 or L4 radicular pain. Differential diagnostic injections and electrodiagnostics can help sort out the differential diagnoses. In diabetic patients, diabetic amyotrophy should be considered. *Diabetic amyotrophy* is a term representing a variety of neurologic injuries. The site of pathology includes polyradiculopathies, lumbar plexopathy, and mononeuropathies.

Neurogenic Claudication

Central or lateral lumbar spinal stenosis occurs frequently in the older population, although congenital stenosis can present with symptoms in a younger population. Central stenosis is narrowing of the central portion of the spinal canal. Lateral stenosis is narrowing around the nerve root canal or intervertebral foramen, or both. Lateral stenosis can be further subdivided into lateral recess stenosis and foraminal stenosis. *Lateral recess* and *subarticular stenosis* refers to narrowing of the anterolateral aspect of the central canal ventral to the medial aspect of the superior articular process and dorsal to the IVD. Foraminal stenosis is narrowing of the intervertebral nerve root canal.[66] Most commonly, stenosis is an acquired process due to soft tissue (i.e., ligamentous and herniated disks) or bony encroachment, or both.

Spinal stenosis patients usually present with neurogenic claudication with or without LBP. Neurogenic claudication is radicular pain that is typically precipitated by standing or walking and relieved with sitting.[67] Neurogenic claudication can be difficult to distinguish from vascular claudication (Table 2.7). Certain specific signs and symptoms associated with postural change can distinguish these two entities. Physical examination in stenotic patients usually reveals limited lumbar extension, which is occasionally painful. Neural tension signs are frequently negative.[68] Katz and others suggest that the 30-second lumbar extension test can have positive predictive value for lumbar spinal stenosis.[29]

The diagnosis of spinal stenosis is usually clinical, but imaging and electrodiagnostic tests can provide important anatomic and functional correlations, respectively. Myelography, CT, and MRI have been used to diagnose anatomic spinal stenosis, with MRI emerging as the study of choice for central and lateral spinal stenosis.[67] Schonstrom has advocated measuring the cross-sectional area of the dural sac, rather than measuring the spinal canal diameter,[69] with less than 10 mm^2 being considered stenotic. Neurophysiologic studies such as needle electromyography, nerve conduction studies, and evoked potentials are useful to assess nerve function, acuteness of nerve injury, levels of involvement, and to rule out other confounding neurologic disorders such as peripheral neuropathy.

Natural history studies reveal that most patients with spinal stenosis treated nonsurgically either improve or remain the same.[70–73] Conservative treatment specific for spinal stenosis includes epidural steroid injections, bracing to prevent extension, and exercise. Therapeutic exercise regimens should focus on decreasing lumbar lordosis, which theoretically increases spinal canal diameter. For example, stretching hamstrings and hip flexors and strengthening glutei and abdominals should promote a reduction in lumbar lordosis. The preceding regimen has shown empiric benefit but has not yet been validated by well-controlled

Table 2.7 Differentiation of Vascular and Neurogenic Claudication

Factor	Neurogenic Claudication (Pseudoclaudication)	Vascular Claudication	Pitfalls and Remarks
Low back pain	Frequently present	Absent	Sometimes, coincidental degenerative joint disease can be present in patients with vascular claudication
Effect of standing	Provokes symptoms	Does not provoke symptoms	—
Direction of radiation	Usually downward	Usually upward	—
Sensory symptoms	Present in 66% of patients	Absent	Some patients may have distal sensory symptoms due to neuropathy
Muscle weakness	Present in more than 40% of patients	Absent	—
Reflex changes	Present in approximately 50% of patients	Absent	In older patients, especially if there is associated neuropathy, reflexes may be decreased or absent
Arterial pulses	Normal	Decreased or absent	—
Arterial bruits	Absent	Frequently present	—
Effect of rest while standing	Does not relieve symptoms	Relieves symptoms	—
Walking uphill	Symptoms produced later	Symptoms produced earlier	—
Walking downhill	Symptoms produced earlier	Symptoms produced later	—
Bicycling (stationary or regular)	Does not provoke symptoms	Provokes symptoms	—

Source: Reprinted with permission from Mayo Foundation. B Mokri, M Sinaki. Lumbar disk syndrome, lumbosacral radiculopathies, lumbar spondylosis and stenosis, spondylolisthesis. In M Sinaki (ed), Basic Clinical Rehabilitation Medicine (2nd ed). St. Louis: Mosby–Year Book, 1993;503–513.

trials.[67] Decompressive laminectomy, with or without a spinal fusion, has been advocated for lumbar spinal stenosis unresponsive to nonsurgical intervention. Surgery appears to have good-to-excellent results initially (approximately 64% per Turner meta-analysis); however, patient satisfaction significantly deteriorates with longer follow-up.[29,74,75]

DIAGNOSTIC TESTING

Diagnostic tests are used in LBP syndromes that typically extend beyond 4–6 weeks, or sooner if red-flag symptoms or signs are present. Reasons for obtaining further testing include ruling out serious illness, planning surgery, determining prognosis, and for medicolegal reasons. As a general rule, diagnostics are ordered only if they affect the treatment plan.

A variety of test options are available, including electrodiagnostics, imaging, diagnostic injections, laboratory tests, and formal assessment of psychosocial functioning. Detailed descriptions of many of these can be found elsewhere in this book.

IMPRESSION AND PLAN

After the history, physical examination, and diagnostics, an impression and plan should be formulated. The impression should be made on three parallel diagnostic axes, as mentioned in the section Making the Diagnosis. First, a functional descriptive diagnosis that includes the acuity of symptoms, symptom provokers, and biomechanical deficits is given. Second, a working pathoanatomic or mechanistic diagnosis should be given if possible. Third, a differential diagnosis should be listed. When relevant, psychological diagnoses should be made using the *Diagnostic and Statistical Manual of Mental Disorders, Fourth Edition.*

A treatment plan then should be tailored to the individual patient, based on the abnormalities identified in the impression. Noninterventional conservative care is appropriate for most LBP disorders for the first 4–6 weeks.[76] This takes into account the favorable natural history of most acute low back conditions. However, urgent surgical referral is appropriate for cauda equina syndrome or rapidly progressive weakness due to radiculopathy.[10] Patients should be educated about the risk to benefit ratio of nonsurgical and surgical care. The choice between surgical and nonsurgical care often becomes an individual issue of expectation, goals, quality of life, and disability. In cases of acute and subacute radiculopathy due to a herniated disk, surgery appears to resolve radicular pain faster than nonsurgical care. Yet, the same functional outcome is achieved in both surgical and nonsurgical groups at 1 year.[77] Furthermore, the presence of nonprogressive weakness does not predict better surgical over nonsurgical outcome.[76]

In general, nonsurgical treatment should be active rather than passive. There is growing evidence against the usefulness of passive treatment such as bed rest and traction. Consequently, a shift has occurred to more active therapy with the involvement of the patient in a home exercise program.[78] Physical therapists can be invaluable partners in initiating an active program. However, the exact time to refer a patient to a therapist is not definitively known. Saal suggests the following approach: for patients with acute, first-time LBP, physical therapy is not necessary; for patients with acute, recurrent LBP, radicular pain, or chronic pain, a referral to physical therapy is appropriate.[79] Exercise treatment ideally is an eclectic and individualized regimen. Treatments can include correcting muscle imbalances, postural retraining, and dynamic lumbar stabilization. At times, pure flexion or extension exercise regimens are appropriate, but frequently, starting with a neutral spine posture is more reasonable, particularly if radicular pain is not well controlled with a flexion- or extension-based approach. For example, it has been consistently demonstrated that flexion exercises should be avoided in most cases of acute LBP.[78] Also, patients with spinal stenosis or a central disk herniation usually do not tolerate extension-based exercises. Finally, back school and an aerobic exercise program complete an active program. Although active treatment is advocated for most LBP conditions, passive treatments may be appropriate in certain clinical scenarios. Table 2.8 shows a list of some passive treatments and when their use is appropriate.

Finally, the clinician should act as a motivator when prescribing the treatment plan. Emphasize to the patient that the natural history of back pain is favorable, but the rate of recidivism can be high if compliance to a therapy program is low. When appropriate, advise the patient that back pain is not a life-threatening problem. Lay terminology should be used when describing the diagnosis. Optimize patient compliance by educating, incorporating exercises within a patient's busy day, and mon-

Table 2.8 Passive Treatments

Passive Treatment	When Appropriate
Bed rest	Acute phase of low back pain (limit to <48 hours)
Acupuncture	Acute or chronic pain
Transcutaneous electrical nerve stimulation	Acute or chronic pain
Orthoses	Acute or chronic pain
Biofeedback	Chronic pain
Medications	See Chapter 7
Trigger point injections	Myofascial pain
Manipulation	Hypomobile joints and acute phase of low back pain
Epidural injections	Acute or subacute radicular pain
Shoe lift therapy	True leg length discrepancy more than one-half inch
Myotherapy	Myofascial pain

itoring through regular follow-up. Moreover, remind the patient that the major goal of treatment is to increase function and that pain control typically follows.[79]

FOLLOW-UP

Follow-up is individualized but usually performed after 4 weeks, or earlier if radicular pain is not well controlled. At this time, the clinician can determine if the treatment plan is actually being instituted. Patient compliance can be assessed by having the patient demonstrate his or her home exercise program. If the proper treatment plan has been instituted and the patient is compliant, the clinician can determine if the treatment plan has had a positive impact. If the goals have not been met, more aggressive care should be considered. Other passive treatments can be used so that pain can be better controlled and subsequently allow patients to progress in their home exercise programs. Persistent radicular pain may be managed with lumbar epidural steroid injections.[20,76,80–90] Surgical referral can be considered if radicular pain and overall function is not improved within 2–3 months. However, patients should be reminded that surgical care is elective and that nonsurgical care is still a viable option even if a referral to a surgeon is made. Finally, if the patient is not responding to the treatment course, the physician should reconsider the working diagnosis. At this point, further diagnostic tests (e.g., MRI) may help revise the diagnosis and therapeutic efforts. However, some patients progress to chronic pain despite a proper treatment course. Treatment for these patients with chronic pain syndrome is discussed in Chapter 14.

REFERENCES

1. Herring SA, Weinstein SM. Assessment and Nonsurgical Management of Athletic Low Back Injury. In JA Nicholas, EB Hershman (eds), The Lower Extremity and Spine in Sports Medicine. St. Louis: Mosby, 1995;1171–1197.

2. Frymoyer JW. Back pain and sciatica. N Engl J Med 1988;318:291–300.
3. Papageorgiou AC, Croft PR, Ferry S, et al. Estimating the prevalence of low back pain in the general population. Evidence from the South Manchester Back Pain Survey. Spine 1995;20:1889–1894.
4. Cypress BK. Characteristics of physician visits for back symptoms: a national perspective. Am J Public Health 1983;73:389–395.
5. Frymoyer JW, Cats-Baril WL. An overview of the incidences and costs of low back pain. Orthop Clin North Am 1991;22:263–271.
6. Spengler DM, Bigos SJ, Martin NA, et al. Back injuries in industry: a retrospective study. I. Overview and cost analysis. Spine 1986;11:241–245.
7. Williams DA, Feuerstein M, Durbin D, et al. Health care and indemnity costs across the natural history of disability in occupational low back pain. Spine 1998;23:2329–2336.
8. Bergquist-Ullman M, Larsson U. Acute low back pain in industry. A controlled prospective study with special reference to therapy and confounding factors. Acta Orthop Scand 1977;170:1–117.
9. Young J, Press J, Herring SA. The disk at risk in athletes: perspectives on operative and nonoperative care. Med Sci Sports Exerc 1997;29[Suppl7]:S222–S232.
10. Weinstein S, Herring SA, Cole AJ. Rehabilitation of the Patient with Spinal Pain. In J DeLisa, B Gans (eds), Rehabilitation Medicine: Principles and Practice. Philadelphia: Lippincott–Raven, 1998;1423–1451.
11. Von Korff M, Deyo RA, Cherkin D, et al. Back pain in primary care. Outcomes at 1 year. Spine 1993;18:855–862.
12. Von Korff M, Saunders K. The course of back pain in primary care. Spine 1996;21:2833–2839.
13. Hides JA, Richardson CA, Jull GA. Multifidus muscle recovery is not automatic after resolution of acute, first-episode low back pain. Spine 1996;21:2763–2769.
14. Bogduk N. Clinical Anatomy of the Lumbar Spine and Sacrum (3rd ed). New York: Churchill Livingstone, 1997.
15. Porterfield J, DeRosa C. Mechanical Low Back Pain: Perspectives in Functional Anatomy (2nd ed). Philadelphia: Saunders, 1998.
16. Cramer G, Darby S. Basic and Clinical Anatomy of the Spine, Spinal Cord, and ANS. St. Louis: Mosby, 1995.
17. Kirkaldy-Willis WH, Wedge JH, Yong-Hing K, et al. Pathology and pathogenesis of lumbar spondylosis and stenosis. Spine 1978;3:319–328.
18. Fardon D. Differential Diagnosis of Low Back Disorders. In JW Frymoyer (ed), The Adult Spine: Principles and Practice. Philadelphia: Lippincott–Raven, 1997;1745–1768.
19. Spitzer WO, Nachemson A. Scientific approach to the assessment and management of activity-related spinal disorders. A monograph for clinicians. Report of the Quebec Task Force on Spinal Disorders. Spine 1987;12:S1–S59.
20. Bigos S, et al. Acute Low Back Problems in Adults: Clinical Practice Guideline. Agency for Health Care Policy and Research (Vol 14). Rockville, Maryland: U. S. Department of Health and Human Services, 1994;81–88.
21. Matsui H, Kanamori M, Ishihara H, et al. Familial predisposition for lumbar degenerative disk disease. A case-control study. Spine 1998;23:1029–1034.
22. Richardson JK, Chung T, Schultz JS, Hurvitz E. A familial predisposition toward lumbar disk injury. Spine 1997;22:1487–1493.
23. Porter RW, Miller CG. Back pain and trunk list. Spine 1986;11:596–600.
24. Nice DA, Riddle DL, Lamb RL, et al. Intertester reliability of judgments of the presence of trigger points in patients with low back pain [see comments]. Arch Phys Med Rehabil 1992;73:893–898.
25. Gerwin RD, Shannon S, Hong CZ, et al. Interrater reliability in myofascial trigger point examination. Pain 1997;69:65–73.
26. Johnson EK, Chiarello CM. The slump test: the effects of head and lower extremity position on knee extension. J Orthop Sports Phys Ther 1997;26:310–317.
27. Slipman CW, Sterenfeld EB, Chou LJ, et al. The predictive value of provocative sacroiliac joint stress maneuvers in the diagnosis of sacroiliac joint syndrome. Arch Phys Med Rehabil 1998;79:288–292.

28. Dreyfuss P, Dryer S, Griffin J, et al. Positive sacroiliac screening tests in asymptomatic adults. Spine 1994;19:1138–1143.

29. Katz JN, Dalgas M, Stucki G, et al. Degenerative lumbar spinal stenosis. Diagnostic value of the history and physical examination. Arthritis Rheum 1995;38:1236–1241.

30. Waddell G, McCulloch JA, Kummel E, Venner RM. Nonorganic physical signs in low-back pain. Spine 1980;5:117–125.

31. Geraci MC, Alleva JT. Physical Examination of the Spine and Its Functional Kinetic Chain. In AJ Cole, SA Herring (eds), The Low Back Pain Handbook. Philadelphia: Hanley and Belfus, 1997;49–70.

32. Jull G, Bogduk N, Marsland A. The accuracy of manual diagnosis for cervical zygapophyseal joint pain syndromes. Med J Aust 1988;148:233–236.

33. Binkley J, Stratford PW, Gill C. Interrater reliability of lumbar accessory motion mobility testing. Phys Ther 1995;75:786–795.

34. Schwarzer AC, Aprill CN, Derby R, et al. The prevalence and clinical features of internal disk disruption in patients with chronic low back pain [see comments]. Spine 1995;20:1878–1883.

35. van den Hoogen HM, Koes BW, van Eijk JT, Bouter LM. On the accuracy of history, physical examination, and erythrocyte sedimentation rate in diagnosing low back pain in general practice. A criteria-based review of the literature [see comments]. Spine 1995;20:318–327.

36. Blower PW, Griffin AJ. Clinical sacroiliac tests in ankylosing spondylitis and other causes of low back pain—2 studies. Ann Rheum Dis 1984;43:192–195.

37. Cole AJ et al. Clinical Presentation and Diagnostic Subsets. In AJ Cole, SA Herring (eds), The Low Back Pain Handbook. Philadelphia: Hanley and Belfus, 1996;71–96.

38. Kuslich SD, Ulstrom CL, Michael CJ. The tissue origin of low back pain and sciatica: a report of pain response to tissue stimulation during operations on the lumbar spine using local anesthesia. Orthop Clin North Am 1991;22:181–187.

39. Nachemson AL. Advances in low-back pain. Clin Orthop 1985;200:266–278.

40. Aprill C, Bogduk N. High-intensity zone: a diagnostic sign of painful lumbar disk on magnetic resonance imaging. Br J Radiol 1992;65:361–369.

41. Fitzsimmons A, Freundlich B, Bonner F. Osteoporosis and rehabilitation. Crit Rev Phys Med Rehabil 1997;9:331–353.

42. Deyo RA. Early diagnostic evaluation of low back pain. J Gen Intern Med 1986;1:328–338.

43. Grobler LJ, Wiltse LL. Classification, and Nonoperative and Operative Treatment of Spondylolisthesis. In JW Frymoyer (ed), The Adult Spine: Principles and Practice. Philadelphia: Lippincott–Raven, 1997;1865–1921.

44. Wiltse L, Rothman L. Classification of spondylolysis and spondylolisthesis. Semin Spine Surg 1989;1:78–94.

45. Schwarzer AC, Aprill CN, Derby R, et al. The relative contributions of the disk and zygapophyseal joint in chronic low back pain. Spine 1994;19:801–806.

46. Helbig T, Lee CK. The lumbar facet syndrome. Spine 1988;13:61–64.

47. Dreyer SJ, Dreyfuss PH. Low back pain and the zygapophysial (facet) joints. Arch Phys Med Rehabil 1996;77:290–300.

48. Schwarzer AC, Derby R, Aprill CN, et al. Pain from the lumbar zygapophysial joints: a test of two models. J Spinal Disord 1994;7:331–336.

49. Revel ME, Listrat VM, Chevalier XJ, et al. Facet joint block for low back pain: identifying predictors of a good response. Arch Phys Med Rehabil 1992;73:824–828.

50. Schwarzer AC, Wang SC, O'Driscoll D, et al. The ability of computed tomography to identify a painful zygapophysial joint in patients with chronic low back pain. Spine 1995;20:907–912.

51. Carette S, Marcoux S, Truchon R, et al. A controlled trial of corticosteroid injections into facet joints for chronic low back pain [see comments]. N Engl J Med 1991;325:1002–1007.

52. Lilius G, Laasonen EM, Myllynen P, et al. Lumbar facet joint syndrome. A randomised clinical trial. J Bone Joint Surg Br 1989;71:681–684.

53. Mixter WJ, Barr JS. Rupture of the intervertebral disk with involvement of the spinal canal. N Engl J Med 1934;211:210.

54. Bernard TN, Cassidy D. The Sacroiliac Joint Syndrome: Pathophysiology, Diagnosis, and Management. In JW Frymoyer (ed), The Adult Spine: Principles and Practice. Philadelphia: Lippincott–Raven, 1997;2343–2366.

55. Fortin JD, Aprill CN, Ponthieux B, Pier J. Sacroiliac joint: pain referral maps upon applying a new injection/arthrography technique. Part I: Asymptomatic volunteers. Spine 1994;19:1475–1482.

56. Fortin JD, Aprill CN, Ponthieux B, Pier J. Sacroiliac joint: pain referral maps upon applying a new injection/arthrography technique. Part II: Clinical evaluation. Spine 1994;19:1483–1489.

57. Grob KR, Neuhuber WL, Kissling RO. [Innervation of the sacroiliac joint of the human]. Zeitschrift fur Rheumatologie 1995;54:117–122.

58. Fortin JD, Falco FJ. The Fortin finger test: an indicator of sacroiliac pain [see comments]. Am J Orthop 1997;26:477–480.

59. Boden SD, Frymoyer JW. Segmental Instability: Overview and Classification. In JW Frymoyer (ed), The Adult Spine: Principles and Practice, Philadelphia: Lippincott–Raven, 1997;2137–2155.

60. Macnab I. The traction spur. An indicator of segmental instability. J Bone Joint Surg Am 1971;53:663–670.

61. Weinstein JN, McLain RF. Primary tumors of the spine. Spine 1987;12:843–851.

62. Frank CJ, Brantigan JW, McGuire MH. Evaluation of patients with spinal column tumors. Spine: State of the Art Reviews 1996;10:13–24.

63. Kirkaldy-Willis WH, Burton CV. Managing Low Back Pain (3rd ed). New York: Churchill Livingstone, 1992.

64. Goupille P, Jayson MI, Valat JP, Freemont AJ. The role of inflammation in disk herniation-associated radiculopathy. Semin Arthritis Rheum 1998;28:60–71.

65. Kostuik JP, Harrington I, Alexander D, et al. Cauda equina syndrome and lumbar disk herniation. J Bone Joint Surg Am 1986;68:386–391.

66. Gundry CR, Heithoff KB, Pollei SR. Lumbar degenerative disk disease. Spine: State of the Art Reviews 1995;9:141–184.

67. Fritz JM, DeLitto A, Welch WC, Erhard RE. Lumbar spinal stenosis: a review of current concepts in evaluation, management, and outcome measurements. Arch Phys Med Rehabil 1998;79:700–708.

68. Sinaki M, Mokri B. Low Back Pain and Disorders of the Lumbar Spine. In RL Braddom (ed), Physical Medicine and Rehabilitation. Philadelphia: Saunders, 1996;813–850.

69. Schonstrom NS, Bolender NF, Spengler DM. The pathomorphology of spinal stenosis as seen on CT scans of the lumbar spine. Spine 1985;10:806–811.

70. Porter RW, Hibbert C, Evans C. The natural history of root entrapment syndrome. Spine 1984;9:418–421.

71. Atlas SJ, Deyo RA, Keller RB, et al. The Maine Lumbar Spine Study, Part III. 1-year outcomes of surgical and nonsurgical management of lumbar spinal stenosis [see comments]. Spine 1996;21:1787–1795.

72. Johnsson KE, Uden A, Rosen I. The effect of decompression on the natural course of spinal stenosis. A comparison of surgically treated and untreated patients. Spine 1991;16:615–619.

73. Johnsson KE, Rosen I, Uden A. The natural course of lumbar spinal stenosis. Clin Orthop 1992;279:82–86.

74. Turner JA, Ersek M, Herron L, Deyo R. Surgery for lumbar spinal stenosis. Attempted meta-analysis of the literature. Spine 1992;17:1–8.

75. Herno A, Airaksinen O, Saari T. Long-term results of surgical treatment of lumbar spinal stenosis. Spine 1993;18:1471–1474.

76. Saal JA, Saal JS. Nonoperative treatment of herniated lumbar intervertebral disk with radiculopathy. An outcome study. Spine 1989;14:431–437.

77. Weber H. Lumbar disk herniation. A controlled, prospective study with ten years of observation. Spine 1983;8:131–140.

78. Deyo R. Nonoperative Treatment of Low Back Disorders: Differentiating Useful from Useless Therapy. In J Frymoyer (ed), The Adult Spine: Principles and Practice. Philadelphia: Lippincott–Raven, 1997;1777–1793.

79. Saal JA, Saal JS. Physical Rehabilitation of Low Back Pain. In JW Frymoyer (ed), The Adult Spine: Principles and Practice. Philadelphia: Lippincott–Raven, 1997;1805–1819.

80. Bush K, Hillier S. A controlled study of caudal epidural injections of triamcinolone plus procaine for the management of intractable sciatica. Spine 1991;16:572–575.

81. White AH, Derby R, Wynne G. Epidural injections for the diagnosis and treatment of low-back pain. Spine 1980;5:78–86.

82. Lutz GE, Vad VB, Wisneski RJ. Fluoroscopic transforaminal lumbar epidural steroids: an outcome study. Arch Phys Med Rehabil 1998;79:1362–1366.
83. Koes BW, Scholten RJ, Mens JM, Bouter LM. Efficacy of epidural steroid injections for low-back pain and sciatica: a systematic review of randomized clinical trials. Pain 1995;63:279–288.
84. Dilke TF, Burry HC, Grahame R. Extradural corticosteroid injection in management of lumbar nerve root compression. BMJ 1973;2:635–637.
85. Ridley MG, Kingsley GH, Gibson T, Grahame R. Outpatient lumbar epidural corticosteroid injection in the management of sciatica. Br J Rheumatol 1988;27:295–299.
86. Breivik H, et al. Treatment of Chronic Low Back Pain and Sciatica: Comparison of Caudal Epidural Injections of Bupivacaine and Methylprednisolone with Bupivacaine Followed by Saline. In JJ Bonica, et al. (eds), Advances in Pain Research and Therapy. New York: Raven Press, 1976;927–932.
87. Mathews JA, Mills SB, Jenkins VM, et al. Back pain and sciatica: controlled trials of manipulation, traction, sclerosant and epidural injections. Br J Rheumatol 1987;26:416–423.
88. Helliwell M. Outpatient treatment of low back pain and sciatica by a single extradural corticosteroid injection. Br J Clin Pract 1985;225–231.
89. Yates DW. A comparison of the types of epidural injection commonly used in the treatment of low back pain and sciatica. Rheumatol Rehabil 1978;17:181–186.
90. Dallas TL, Lin RL, Wu WH, Wolskee P. Epidural morphine and methylprednisolone for low-back pain. Anesthesiology 1987;67:408–411.

Chapter 3
Geriatric Lumbar Spine Disorders

Robert G. Viere

When an elderly patient enters the office complaining of back or leg pain, or both, a multitude of factors play a role in the diagnostic decision-making process. A large component of the process occurs during the history and physical examination. Ancillary tests generally play only a confirmatory role. Therefore, it is vitally important to approach the history and physical examination in a systematic and thorough fashion. Careful attention to detail, starting with the chief complaint and progressing through the history of present illness, past medical history, review of systems, medications, family history, social history, and a thorough physical examination, are all clues that help to make an accurate diagnosis. Diagnostic testing helps to confirm and guide treatment decisions.

HISTORY OF PRESENT ILLNESS

The patient's age, sex, and ethnic background start the history and play a role in the decision-making process. Malignancies, Paget's disease, osteoporosis, osteomalacia, and degenerative changes of the spine all occur more frequently with increasing age. Females are twice as likely to have osteoporotic compression fractures than males; and fair-skinned white females are four times as likely to have osteoporotic compression fractures than black females.[1] The second part of this history is to determine where the pain is located. Is the pain in the upper back or the lower back? Osteoporotic compression fractures are less common above T8 and pain in the upper thoracic region is generally caused by other sources. Does the pain radiate into the lower extremities, and, if so, does it radiate into both lower extremities or only one lower extremity? Sixty-nine percent of patients with spinal stenosis have bilateral lower extremity symptoms.[2] Does the pain involve the whole limb or only above the knee or below the knee? Seventy-eight percent of patients with spinal stenosis have pain involving the entire limb, and 7% have pain below the knee only.[2] How did the pain start? Was it of insidious onset or abrupt onset? Was there trauma involved? Abrupt onset of symptoms, especially precipitated by trauma, indicates the possibility of fracture. However, polymyalgia rheumatica commonly starts with an abrupt onset, as do several other nonspinal etiologies of back and leg pain (Table 3.1).

Table 3.1 Nonspinal Etiologies of Back and Leg Pain

Conditions	Key Points
Vascular	
Abdominal aortic aneurysm	Age >50 years, more common in males
	Abdominal and back pain
	Familial tendency
	Pulsatile mass in abdomen
Genitourinary	
Kidney stones	Flank pain, hematuria
	Cerebrovascular accident tenderness
Prostasis	Can cause ileus, nausea, and vomiting
	Pelvic pain radiation to low back and perineal area
	Dysuria—low-grade fever
Rheumatologic	
Polymyalgia rheumatica	Age >50 years
	Acute onset
	Hip and shoulder girdle pain and severe morning stiffness
	Elevated erythrocyte sedimentation rate
	Dramatic response to corticosteroids
Diffuse idiopathic skeletal hyperostosis	Age >50 years
	Diffuse spinal stiffness
	Anterior vertebral calcification
	Occasional dysplasia
Piriforms syndrome	Buttock and leg pain
	Pain on resisted external rotation or full internal rotation
	Transgluteal tenderness
Trochanteric bursitis/iliotibial band tendonitis	Pain on palpation over greater trochanter
	Pain may increase lying on involved side at night
	Pain with hip rotation
Metabolic	
Osteomalacia	Diffuse skeletal pain or tenderness even without fracture
	Increased alkaline phosphatase
	Bone biopsy—wide osteoid seams
	Antalgic waddling gait
	May be related to malabsorption syndromes
Paget's disease	More common as population ages
	Ten percent in people older than age 80 years
	Can lead to increased skull size and hearing loss
	May be associated with acute spinal stenosis
Diabetic radiculitis	Typically seen in older patients
	More common in males than females
	Not related to severity of diabetes
	Often occurs in mid-adult onset diabetes of recent onset
	May be diffuse or dermatomal leg pain, worse at night
Gastrointestinal pancreatitis	Abdominal pain radiates to back; deep boring quality
	Systemic signs (e.g., nausea)
	Elevated serum amylase
	May be associated with chololithiasis or alcohol abuse
Perforated gastric or especially duodenal ulcer	Abdominal pain radiating to back
	May be associated with nonsteroidal anti-inflammatory drug use
	May see blood on hemoccult test

How long has the pain been ongoing? Symptoms that have been ongoing for longer than 1 month, or are progressively getting worse, cause more concern than short-term symptoms. Has this pain been present before? If the patient has had episodes like this previously that have resolved spontaneously or with treatment, this can help guide the treatment plan. Lifetime prevalence of benign low back pain exceeds 70% in all industrialized countries and tends to be episodic in nature.

What is the quality of the pain? Is the pain worse at night or associated with morning stiffness? What makes the pain better or worse? A deep aching pain in the low back without radiation suggests that there is no neurologic impingement. However, low back pain associated with a sharp radiating pain down the lower extremities could suggest neurologic involvement. A pain that is worse at night could indicate a malignancy. A pain that is worse in the early morning hours or associated with severe morning stiffness suggests an inflammatory etiology for the pain. Are there any associated constitutional symptoms? A patient with fever, chills, and weight loss suggests a systemic abnormality that is presenting as back pain.

Is there any associated weakness, numbness, paresthesias, or dysesthesias? All of these suggest neurologic involvement. Is the pain, weakness, or numbness, or any combination of these symptoms, associated only with activity, or is it also present with recumbency? Patients with spinal stenosis often have symptoms in the lower extremities only with ambulation or standing. If the pain is not positional or affected by activity, but radiates into the lower extremity, it is more suggestive of a neuropathy or a causalgia type of pain.

Has the problem been affecting the patient's sleep? If the patient is not getting adequate rest at night, that tends to increase the patient's overall pain perception. Has the patient noticed any discreet areas of tenderness? Patients with trochanteric bursitis may tell you that they cannot lie on one side without getting severe pain that does not allow them to sleep. Has there been any bowel or bladder dysfunction or increased urination? Bowel and bladder dysfunction is generally a late neurologic finding, except in a setting of acute neurologic compression. Increased urinary frequency may be a sign of bladder obstruction, which can sometimes lead to genitourinary infections, which can present as back pain. Additionally, patients with undiagnosed diabetes present with increased urination. The components of the present history should be put in the context of the patient's previous medical history.

PAST MEDICAL HISTORY

A thorough evaluation of the patient's previous medical problems is vitally important. Does the patient have a history of hypertension? This tends to increase risk of abdominal aortic aneurysm, which can present as back pain. Does the patient have a history of diabetes? Acute diabetic radiculitis can present as severe back and leg pain. This can be monoradicular or polyradicular. It does not appear to be related to the severity of the diabetes itself and often can be the initial presenting symptom of new onset diabetes. Does the patient have a history of peripheral vascular disease? Vascular claudication presents as buttock or leg pain, or both. Vascular claudication generally is noted with activity, such as walking, and is relieved by standing still. Neurogenic claudication, on the other hand, is generally brought on by walking, but to relieve the symptoms, patients either lean forward or sit down; simply standing still does not help their leg pain. Many patients with spinal stenosis note that as they

Table 3.2 Estimated New Cases of Metastatic Malignancy
to the Spine—Most Common Tumors

Site	Number of Cases Metastatic to Spine	Percentage of Total Malignancy
Breast	61,000–86,000	50–70%
Prostate	45,000–72,000	50–80%
Lung	15,000–45,000	10–30%
Colon/rectal	28,000–42,000	20–30%
Urinary tract	6,000–15,000	10–25%

walk further, they find themselves leaning more forward, or, for example, when they go grocery shopping, they need a grocery cart to support them if they are on their feet for longer than short periods.

Is there is any history of hematologic disorders (e.g., myelodysplasia)? Patients with myelodysplastic disorders are more prone to occult infections, which can commonly present as low back pain.

Does the patient have a history of cancer? What kind of cancer did he or she have and what treatment regimen did he or she undergo? Patients with previous radiation to the lumbar spine can present with osteitis or osteonecrosis with subsequent fracture. Certain malignancies are associated with bony metastasis, which frequently involves the spinal column and more often involves the lumbar spine than any other area of the spine (Table 3.2).

Does the patient have a history of asthma or nasal polyps? The most common medication regimen for patients with benign low back pain is nonsteroidal anti-inflammatory drugs (NSAIDs). Patients with a history of asthma or nasal polyps may be sensitive to NSAIDs (Table 3.3). NSAIDs also should be used with some caution in the elderly due to possible decreased renal filtration, as well as a greater incidence of hepatitis. Patients who are taking nonsteroidal anti-inflammatories on a continuous basis should be monitored with blood urea nitrogen, creatinine, and liver function tests approximately every 3 months. The NSAIDs also tend to affect platelet function and, in the elderly, who are susceptible to falls, could increase the risk for developing clinically significant hematomas.

The previous surgical history is vitally important. Has the patient had any previous back surgery? Previous surgery can make the patient more susceptible to occult infection, iatrogenic instability of the spine, such as degenerative scoliosis or spondylolisthesis, as well as progressive degeneration above the site of previous surgery. Patients with a partial sacralization of L5 have four times the incidence of degenerative spondylolisthesis at L4–L5.[3] Patients with previous lumbar fusions often have degenerative spondylolisthesis above their fusion based on the same increased mechanical stress at the interface between a mobile and nonmobile segment. Other previous surgeries may also play a role. Has the patient had thyroid surgery? Excess thyroid replacement can lead to osteoporosis. Injury to the parathyroid gland can affect the calcium metabolism. Patients with previous biliary surgery may have a higher incidence of pancreatitis, which can present as back pain. Previous gastric procedures, especially Billroth II gastric bypasses, can lead to malabsorption syndrome, which can lead to osteomalacia (Table 3.4).

Table 3.3 Nonsteroidal Anti-Inflammatory Drugs

	Name	Starting Dose	Maximal Dose
Short half life (4–6 hrs)			
	Aspirin	650 mg q4–6 hrs	4,000–5,000 mg
	Ibuprofen (Motrin)	400 mg q6 hrs	3,200 mg
	Ketoprofen (Orudis)	50 mg q6 hrs	300 mg
	Flurbiprofen (Ansaid)	50 mg q6 hrs	300 mg
Intermediate half life (8–12 hrs)			
	Etodolac (Lodine)	400 mg q12 hrs	1,200 mg
	Sulindac (Clinoril)	100 mg q12 hrs	400 mg
	Diflunisal (Dolobid)	500 mg q12 hrs	1,500 mg
	Naprosyn	375 mg q12 hrs	1,000 mg
	Diclofenac (Voltaren)	50 mg q8 hrs	200 mg
	Trisalicylate (Trilisate)	1,000 mg q12 hrs	3,000 mg
	(Celebrex)	100 mg q12 hrs	400 mg
	Indomethacin (Indocin)	25 mg q8 hrs	150 mg
Longer half life (up to 24 hrs)			
	Piroxicam (Feldene)	20 mg q24 hrs	20 mg
	Nabumetone (Relafen)	1,500 mg q24 hrs	1,500 mg
	Oxaprozin (Daypro)	1,200 mg q24 hrs	1,200 mg
	Etodolac (Lodine XL)	800 mg q24 hrs	1,000 mg
	Naprelan	1,000 mg q24 hrs	1,000 mg
	Indomethacin (Indocin SR)	75 mg q24 hrs	75 mg

Rheumatologic disorders typically present with axial skeletal pain. Rheumatoid arthritis, ankylosing spondylitis, psoriatic arthritis, polymyalgia rheumatica, and disseminated idiopathic skeletal hyperarthrosis, typically have back pain as a major component of the disease process. Certain endocrine states can lead to osteoporosis and increased risk of spinal fracture (Table 3.5). Diseases themselves, as well as the treatment of various disease states, affect the patient's risk for clinical abnormalities that can lead to back pain.

MEDICATIONS

Corticosteroid usage, including inhalational corticosteroid usage, has been shown to increase the risk of osteoporosis. Certain antilipid medications, especially cholestyramine, can lead to an increased risk of biliary obstruction and, therefore, pancreatitis. Certain anticonvulsive medications can lead to osteomalacia (see Table 3.3). For a female, estrogen replacement in the postmenopausal period appears to play a significant role in the possible development of osteoporosis later in life (Table 3.6). NSAIDs increase the risk of gastric perforation, which can present as back pain.

Table 3.4 Major Causes of Osteomalacia

Deficiency states
Scurvy
Malnutrition
Gastrointestinal malabsorption
Gluten sensitive enteropathy
Regional enteritis
Resection or bypass of small intestine
Liver disease
Chronic biliary ducal and hepatocellular disorders
Cirrhosis
Cholestyramine therapy
Anticonvulsant drugs
Phenobarbital and phenytoin most common
Renal osteodystrophy

REVIEW OF SYSTEMS

Careful review of systems to ascertain whether any other medical processes are affecting the patient's back pain is important. The review of systems starts with a general overview, emphasizing any patient reports of constitutional symptoms for overall health, followed by a systematic review of various systems of the body.

Head, Ears, Eyes, Nose, and Throat

Has the patient noticed any visual disturbances? Multiple sclerosis, which can present as neurologic disturbances into the hands and legs, also commonly has associated visual symptoms. Has the patient had any other cranial nerve symptoms

Table 3.5 Major Causes of Osteoporosis

Senile and postmenopausal states
Medications
Corticosteroids
Thyroid hormone excess
Heparin
Antacids containing aluminum
Isoniazid
Endocrine states
Hyperthyroidism
Hyperparathyroidism
Cushing's Disease
Acromegaly
Pregnancy
Diabetes
Hypogonadism

Table 3.6 Risk Factors for Low Bone Mass in Postmenopausal Women

---

Female
White or Asian ethnicity
Fair skin
Thin body habitus
Low calcium intake
Positive family history
Oophorectomy
Early menopause
Nulliparity
High sodium intake
High caffeine intake
High phosphate intake
Alcohol abuse
Cigarette smoking
Sedentary lifestyle

---

or has the patient noticed any increase in hat size? Paget's disease can cause enlargement of the skull, which can cause narrowing of the foramen through which the cranial nerves exit. This most often affects the acoustic nerve and can lead to hearing loss. Paget's disease affects the low back and pelvis and can lead to isolated low back pain, as well as spinal stenosis, sometimes precipitating an acute neurologic emergency (see Table 3.1).

Neck

Does the patient have any stiffness of the neck or dysphasia? Large osteophytes that can form anteriorly in disseminated idiopathic skeletal hyperarthrosis can cause dysphasia. There is also a high correlation between the incidents of degenerative disease of the cervical spine and degenerative disease of the lumbar spine.

Chest

Has the patient had any recent cough or upper respiratory illness? Patients with osteoporosis can have spontaneous rib and vertebral fractures with coughing episodes. Has the patient had any shortness of breath or dyspnea on exertion? If this has led to the patient pursuing a sedentary lifestyle, it can lead to increased incidence of chronic low back pain on a multifactorial basis.

Heart and Vascular

Patients with a history of abdominal aortic aneurysm can sometimes present with acute low back pain. This may be a sign of acute rupture and constitutes a medical emergency.

Musculoskeletal

Has the patient noticed any change in posture? Degenerative scoliosis often relates to back pain and spinal stenosis and is noted as a change in the sagittal and coronal plain posture of patients. Increased thoracic kyphosis can occur due to multilevel disk degeneration (e.g., Dowager's hump), or can be due to thoracic-level compression fractures. Has the patient noticed any deformity of the lower extremities? Paget's disease can sometimes present as a bowing deformity of the lower extremities. Has the patient noticed any other joint swelling? Psoriatic arthritis, which can affect the spine, can also affect the digits of the hand, causing what is classically called a *sausage digit*.

Has the patient noticed any recent deformity of the foot? Abnormalities of the foot, such as posterior tibial tendon rupture, can lead to an alteration in gait, which, in a patient with a stiff osteoarthritic spine, can be a contributory factor to back pain.

Genitourinary

Has the patient noticed any painful urination, any change in urine color, or any blood in the urine? Blood in the urine can be a sign of kidney infection or kidney stone, or both, which can be a cause of back pain. Change in color or smell of the urine can be a sign of infection, either bladder infection or, in males, a prostate infection, which can also radiate pain to the low back. In a female it is important to find out if the patient had amenorrhea as a young woman as this increases her risk of osteoporosis. When did the patient go through menopause? Was it a natural menopause or a surgically induced menopause? Did the patient have hormone replacement at the onset of menopause? Patients who experience menopause at a young age, especially those in whom it has been surgically induced, have a higher incidence of osteoporosis. Hormone replacement in the first 6 years after menopause can significantly reduce the rapid bone loss that follows menopause (see Tables 3.4 and 3.5).[1,4]

Gastrointestinal

Gastrointestinal and dietary history is important. Does the patient have any food allergies? Do the types of foods the patient eats provide him or her with adequate calcium intake. Diets high in phytate and lignin, such as rhubarb, tend to bind calcium and decrease calcium absorption. Does the patient get adequate vitamin D intake? Patients with lactose intolerance who do not supplement their calcium intake with other sources of calcium may be getting deficient calcium in their diet. This can lead to an increased incidence of osteoporosis. Patients who do not get adequate vitamin D intake, especially institutionalized or home-bound elderly patients, are at a higher risk for osteomalacia.

Does the patient have any history of biliary disease, Crohn's disease, or gluten-sensitive enteropathy? These entities can lead to malabsorption syndrome of the intestines and lead to possible osteomalacia. Crohn's disease can be associated with peripheral-joint arthritis. Does the patient have a history of peptic ulcer disease? A perforated peptic ulcer, either gastric or duodenal, can present as acute low back pain. Does the patient have a history of liver disease? Vitamin D metabolism occurs in the liver; therefore, patients with hepatocellular or hepatobiliary disease of the liver can become vitamin D deficient because they are unable to complete the full metabolic construction of the vitamin D molecule. This can lead to osteomalacia.

Neurologic

Does the patient have a history of cerebrovascular accident, which can lead to spasticity, decreased ability to ambulate, and joint stiffness, all of which can lead to back and extremity pain? Does the patient have any difficulty with balance? This can make the patient more susceptible to falls, suggestive of a more traumatic etiology for back pain. This also could be a sign of neural compression, such as lumbar stenosis or compression of the spinal cord in the cervical or thoracic region.

SOCIAL HISTORY

The patient's social activities also play a role in the etiology of back pain. It is important to take a careful work history because patients who have a job that requires repetitive heavy lifting or patients who have to do a lot of vehicular driving, because of the vibration involved in driving, have a higher incidence of back pain on a diskogenic or degenerative basis.

Does the patient smoke cigarettes? Cigarette smoking increases the risk of lung cancer, but also decreases the pH inside the disk, increasing the risk of diskogenic pain. Cigarettes also increase the rate with which NSAIDs cause ulcer disease, which can be a cause of back pain.

Does the patient drink alcohol? Alcohol use increases the risk of nutritional deficiency, causing increased rate of osteoporosis and osteomalacia. Alcohol use also increases the risk of hepatobiliary disease, increasing the risk of pancreatitis, which can present as back pain. Alcohol use also increases the risk of ulcer production with NSAIDs.

FAMILY HISTORY

Several medical conditions have familial tendencies of which back or leg pain, or both, may be the presenting complaint. Patients with a family history of diabetes are statistically more likely to be diagnosed with the disease. Diabetes can present as acute polyradiculitis or monoradiculitis, which can mimic a nerve root compression and cause severe back or leg pain, or both.

Studies show an increased risk of aortic aneurysm in first-degree relatives of patients with a documented diagnosis of an aortic aneurysm; therefore, this should be noted in the family history. Patients are more likely to develop spondyloarthropathies or psoriatic arthritis if relatives have been diagnosed with the disease. The spondyloarthropathies, particularly in women, can have a variable presentation and may not have the associated diagnostic changes of the sacroiliac joints and vertebral bodies that are noted in the majority of males with ankylosing spondylitis.

Rheumatoid arthritis tends to pass a generation, transmitted from grandmother to granddaughter, and is more common in females. Rheumatoid arthritis can have a variable presentation. At least 30% of patients have minimal obvious joint involvement with their rheumatoid disease and may have only occasional flares of variable lengths.

Certain malignancies tend to have a higher incidence in family groups. In particular, breast cancer is noted to have a significant increased risk in first-degree female relatives of patients with breast cancer. In approximately 30% of cases, the initial presentation for malignancy is metastatic disease of which metastases to the spine are common (see Table 3.2).

PHYSICAL EXAMINATION

After taking a thorough history, have in mind a list of possible diagnoses. The physical examination helps to eliminate certain possibilities and brings to the forefront other possible diagnoses. The physical examination begins with taking the vital signs. By the time a patient is placed in a room, he or she should have had his or her height, weight, blood pressure, pulse, and respiration documented.

A good physical examination begins with a general observation of the patient. If possible, watch the patient walk down the hallway as he or she is led to an examination room because this may provide insight to his or her level of function. Observe the patient to see if he or she appears pale or robust, overweight or underweight, or has any obvious deformities. Whenever possible, have the patient wear an examination gown to have complete access to visualize the involved body parts.

After general observation of the patient, examine the patient's gait with the gown on and with shoes and socks off. Watch for a limp, as this may suggest the degree of pain or muscular weakness the patient has; and evaluate the patient for a Trendelenburg gait or a foot drop. A Trendelenburg gait in a patient who has not had previous hip surgery may suggest weakness of the hip abductors on a neurologic basis due to lower nerve root impingement. Observe whether the patient leans forward when walking. Again, patients with spinal stenosis tend to lean forward progressively with gait because this allows them to walk further without severe leg pain.

Does the patient have any balance difficulties? Again, muscle imbalance can be a sign of neurologic involvement and should be evaluated carefully. Can the patient elevate his or her weight on toes and heels? This is a quick way to evaluate for general strength of the muscles below the knees.

A closer inspection of the spine should be made. Determine if there is any deformity within the spine or any increased kyphosis in the thoracic spine suggestive of possible compression fracture. Is there any scoliosis of the thoracic or lumbar spine, and are these deformities of a gentle nature, or is there an abrupt change in curvature to suggest a more traumatic etiology to the curvature? In the lumbar spine, has the patient lost normal lordosis? This occurs with advancing disk degeneration, and this postural abnormality may be the cause of the patient's back pain. With increased thoracic kyphosis due to fracture or disk degeneration and loss of normal lumbar lordosis, the patient is placed in a forward flexed posture, which puts significantly increased stress on the paraspinal musculature. The normal spine and its sagittal curve is such that the spine is balanced, and the muscles have to simply fire periodically to maintain an upright position. If the muscles have to hold the trunk in an upright position continuously throughout the day they fatigue, and this fatigue can be a cause of significant back pain. Palpate for tenderness along the thoracic or lumbar area. Are there any palpable trigger points in the paraspinal muscle? Are there any nodules over the sacroiliac joint that are painful? Occasionally, patients have fibrofatty nodules over the sacroiliac joints that have become inflamed and, because they can become easily irritated in the sitting position, they can be a cause of low back and buttocks pain. Evaluate range of motion to determine if there are any segmental areas of the spine that are limited in motion. This also helps to determine if in forward flexion there is a list to one side, or whether the patient may be trying to open the neuroforamen on one side of the spine by listing in the opposite direction. Patients with nerve root impingement do this to relieve pressure on the involved nerve. Also, severe generalized stiffness can be seen in conditions such as ankylosing spondylitis and disseminated idiopathic skeletal hyperarthrosis. Occasionally, a palpable step-off between the spinous processes of the lumbar area can be indicative of a spondylolisthesis.

Does the range of motion in any plane increase that pain? In patients with spinal stenosis, lumbar extension can aggravate that pain and cause radiating pain into the lower extremities. Classic teaching suggests that it takes a leg length discrepancy of an inch or more to be considered the cause of back pain. This may be the case in a younger population; however, the elderly, because of the stiffness in the spine that occurs with age, are unable to compensate for a leg length discrepancy to the same degree, and that compensation may produce increased stress on osteoarthritic disks and joints that can present as back or leg pain, or both.

Have the patient sit on the examining room table and examine his or her neck to make sure there are no masses in the neck, as well as check range of motion of the neck. Again, there is a direct correlation between significant spondylosis of the neck and significant spondylosis of the lumbar spine. Check for tenderness in the temporal area. Patients with polymyalgia rheumatica have severe tenderness and possible temporal arteritis. Evaluate for trigger points in the neck and parascapular region, evaluating for a possible myofascial etiology for the patient's pain. Check range of motion of the joints of the lower extremities. Are there any hip flexion contractures? Hip flexion contractures can cause a person to lean forward, leading to fatigue pain in the low back. Does the patient have pain with resisted external rotation or with full internal rotation, suggesting a possible piriformis syndrome? Does the patient have limited internal rotation, suggestive of possible hip disease as a contributing factor to his or her back pain? Do the joints of the lower extremities have any thickening or swelling that suggest a possible rheumatologic disease process? Is there any bowing of the long bones? Again, Paget's disease may present as a bowing deformity of the long bone of the leg. Does the patient have any evidence of rotator cuff tendonitis or tear? Patients with shoulder pathology often have upper back pain as well, and the pain from the shoulders at night may affect their sleep, thereby increasing their risk of back pain due to fatigue.

Does the patient show any signs of hypersensitivity to palpation of the back or significant increasing pain with rotation of the hips and shoulders as a unit, or any increased pain with minimal compression of the top of the head? These and the other Waddell's signs can suggest symptom magnification with somatization, which may require the assistance of a psychologist in the patient's treatment regimen.

Does the patient show any signs of atrophy of the lower extremities, atrophy of the skin, or hair loss of the lower extremities. Patients with causalgias commonly have an atrophy of the skin with a shiny nature to the skin, hair loss, and hypersensitivity to palpation. Patients with peripheral vascular disease may also have loss of hair growth on the feet due to vascular insufficiency. Vascular insufficiency can also cause skin changes, and these should be evaluated carefully. Does the patient have palpable pulses bilaterally, or are they diminished from one side to the other? Atrophy of the lower extremities can also be a sign of neurologic involvement with muscle atrophy due to denervation.

A complete neurologic examination is imperative. Begin the examination with straight leg raising, both in the supine and sitting position. Positive straight leg raising below 30 degrees is highly predictive of nerve root impingement or inflammation, or both, which can be caused by a herniated nucleus pulposus. A positive straight leg raising above 50 degrees loses its diagnostic significance. Contralateral straight leg raising causing pain down the involved limb is specific to nerve root impingement. A complete motor examination should be done. Does the patient have any weakness on static testing? Sometimes this weakness may be subtle, and muscle strength should be tested in several different ways. It should be tested with maximal resistance, which can sometimes pick up a subtle change from one side to the other. The strength of lower extremities can be checked by having the patient do repetitive toe raises. On the involved limb, the patient is able to elevate his or her weight on his or her toes significantly less often than on the uninvolved limb. Patients with spinal stenosis may not have any static neurologic loss; however, with walking down the hallway back and forth they may start to have increased pain and significant weakness on examination.

Patients with diabetic polyradiculopathy (amyotrophy) may have significant proximal muscle weakness and muscle wasting, which often presents as difficulty rising from a chair or Bower's sign when they try to rise from the floor.

A careful sensory examination is necessary. Does the patient have normal light-touch sensation equal from side to side in all dermatomes? Does he or she have normal pinprick sensation in all dermatomes? If there is sensory loss, what is its distribution? Is it in a dermatomal distribution, suggestive of a nerve root impingement? Does it involve an entire extremity, suggestive of a cord-level lesion or central nervous system abnormality? Is the sensory loss in a stocking-glove distribution, suggestive of a peripheral neuropathy? Does the patient have normal vibratory sense and proprioception? Again, these can be affected by a peripheral neuropathy or posterior column of the spinal cord abnormality. Are the reflexes symmetric from side to side and also from knee to ankle? A loss of an ankle jerk on one side suggests an S1 nerve root dysfunction on that side. Loss of bilateral ankle jerks with intact knee reflexes suggests distal nerve root impingement, such as spinal stenosis or, perhaps, a peripheral neuropathy. How do the patient's upper extremity reflexes compare to the lower extremity reflexes? The reflexes at the knee are reduced or absent in 18% of patients with spinal stenosis. Ankle reflexes are reduced or absent in 43% of patients with spinal stenosis, and upper extremity reflexes should be normal. Evaluate the patient for any long track signs. Does he or she have a positive crossed adductor reflex. Is it bilateral or unilateral? Does the patient have clonus or upgoing plantar reflexes, suggesting upper motor neuron impingement? Occasionally, a patient may have myelopathy from upper motor neuron impingement, but his or her reflexes are depressed due to concomitant lumbar spinal stenosis; therefore, the hyperreflexia of the lower extremities typically seen in myelopathy are not present. If the patient's long track signs are positive, even on only one sign, it suggests a more central etiology for the patient's neurologic dysfunction.

At the completion of the physical examination you should have a clear list in your head of the possible etiologies for the patient's symptoms, and the symptoms should be ranked from most to least probable. If, after the history and physical examination, you are convinced of the cause of the patient's symptoms, treatment may begin. If, however, there are several remaining possibilities for the etiology of the patient's pain, then ancillary testing can be performed to further confirm or rule out diagnoses and to focus the treatment regimen.

ANCILLARY TESTING

After completion of a thorough history and physical examination, various ancillary tests can be beneficial in confirming your clinical impression.

Plain Radiographs

Numerous studies have suggested that the changes noted on plain radiographs have limited use regarding correlation with the etiology of back pain. Plain radiographs can, however, confirm certain clinical suspicions. For patients who have not had x-rays in the recent past, at least a baseline anteroposterior and lateral x-ray of the spine can be helpful. For patients who have subtle signs of instability, such as retrolisthesis, on a standard anteroposterior and lateral film, flexion and extension radiographs can be helpful. Plain x-rays can confirm the possible presence of compression fractures in an area correlating with a site of the patient's pain. Irregularities on plain x-ray sometimes show an area suspicious for possible metastatic lesion or infection. Degenerative spondylolisthesis visible on a plain x-ray may be the cause of the patient's symptoms of spinal stenosis (Figure 3.1).

Although plain x-rays are not diagnostic, their correlation with history and physical findings can be diagnostic. In those cases in which the films may not be diagnostic, such as with a degenerative spondylolisthesis, they may lead to further testing to confirm suspicion of spinal stenosis at that level.

Bone Scans

Radionucleotide bone imaging studies can be helpful in evaluating occult fractures. Patients with significant osteoporosis may have insufficiency fractures that are not evident on plain radiographs. They may also have compression deformities of the spine of varying ages and the presence of a wedge compression deformity of the vertebral body noted on previous radiographs. This does not preclude the possibility that further subtle compression could lead to a new onset of pain. In patients with a history of malignancy and back pain of unclear etiology, a bone scan may be beneficial to evaluate the possibility of metastatic disease. It should be remembered, however, that in multiple myeloma the bone scan can be normal even in the presence of spinal lesions. Insufficiency fractures of the sacrum can present as back pain and are most easily appreciated on bone scan (Figure 3.2).

Vascular Studies

For the patient who presents with claudication-type symptoms, it may be unclear whether the origin is neurogenic or vascular. In some cases, an elderly patient may have concurrent disease of both neurogenic and vascular origin. Vascular studies,

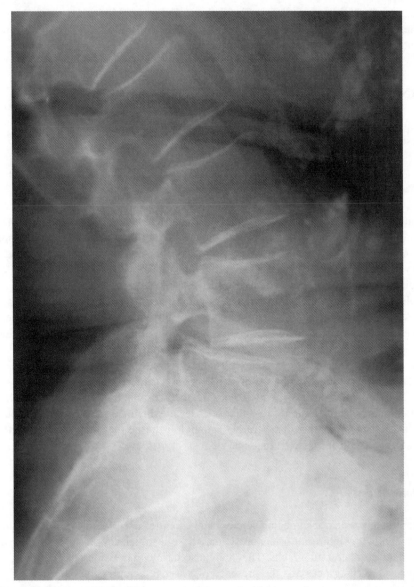

Figure 3.1 This is a 68-year-old woman who presented with progressive increasing neurogenic claudication until she was ambulatory for only a few feet. Plain x-rays show a degenerative spondylolisthesis at the L4–L5 level.

including Doppler flow and toe pressures, can provide a baseline to ascertain whether the patient does have adequate flow into the lower extremities to preclude vascular claudication. Dopplers are also useful in evaluation of deep venous thrombosis. Patients can commonly present with edema of the lower extremities. Generally this can be from a multitude of causes, including cardiac, renal, water retention, and simple benign dependent edema. However, the sedentary nature of the elderly also makes them more prone to deep venous thrombosis, and venous Doppler studies are the most common initial evaluation for that diagnosis.

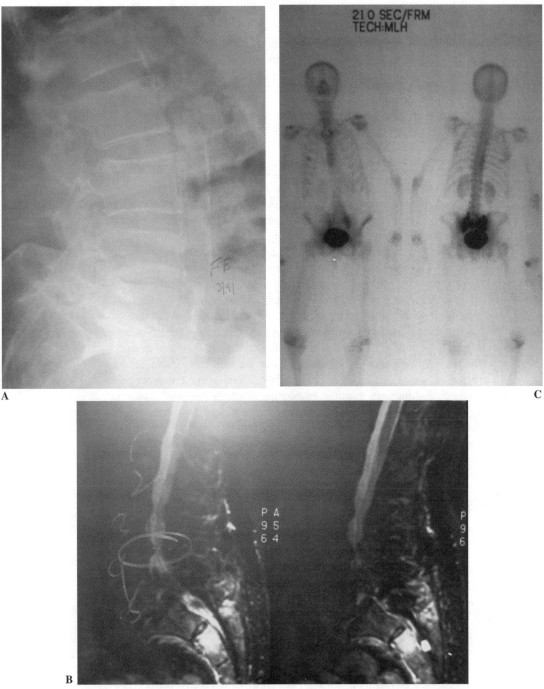

Figure 3.2 (**A**) A lateral x-ray of a 77-year-old woman with acutely exacerbated long-term back pain. Lateral x-rays show a grade II spondylolisthesis of L5 and S1. They also show a wedged deformity of the L4 vertebral body of indeterminate age. (**B**) Magnetic resonance imaging shows multilevel advanced degenerative disk disease, including a fairly significant bulge at the L3–L4 level causing moderate spinal stenosis in the same patient. We also see the grade II spondylolisthesis at L5–S1. Attention, however, should be directed to the area of increased signal intensity within the sacrum, which is consistent with a sacral insufficiency fracture. (**C**) A bone scan of the same patient confirms bilateral sacral insufficiency fractures as the cause of this woman's acute exacerbation of her long-term back pain.

For patients who have evidence of possible aortic aneurysm, either on physical examination or when plain radiographs suggest dilatation of the distal aorta, an abdominal ultrasound can provide a picture of the degree of dilatation. Abdominal ultrasound can also be beneficial in evaluation for possible intra-abdominal masses, as well as for cholelithiasis and kidney stones, all of which can be the possible cause of back pain.

Laboratory Evaluation

Laboratory tests can be beneficial in providing diagnostic information as well. The standard panel of electrolytes, for example, can indicate whether the patient's glucose is elevated, possibly leading to confirmatory tests and a diagnosis of diabetes. A blood cell count can be helpful in evaluating for possible occult infection; an erythrocyte sedimentation rate and C-reactive protein also are useful nonspecific tests that may indicate a more vigorous investigation is warranted for possible infection or inflammatory disease. The erythrocyte sedimentation rate is generally extremely high for patients with polymyalgia rheumatica. Elevated creatine phosphokinase is present in patients with myositis. Urinalysis can be helpful with blood in the urine or protein in the urine, sometimes being a sign of more proximal renal disease, which can present as back pain and can give an indication of possible renal or bladder infection, or both. Elevated hydroxyproline in the urine is seen in cases of Paget's disease. Elevated alkaline phosphatase can be seen in cases of biliary obstruction as well as cases of Paget's disease. A monoclonal spike on serum protein electrophoresis can indicate multiple myeloma, which is the most common metastatic carcinoma in the elderly. Thyroid function tests can be diagnostic of hyperthyroidism which can be a cause of osteoporosis. Parathyroid hormone also in excess can cause osteomalacia. Deficiency of vitamin B_{12} can cause pernicious anemia, which is a cause of peripheral neuropathy.

Bone biopsies can be useful for evaluating patients to make the differential diagnosis between osteomalacia and osteoporosis and to evaluate the patient's response to treatment regimens for these entities.

Electromyography and Nerve Conduction Velocities

Electrophysiologic testing can be helpful in the differential diagnosis of leg pain. It is not uncommon for elderly patients to have concomitant disease problems. Patients with evidence of neurogenic claudication and spinal stenosis may have some symptoms that are inconsistent with the diagnosis, such as burning pain into the lower extremities, especially in the feet, that may persist even at night or at rest. Patients with diabetes may have some concomitant spinal stenosis, but the spinal stenosis may not be the true cause of their leg pain. In these settings, electromyelogram and nerve conduction velocities can help differentiate between an acute radiculitis, an acute or chronic radiculopathy, or both, and peripheral neuropathy. The type of neuropathy present, whether it be primarily motor or sensory, or both, also may provide a clue to the etiology. For patients who have subtle changes on their radiographic imaging that may suggest, but not confirm, compression of a nerve root, findings on electromyelogram consistent with nerve root dysfunction in that dermatome can be helpful.

Differential Blocks

For patients who have leg pain with nonconfirmatory changes on their imaging studies, differential blocks can be beneficial. Patients whose symptoms suggest an L4 nerve root radiculopathy may have some subtle compression on imaging studies, but have diffuse degenerative changes. It may be impossible to determine on the imaging studies alone that this is the cause of the patient's leg pain. An L4 nerve root block that completely relieves the patient's leg pain can confirm the etiology of his or her pain. Differential blocks of the facet joints can also be helpful, although they are generally less specific than individual nerve root blocks. Patients who have significant spondylosis involving the facet joints may sometimes obtain significant relief from a block of the facet joint that incorporates local anesthetic and cortical steroid, which may help them get through an acute painful episode, as well as give the physician some diagnostic information.

Computed Tomography Scans

Plain computed tomography (CT) scans without intrathecal or intravenous contrast can be beneficial for looking at bony anatomy, and, therefore, for patients who may have an infection of the sacroiliac joint, a lytic lesion within a particular vertebra, or a subtle insufficiency fracture of the sacrum, the CT scan can be a diagnostic examination. The CT scan also can be helpful looking for intra-abdominal pathology such as evaluation of an abdominal aortic aneurysm. A CT scan can indicate the presence of possible spinal stenosis, either central or neural foraminal. However, it is less accurate when done without intrathecal contrast. CT scans are used primarily for evaluation of possible fractures. For evaluation of status of fusion and when patients cannot have intrathecal contrast due to a dye allergy, CT scans can be used in conjunction with a magnetic resonance imaging (MRI) scan to obtain a more complete picture of the bony anatomy than is available with an MRI scan alone.

The addition of myelography to the CT scan can significantly increase its diagnostic capacity for evaluation of nerve root impingement or spinal stenosis, or both. For patients who have a significant deformity of the spine, or for patients who have advanced spondylosis with significant osteophytosis, myelography combined with CT scanning is the gold standard for evaluation of nerve root impingement. A myelogram also allows the physician to observe any changes of nerve root impingement in the upright position as opposed to the supine position and can also provide flexion extension views with some myelographic dye in place, which can give some dynamic information about postural changes causing nerve root impingement.

Magnetic Resonance Imaging

MRI has revolutionized the ability to diagnose abnormalities within the spine. MRI is the imaging modality of choice when evaluating for possible infection or possible metastatic disease (Figure 3.3). It can also provide information about the age of fractures because of the change in the edema pattern as the fracture heals. In patients who have no significant deformity of the spine, MRI is the diagnostic imaging modality of choice for the diagnosis of spinal stenosis. MRI can be diag-

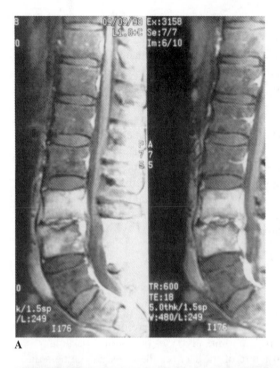

A

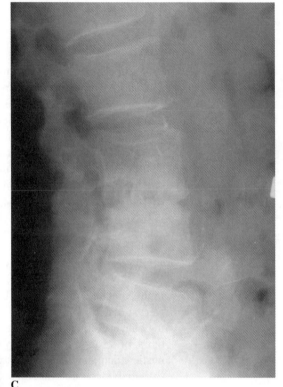

C

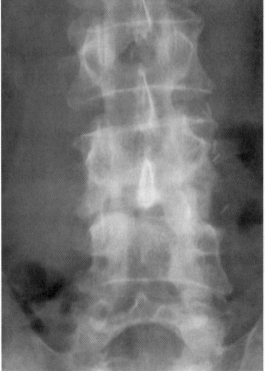

B

Figure 3.3 (**A**) Magnetic resonance imaging of a 63-year-old man who presented with spontaneous onset of severe progressive increase in back pain. The MRI shows a disk-space infection with associated irregularities of the vertebral end plates with a small fluid collection in what was the previous L3–L4 disk space. Please notice the significantly increased bone marrow signal of the vertebral bodies. (**B**) Anteroposterior and (**C**) lateral view of the patient after undergoing complete débridement of the disk space, and interbody fusion with dowel autographs taken from the iliac crest.

nostic for Paget's disease if used in correlation with plain x-rays. It allows imaging of the entire neuraxis in a noninvasive manner.

The addition of gadolinium helps the MRI become a more accurate tool in the evaluation of infection (Figure 3.4), or possible occult metastasis, or both. Gadolinium enhancement also helps to differentiate in the patient who has had previous surgical procedures of the spine between scar tissue and new pathology that may be causing neural impingement. With the advent of MRI spectroscopy in the future, physicians will be able to better delineate possible metabolic irregularities that may present as pain syndromes.

Treatment

Treatment of elderly patients with back pain is multifaceted and should be tailored to the individual patient's needs. Some of the techniques already mentioned, such as epidural steroid injections and facet blocks, can be useful adjuncts to get patients through the acute phase of pain. Some general concepts can be used in the treatment of specific disorders.

DEGENERATIVE CONDITIONS OF THE SPINE

Degenerative conditions of the spine compose the most common etiologies and generally fall within four separate subheadings: disk degenerations, spinal stenosis, degenerative spondylolisthesis, and degenerative adult scoliosis.

Disk Degenerations

Disk degenerations although relatively uncommon in elderly patients at age 65 years, can still occur in that subgroup. The treatment initially is nonoperative, starting with limited bed rest. Generally, patients who have back pain alone are put on bed rest for 2 days. Patients who have associated severe sciatica may be allowed to have bed rest up to 7 days. Although limited bed rest is generally preferred for those patients with severe nerve root pain, longer periods of rest up to 7 days may be indicated to limit irritation to the inflamed nerve root. A progressive increase in activity-McKenzie extension exercises and aerobic low-impact exercise programs are then started. Aquatic therapy also can be helpful for elderly patients. Epidural cortisone injections can be beneficial. They have been proved to be of short-term benefit in controlling acute symptoms, but have not been proved to be of any long-term benefit or to affect the long-term outcome. Aggressive physical therapy can also benefit the elderly as improvement progresses. Surgery should be considered for patients who do not respond to nonoperative management.

For disk herniations isolated to single segments, microdiskectomies are the treatment of choice. Studies have shown a 60% pain-free, long-term follow-up.[5] When comparing patients who were treated surgically versus those who were treated non-surgically for disk herniations and sciatica, approximately 87% of patients who had surgery were satisfied with their care versus 68% in the nonoperative group. Approximately 5–15% of patients require further surgery due to leg degenerative changes and developmental spinal stenosis.

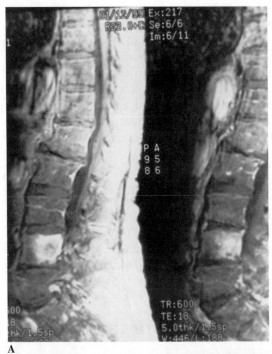

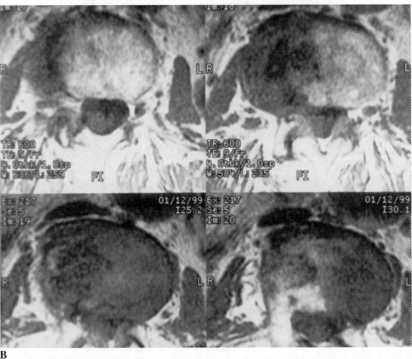

Figure 3.4 (A) A sagittal magnetic resonance imaging scan of an 87-year-old woman with long-standing back pain who had gradually increasing symptoms over the span of 6 months. The image shows an area of significant increase in signal intensity in the body of L4 on the left side. **(B)** Axial images of the same magnetic resonance imaging scan show significant signal enhancement in the body of L4 consistent with metastatic carcinoma. This patient had metastatic adenocarcinoma of the lung, the primary for which was diagnosed after biopsy of the metastatic lesion, and was otherwise not clinically evident.

Spinal Stenosis

For patients with spinal stenosis, the initial treatment regimen should be nonoperative, starting with lumbar flexion–type exercises. Flexion increases the size of the neural canal, alleviating the patient's symptoms to some degree. Aquatic exercise can be beneficial to patients with spinal stenosis because it takes weight off their spine and allows them to be more physically active, improving the endurance of their muscles, gradually allowing them to increase their activity level on land. Once they have gotten beyond the initial stages of therapy, low-impact aerobic conditioning is important to continue to build endurance in the available muscles. Bicycling may benefit patients with stenosis in determining the onset of neurogenic claudication. Bicycling tends to put the patient in a flexed posture to the lumbar spine, which increases the size of the neural canal, which allows more vigorous exercise. Epidural cortisone injections can give symptomatic relief in the short-term, but long-term benefit is unclear. Patients with spinal stenosis often go through a step cycle in which their symptoms show classic periods of exacerbation and remission. However, during the remissions, patients tend to never quite get back up to the level of their previous function before the exacerbation. Calcitonin has been shown to reduce symptoms of stenosis in studies, and may be helpful in patients who medically are not candidates for other options. Doses are similar to those used in osteoporosis.

Surgical intervention is reserved for patients who are unresponsive to conservative management; patients who have not responded to medication management, physical rehabilitation, epidural steroid injections, and continue to have debilitating symptoms. Lumbar laminectomy and foraminal decompression have approximately 80–85% rate of significant improvement in symptoms. However, a reoperation rate of approximately 15–20% is related to the development of stenosis at other levels, possible recurrent stenosis, or development of iatrogenic instability requiring secondary fusion. If the spinal stenosis is due to instability (spondylolisthesis or degenerative scoliosis), concomitant fusion is necessary.

Degenerative Spondylolisthesis

Patients who present with degenerative spondylolisthesis without symptoms of spinal stenosis have primarily back pain. Nonoperative treatment consists of exercise programs, such as low-impact aerobic conditioning, truncal strengthening program, flexion exercises and abdominal strengthening programs. Bracing may be intermittently necessary to control symptoms during acute exacerbations. NSAIDs and analgesics are sometimes necessary for short periods when patients are having acute exacerbations. The NSAIDs are the medication of choice; however, in the elderly, caution is required with dosing regimens and monitoring of liver and kidney function. Facet joints and epidural blocks may give symptomatic relief (with unknown long-term efficacy). Facet rhizotomies in patients who respond well to localized facet blocks are another treatment option.

Surgical intervention is necessary in approximately 10–15% of patients with degenerative spondylolisthesis. Patients presenting with neurologic complaints do better than patients with back pain alone. Patients treated with decompression and fusion clinically and statistically do better than patients with decompression alone or fusion alone. The need for spinal instrumentation depends on the degree of instability of the spondylolisthesis. In patients with a mobile spondylolisthesis, instrumentation to stabilize the segment is used while the fusion is ongoing.

Degenerative Scoliosis

In patients with degenerative scoliosis, it is important to determine if the scoliosis is related to simple disk degeneration or associated fractures due to osteoporosis or osteomalacia. There is a 32–38% prevalence of degenerative adult scoliosis in patients with osteoporosis and osteomalacia, and it is important to treat the underlying problem before treatment of the deformity.[2] Nonsurgical treatment includes NSAIDs and flexion exercises, as well as a general aerobic conditioning program.

Braces and corsets are used temporarily during acute exacerbations, and it is important to treat coexistent osteoporosis or osteomalacia. Many of these patients have severe muscle fatigue pain because the deformity requires their paraspinal muscles to hold them up continuously during the day. For these patients, it is important to regiment rest periods such as length, frequency in their daily routine, and to try and improve the endurance of their paraspinal muscles. These rest periods should be short (15–30 minutes) and interspersed throughout the day, taking approximately two to three rest periods in the course of 1 day.

Nerve root symptoms and spinal stenosis are the major indications for surgical intervention. Decompression alone should only be used for patients in whom the disease is limited to one nerve root and the facets can be preserved. Under those conditions, a microlaminotomy decompression of an individual nerve root can be performed with a high success rate and low risk of progressive deformity. For those patients who require multilevel decompression or wide laminectomy, it is important that the areas involved be fused as well as decompressed. The fusion should incorporate all levels with full to trace subluxation, disk-space narrowing, and wedging. It is important to maintain or obtain lumbar lordosis, and, therefore, sometimes osteotomies or concomitant anterior fusion may be necessary in those patients who have significant kyphotic deformity. Eighty-five percent to ninety percent positive results in adult scoliosis can be obtained if the preceding criteria are followed.[6]

NEOPLASTIC CONDITIONS OF THE SPINE

In patients older than age 21 years, more than 70% of primary spinal neoplasms are malignant. The most common presenting complaint is back pain, occurring in 85% of patients, and approximately 40% of patients present with associated weakness. Benign tumors of the spine such as osteochondroma, osteoblastoma, and giant cell tumor and aneurysm of bone cyst are all uncommon in the elderly. The most common benign tumor is a hemangioma that occurs in approximately 10% of patients, is rarely symptomatic, and is considered to be an incidental finding in many patients. The most common malignant tumors involving the spine are multiple myeloma and isolated plasmocytoma. Patients with solitary plasmocytoma may have prolonged survival despite eventual progression to multiple myeloma. Prognosis for survival in disseminated multiple myeloma is poor, with a 5-year survival rate of 18%. Spinal column involvement denotes an even worse prognosis. Solitary plasmacytoma of the spine has approximately a 60% 5-year disease-free survival rate. The treatment of solitary plasmacytoma is initially radiation. Surgery is reserved only for the refractory cases and those patients who have progressive neurologic deterioration. These diagnoses should be considered in patients who present with vertebral column compression fractures. Chordomas are another relatively rare primary malignant tumor in the spine, predominantly found in patients in the fifth and sixth decades of life. Chordomas tend to occur in the suboccipital or sacral coccygeal regions of the spine and are unresponsive to radiation; surgical extirpation with wide margins is the only curative procedure. Other primary malignant tumors include osteosarcoma, which may occur in pagetoid bone, chondrosarcoma, and Ewing's sarcoma, all of which are rare in the spine and especially in the elderly.

Metastatic tumors to the spine are much more common than primary tumors (see Table 3.2). The primary treatment options are radiation and chemotherapy. The majority of spinal metastasis are radial sensitive. Even patients with neurologic involvement should be given radiation as an initial prescription, except for specific circumstances. Bracing can be performed to maintain spinal alignment as radiation therapy is ongoing. The majority of bony lesions heal after radiation. Surgery is reserved for patients who have tumors known to be radial sensitive, patients who have progressive neurologic deficit while undergoing therapy, and patients whose neurologic deficits are due to deformity or fracture caused by the tumor, not to the tumor itself. Patients with a limited life span who are not able to function without surgical stabilization to decrease pain or stabilize the spine are also candidates for surgical intervention.

METABOLIC CONDITIONS OF THE SPINE

Osteomalacia

Treatment of osteomalacia is dependent to some degree on the specific etiology of the osteomalacia. Therefore, it is important to determine the underlying cause, whether it is vitamin D deficiency, whether that vitamin D deficiency is related to gastrointestinal malabsorption or liver disease, or both, or whether it is related to anticonvulsant medications or renal osteodystrophy. If this specific etiology can be determined, then specific intervention geared toward those particular problems should be undertaken. In general, vitamin D deficiency can generally be cured by an intake of 1,600 IU (400 IU is the recommended daily requirement) per day. In patients with renal osteodystrophy, the active metabolite 1,25 Dihydroxy vitamin D 3 should be given for it to have any beneficial effect. Dosages are generally in the range of 5,000–10,000 IU per week for patients with osteomalacia due to anticonvulsant medications. Dosages from 2,000–10,000 IU may be necessary to treat patients with liver disease.

Osteoporosis

The major battle in the treatment of osteoporosis should be geared toward the actual prevention of the development of osteoporosis. This should begin early in life. There is a direct relationship between weightbearing exercise and bone mass. It is important that people get adequate calcium intake. Adolescents should have an average daily intake of 1,500 mg of calcium. Premenopausal women should receive

1,000 mg of calcium per day, and postmenopausal women should receive 1,500 mg of absorbable calcium per day. It is important to replace deficient sex hormones if there are no contraindications to that replacement. Vitamin D supplementation is important in the elderly. They should receive 800 IU, which is twice the daily recommended allowance. It is important to evaluate patients who are at risk for osteoporosis. Premenopausal women who have other significant risk factors and who have a bone density one standard deviation below the norm should receive estrogen therapy at the time of menopause. Estrogen therapy is most important in the first 3–6 years after menopause. During this period, there is accelerated bone loss; however, bone loss related to low estrogen may continue for up to 20 years. Prolonged amenorrhea in young women should be treated. Estrogen therapy should begin soon after onset of menopause or during menopause. It has been shown that patients require at least 0.625 mg of conjugated estrogen to retard bone loss. Transdermal beta estradiol 0.1 mg has been shown to retard bone loss as well. Estrogen can have other beneficial side effects. It may decrease the incidence of cardiovascular disease up to 50%. However, estrogen replacement is contraindicated in patients with a history of breast cancer or uterine cancer. Medroxyprogesterone acetate, either cycled through days 11–21 or used continuously, eliminates increased risk of endometrial cancer. With continuous medroxyprogesterone, spotting generally stops after 2–6 months. This regimen may cut the incidence of fracture by 50% within early menopause. In patients with family history of breast cancer, annual mammography and physical examination is important.

For those patients who do not have adequate calcium intake in their diet, it is important for calcium supplementation to be undertaken. Postmenopausal women should receive 1,500 mg of calcium per day. Calcium citrate has better bioavailability than other calcium compounds. Generic brands may have less bioavailability than name brands. In the elderly, estrogen may be discontinued in patients treated with adequate calcium and adequate vitamin D alone. It is also important to remember that dietary factors can also affect the absorption and excretion of calcium. Phosphates such as seltzer and carbonated beverages can bind calcium in the gastrointestinal tract. High levels of fiber in the diet can decrease the transient time, decreasing the calcium available for absorption. Caffeine tends to increase the renal excretion of calcium, and chocolate affects the availability of calcium in the gastrointestinal tract.

Calcitonin decreases the loss of trabecular bone, but may not reduce the loss of cortical bone. It may be a useful adjunct in patients who cannot take estrogen. Calcitonin is available in nasal spray form, which is taken one spray each day, alternating nostrils. Resistance to calcitonin is less common if given nasally or continuously. New biphosphates, such as alendronate (Fosamax), have been helpful in the treatment of patients with osteoporosis and fracture. They inhibit bone resorption at much lower dosages than they inhibit bone formation. The diphosphonate can also be taken continuously, as opposed to the etidronate, which should be cycled, given for 14 days on and 76 days off. It is important that alendronate be given with adequate oral intake of water, and there is a subset of patients who cannot tolerate alendronate and other selective diphosphonate due to gastrointestinal side affects.

Sodium chloride has been used with variable success, but has not gained widespread use due to significant side effects. New soil release fluorides plus continuous calcium citrate have been shown to increase bone density and inhibit vertebral fracture. The slow-release fluorides tend to have lower incidence of side effects.

Surgery should be reserved for those patients who present with progressive deformities and impending neurologic loss due to collapsing osteoporotic fractures. The goal of surgery should be decompression of dural elements and stabilizing of the vertebral column. This requires getting the spine back into a normal balanced alignment. Surgery should not be attempted unless the surgeon is prepared to achieve this goal by whatever means is necessary.

Paget's Disease

Some patients with Paget's disease have only intermittent symptoms. These patients still require follow-up if the Paget's disease involves the spine because of the risk of enlargement of the vertebral body and the development of possible acute neurologic deterioration. In general, the treatment of Paget's disease is consistent use of diphosphonate or calcitonin. The diphosphonate should be used in a 20 mg/kg per day regimen for a month, progressing to lower dosages for long-term suppression. Calcitonin should be used 1.5–2.0 IU/kg per day in divided doses; however, relapses have occurred with discontinuation of calcitonin treatment. Erythromycin 15–25 µg/kg per day intravenously for 10 days should be used for cases of impending paraplegia without fracture. Surgery should be reserved for cases of progressive spinal stenosis or impending paraplegia due to vertebral expansion or vertebral fracture. Pretreat the patient for a period preoperatively with diphosphonate. Etidronate decreases blood flow and makes surgery safer in elective decompression of spinal stenosis. The new diphosphonates are under investigation at this time, with more selective decrease in bone resorption possible; it may be beneficial in the treatment of Paget's disease in the future.

Medication Issues

The elderly comprise approximately 12% of the U.S. population, but consume approximately 33% of all prescription drugs. The incidence of adverse drug reactions is higher in people older than age 65 years due to the decreased renal function and higher incidence of liver disease both premedication and related to medication use. In prescribing medications for the elderly, it is important to keep this in mind, especially with medications that may affect cognitive function, such as certain analgesics. Certain risk factors have been identified that increase the elderly's risk for falling, and modification of these factors may decrease that risk. Patients with postural hypertension; who use sedatives; who use at least four prescription drugs; who had impairment in arm strength, range of motion, or the ability to move safely in transfers; and who were on diazepam, diltiazem, diuretics, and laxatives were found to be at higher risk for multiple falls.

SUMMARY

Elderly patients present a unique subset of individuals who present with a relatively high incidence of back pain. It is less common for the elderly to present with back pain due to muscular strain, although the elderly are a much more active subset of the population today than in years past. Acute attention to detail in the patient's history on physical examination is vital in determining the etiology of the elderly patient's back pain. Intervention should be initiated cautiously, using conservative methods that do not require the use of cognitive effects of medications before more aggressive regimens. The judicious use of surgery can be successful and rewarding in select elderly patients, and one should not hesitate to proceed with necessary surgical intervention if other conservative options are not successful.

REFERENCES

1. Jenkins EA, Cooper C. Epidemiology of osteoporosis: who is at risk? Musculoskel Med 1993;18–33.
2. Duffy JD. Spinal Stenosis. In JW Frymoyer, TB Ducker, NM Hadler, et al. (eds), The Adult Spine: Principles and Practice. New York: Raven Press, 1991;1811–1820.
3. Anderson GBJ. Epidemiology of Spinal Disorders. In JW Frymoyer, TB Ducker, NM Hadler, et al. (eds), The Adult Spine: Principles and Practice. New York: Raven Press, 1991; 107–146.
4. Kane WJ. Osteoporosis, Osteomalacia, and Paget's Disease. In JW Frymoyer, TB Ducker, NM Hadler, et al. (eds), The Adult Spine: Principles and Practice. New York: Raven Press, 1991;637–660.
5. Frymoyer JW. Radiculopathies: Lumbar Disk Herniation and Recess Stenosis. In JW Frymoyer, TB Ducker, NM Hadler, et al. (eds), The Adult Spine: Principles and Practice. New York: Raven Press, 1991;1719–1732.
6. Simmons EH, Jackson RP. The management of nerve root entrapment syndromes associated with collapsing scoliosis, radiopathic lumbar and thoracolumbar curves. Spine 1979;4:533–541.

RECOMMENDED READINGS

Babbit AM. Osteoporosis. Orthopedics 1994;17:935–941.
Cats-Baril WM, Frymoyer JW. The Economics of Spinal Disorders. In JW Frymoyer, TB Ducker, NM Hadler, et al. (eds), The Adult Spine: Principles and Practice. New York: Raven Press, 1991;1145–1164.
Cummings RG, Mill JP, Kelsey JL, et al. Medications and multiple falls in elderly people: The St. Louis OASIS study. Age Ageing 1991;20:455–461.
El-Choufi L, Nelson J, Kleerekoper M. Therapeutic options in osteoporosis. Musculoskel Med 1994;15–21.
Epstein JA, Epstein BS, Jones MD. Symptomatic lumbar scoliosis with degenerative changes in the elderly. Spine 1979;4:542–547.
Grobler LJ, Wiltse LL. Classification, Non-Operative, and Operative Treatment of Spondylolisthesis. In JW Frymoyer, TB Ducker, NM Hadler, et al. (eds), The Adult Spine: Principles and Practice. New York: Raven Press, 1991;1655–1704.
Grubb SA, Lipscomb HJ, Koonrad RW. Degenerative adult onset scoliosis. Spine 1988;13:241–245.
Jacobsen SJ, Cooper C, Gottlieb MS, et al. Hospitalization with vertebral fracture among the aged: a national population-based study, 1986–1989. Epidemiology 1992;3:515–518.
Kostuik JP. Adult Scoliosis. In JW Frymoyer, TB Ducker, NM Hadler, et al. (eds), The Adult Spine: Principles and Practice: New York: Raven Press, 1991;1405–1441.
Kostuik JP. Compression Fractures and Surgery in Osteoporotic Patient. In JW Frymoyer, TB Ducker, NM Hadler, et al. (eds), The Adult Spine: Principles and Practice. New York: Raven Press, 1991;661–678.
Kostuik JP, Weinstein JM. Differential Diagnosis in Surgical Treatment of Metastatic Spine Tumors. In JW Frymoyer, TB Ducker, NM Hadler, et al. (eds), The Adult Spine: Principles and practice. New York: Raven Press, 1991;861–888.
Lindsey R. Osteoporosis: a clinical overview of diagnosis and therapy. Musculoskel Med 1993; 31–41.

Lufkin EG, Wahner HW, O'Fallon WM, et al. Treatment of post-menopausal osteoporosis with transdermal estrogen. Ann Intern Med 1992;117:1–9.

Lukert BP. Vertebral compression fractures: how to manage pain, avoid disability. Geriatrics 1994;49:22–26.

Melton LJ 3rd, Atkinson EJ, O'Fallon WM, et al. Long-term fracture prediction by bone mineral assessed at different skeletal sites. J Bone Miner Res 1993;8:1227–1233.

Nash CL, Goldstein JM, Wilham MR. Selection of lumbar fusion levels in adult idiopathic scoliosis patients. Presented at the Scoliosis Research Society Meeting, Amsterdam, 1989.

Pak CY, Sakhaee K, Piziak V, et al. Slow-release sodium fluoride in the management of postmenopausal osteoporosis: a randomized controlled trial. Ann Intern Med 1994;120:625–632.

Patel U, Skingle S, Campbell GA, et al. Clinical profile of acute vertebral compression fractures in osteoporosis. Br J Rheumatol 1991;30:418–421.

Pitt MJ. Rickets and Osteomalacia. In D Resnick. Diagnosis of Bone and Joint Disorders. Philadelphia: Saunders, 1995;1885–1922.

Prestwood KM, Raisz LJ. Using estrogen to prevent osteoporosis. Musculoskel Med 17–24.

Resnick D, Niwayama G. Osteoporosis. In D Resnick. Diagnosis of Bone and Joint Disorders. Philadelphia: Saunders, 1995;1781–1853.

Resnick D, Niwayama G. Paget's Disease. In D Resnick. Diagnosis of Bone and Joint Disorders. Philadelphia: Saunders, 1995;1923–1968.

Riggs BL, Melton AJ 3rd. Prevention and treatment of osteoporosis. N Engl J Med 1992;327:620–628.

Sundaresan N, Kroll G, Digiacinto GJ, Hughes JEO. Metastatic Tumors of the Spine. In N Sundaresan. Tumors of the Spine: Diagnosis and Clinical Management. Philadelphia: Saunders, 1990.

Tinetti ME, Baker BI, McAvay G, et al. A multi-factorial intervention to reduce the risk of falling among elderly people living in the community. N Engl J Med 1994;331:821.

Valkenburg HA, Haanen HCM. The Epidemiology of Low Back Pain. In AA White, SL Gordon (eds), Proceedings of the American Association of Orthopedic Surgeons Symposium on Low Back Pain, 1982;9–22.

Van Kuijk C, Hagiwara S, Genant HK. Radiologic assessment of osteoporosis. Musculoskel Med 1994;25–32.

Weinstein JN. Differential Diagnosis and Surgical Treatment of Primary Benign and Malignant Neoplasms. In JW Frymoyer, TB Ducker, NM Hadler, et al. (eds), The Adult Spine: Principles and Practice. New York: Raven Press, 1991;829–860.

PART II
Assessment

Chapter 4

Biomechanical Assessment
of Low Back Pain

Mark R. Bookhout

On completion of a thorough history and physical examination to rule out a non-musculoskeletal pathologic condition, a biomechanical examination should be undertaken for patients presenting with low back pain with or without leg pain. From the patient's history, the postures, movements, and activities that seem to increase or decrease the patient's symptoms are recorded; during the biomechanical examination, the examiner attempts to replicate these activities with testing maneuvers designed to provoke the patient's pain either partially or wholly. If pain is present before movement, the test motions may increase or decrease its intensity and change or alter its location. If the patient is asymptomatic at the time of the assessment, the test movements may elicit the pain he or she has described or identify areas of abnormal function, or both.

BIOMECHANICAL MODEL

Traditionally, the physician has used the neurologic model as the basis for the assessment of low back and leg pain. The objectives of the classic neurologic examination are to identify motor weakness, objective sensory deficits, and absent or diminished reflexes in a corresponding spinal segmental level (e.g., foot drop [weakness of the tibialis anterior] with objective loss of sensation to pinprick in the L4 dermatome and absent or diminished knee jerk reflex).

The vast majority of patients presenting with low back pain with or without leg pain, however, have minimal, if any, objective neurologic signs.[1] Therefore, there is a need for a supplemental biomechanical model for assessment of low back pain to help in determining a definitive diagnosis and treatment plan. The three-joint complex, as described by Kirkaldy-Willis,[2] serves as the foundation for the biomechanical model. The three-joint complex is defined as the intervertebral disk and its corresponding posterior facet joints.

Three distinct pathophysiologic phases may occur as a result of injury or repetitive trauma and the normal aging process of the lumbar spine. Phase 1, dysfunction, is the earliest. A minor pathologic condition may result in abnormal function of the

posterior facet joints and the intervertebral disk; this would include disk herniations. Phase 2, instability, is characterized by progressive degeneration due to
repeated trauma, producing laxity of the posterior joint capsules and the annulus.
Phase 3, restabilization, is the final stage in the process. Fibrosis of the posterior
joints and the capsule, loss of disk material, and formation of osteophytes render
the segment stable as movement is reduced.[3] The goal of the biomechanical assessment is to decide where the patient fits in this pathophysiologic model, correlating
the patient's clinical presentation with results of other tests, such as computed
tomography or magnetic resonance imaging, that may be available.

Most patients with low back pain are in the dysfunction phase and lack definitive
neurologic and radiologic signs. Dysfunction has been defined by Paris[4] as either an
increase or decrease in motion from the expected normal, or the presence of aberrant movement of a spinal segment. Hypermobility, not to be confused with instability, is defined as an increase in motion from the expected normal when
comparing the mobility of a spinal segment with that of neighboring spinal or
peripheral joints. A decrease in motion at a given joint is known as *hypomobility*.
Either condition may produce pain, although the exact mechanism for pain production has not been clearly explained.

ASSESSMENT

To assess spinal function, the examiner must have some understanding of the normal
biomechanicals of spinal movement. The following section describes the biomechanical assessment of the patient with low back pain in the standing, sitting, supine, and
prone postures. Objectives of the biomechanical examination are to (1) determine the
phase of the pathologic condition, (2) determine the area(s) of greatest dysfunction,
(3) reproduce the patient's symptoms partially or wholly, and (4) determine, if possible, the tissue(s) at fault.

Standing

First, the patient's standing posture is observed for the presence or absence of a normal lumbar lordotic curve. Loss of normal lumbar lordosis and the presence of a list
or lateral shift is a frequent finding in patients with low back pain, especially those
in the acute stages (Figure 4.1). Presuming the pain is unilateral, the lateral shift
may be toward the side of pain or, more frequently, away from the side of pain (i.e.,
a contralateral list). The list has been explained as an attempt by the body to avoid
further irritation of a nerve root by disk protrusion.[5] This assumes that the list represents an antalgic posture. Disk protrusions lateral to the nerve root tend to produce
a contralateral list, whereas those medial to the nerve root produce an ipsilateral list
(Figure 4.2).[5] However, Porter and Miller[6] found, during surgical excision of herniated disks in 20 patients, that the direction of the list was not related to the side of
the disk protrusion, nor was it related to the topographic position of the disk relative
to the nerve root. More recently, Matsui et al.[7] reported in a series of 40 patients
who had a sciatic scoliosis before surgery that 80% of the patients were found to
have a lumbar disk herniation on the convex side of the scoliosis at the time of surgery, irrespective of the location of the herniation to the nerve root. Clinically, in
my experience, correction of the lateral list, or shift, especially a contralateral list,

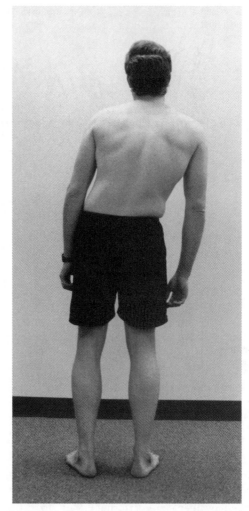

Figure 4.1 Patient with loss of lumbar lordosis and right lateral shift.

frequently improves patients' symptoms, which implies that the majority of lists are not antalgic and some other neurophysiologic explanation is necessary. McKenzie[8] believes that the lateral shift represents the body's response to internal posterolateral disk herniation with a fluid shift of the nucleus and proposes attempted shift correction and restoration of the lumbar lordosis as the primary mode of treatment. Farfan and Kirkaldy-Willis[9] have explained the kyphotic deformity with the lateral shift in the absence of muscle spasm as the result of a torsional injury to the facet joint and annulus.

From the foregoing discussion, it should be obvious that when a patient presents with a kyphotic lumbar spine and a lateral shift, shift correction must be attempted before its cause can be determined. It cannot be assumed that the posture is truly antalgic until shift correction is attempted. A desirable response to attempted shift correction is centralization of the patient's pain, first noted by McKenzie.[8] Centralization of symptoms occurs when pain arising from the spine and felt laterally from the midline or distally in the extremity is reduced or transferred to a more central or

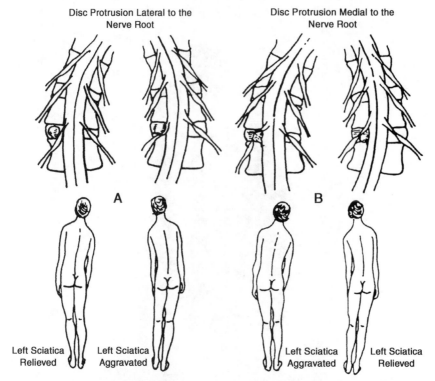

Disc Protrusion Lateral to the Nerve Root

Disc Protrusion Medial to the Nerve Root

A   B

Left Sciatica Relieved   Left Sciatica Aggravated   Left Sciatica Aggravated   Left Sciatica Relieved

Figure 4.2 Contralateral and ipsilateral lists. (**A**) Disk protrusion lateral to the nerve root. (**B**) Disk protrusion medial to the nerve root. (Reprinted with permission from BE Finneson. Low Back Pain. Philadelphia: JB Lippincott, 1980.)

near midline position, or both. The patient may actually experience an increase in low back pain while noting a decrease or reduction in the lateral or distal (extremity) pain when certain movements are performed. McKenzie[8] believes that centralization of pain occurs only with disk herniations (derangements) and that such centralization is absolutely reliable in indicating the movements that should be chosen to reduce the mechanical deformation. Donelson et al.'s[10] study supports the ability to centralize a patient's pain as a favorable prognosis for improvement with conservative care, but their patient population tended to be more acute (i.e., 78% of patients reported onset of symptoms of less than 12 weeks' duration). More recently, Long[11] reported the usefulness of centralization in chronic low back pain patients, noting a significant decrease in maximum pain ratings and a higher return to work rate in subjects able to centralize their pain compared to noncentralizers. Sufka et al.[12] further defined complete centralization as the movement of symptoms to a central location within 2.54 cm (1 in.) adjacent to the spinous processes of the lumbar spine and reported improved functional outcomes in patients who achieved complete centralization within 14 days of initiation of treatment. If attempted shift correction increases the patient's low back pain and leg pain (peripheralization of symptoms) when he or she is standing (Figure 4.3), the procedure should be attempted in the prone position (Figure 4.4), as intradiskal pressure has been shown to diminish in the recumbent position.[13] In my experience, failure to achieve shift correction after several days' trial, coupled with an increase in the patient's pain or

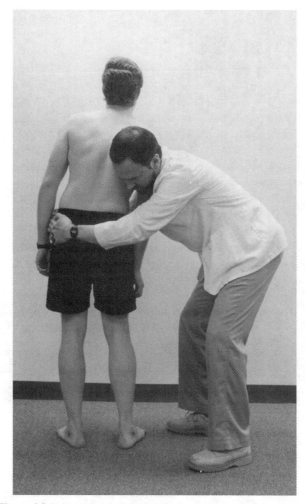

Figure 4.3 Attempted right lateral shift correction in standing position.

peripheralization of symptoms, or both, is often due to a large disk herniation, including free fragment or lateral disk herniations, or both, often with subarticular recess stenosis confirmed by computed tomography or magnetic resonance imaging and surgical reports.

The clinical setting largely determines the type of patient seen. In an industrial outpatient clinic, for example, a patient with acute pain who presents with a kyphotic lumbar spine and lateral shift often is unable to tolerate or perform part or all of the biomechanical examination. Therefore, the initial assessment might conclude with notation of the patient's response to attempted shift correction in the standing and prone postures. Appropriate neurologic tests can be administered to determine which, if any, spinal nerve root is involved. If centralization of symptoms occurs with attempted shift correction, referral should be made to a physical therapist for instruction in self-mobilization exercises to be repeated until permanent correction is achieved. Failure to achieve centralization of symptoms with shift correction, even with the patient prone, may eventually necessitate further diagnostic

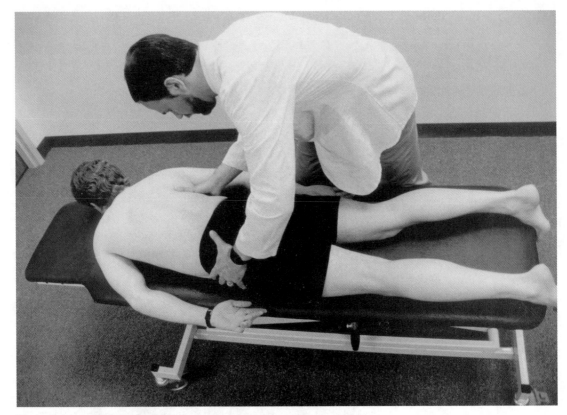

Figure 4.4 Attempted right lateral shift correction in prone position.

tests, such as computed tomography or magnetic resonance imaging, to rule out a large or sequestrated disk fragment before referral to physical therapy. Bowel and bladder signs and progressing neurologic deficits demand an immediate referral to a surgeon who specializes in lumbar spine surgery.

The patient with a less irritable condition should be able to tolerate continuation of the biomechanical examination. Palpation of the iliac crests and greater trochanters while the patient is standing with shoes off is a functional test for leg length inequality. If the iliac crest and greater trochanter are both lower on one side than the other, the patient has a short leg. Observation of the lower extremity may indicate whether the cause of the inequality is structural or functional (i.e., an excessively pronated foot could result in a functionally short leg on that side). In 1959, Stoddard[14] reported that a short lower extremity and resulting pelvic tilt occurred twice as often in patients with low back pain than in a controlled asymptomatic population. Giles and Taylor[15] found that leg length inequality of 10 mm or more appears to be twice as common in patients with low back pain than in a normal asymptomatic population.

Movement analysis in the standing posture includes observation of the range and quality of motion with forward and backward bending of the spine. Biomechanically, several events occur as forward bending and backward bending place mechanical stresses, primarily compression, tension, and shear, on different vertebral tissues (Table 4.1).

Table 4.1 Events That Occur with Forward and Backward Bending of the Spine

Forward bending
  Facets slide up and open, facet capsules stretched
  Anterior translation of superior vertebral body on inferior vertebral body
  Increased tension on posterior ligamentous structures
  Increased tension on posterior aspect of intervertebral disk
  Increased opening in intervertebral foramen and central canal
  Increased tension on dural sac
  Lengthening of erector spinae and hamstring musculature
Backward bending
  Facets slide down and close, facet capsules placed on slack
  Posterior translation of superior vertebral body on inferior vertebral body
  Decreased tension on posterior ligamentous structures
  Increased compression on posterior aspect of intervertebral disk
  Narrowing of intervertebral foramen and central canal
  Decreased tension on dural sac
  Relaxation of erector spinae and hamstring musculature

Observation of recruitment of motion in forward bending should include notation of flat spots, areas of increased kyphosis, and the ability to reverse the lumbar lordosis. On return to upright standing, a reversal of the normal lumbopelvic rhythm[16] (Figure 4.5) and late derotation of the pelvis[17] (Figure 4.6) may indicate spinal instability, the second phase in the Kirkaldy-Willis[2] pathophysiologic model. Typically, these patients report an increase in low back pain when returning to upright stance from the forward bent position and often are relatively pain-free and unlimited during forward bending. This symptomatic response is distinctly different from the patient with an acute herniated disk who reports an accentuation of pain during forward bending with a significant limitation in forward flexion mobility. A deviation from the midline on forward bending may be suspect for abnormal unilateral nerve root tension, especially if the deviation is accompanied by flexion of the ipsilateral knee.[18] If, during the history, the patient reported problems with forward bending or lifting, repetitive forward bending or forward bending with overpressures or with weights held in the hands may be necessary to provoke symptoms.

A sacroiliac screening test is also done while the patient is standing. The examiner places his or her thumbs on the inferior slope of the posterior superior iliac spine and notes the relative excursion of each thumb while the patient bends forward fully (Figure 4.7).[19,20] The thumb that travels further (has the greatest excursion) usually indicates either that the sacroiliac joint is hypomobile on that side or that the hamstring musculature is tight on the opposite side. The standing hip flexion test, or stork test (Figure 4.8), is another sacroiliac joint screening test that can be done to complement the forward bending test and is thought to be more sensitive in detecting sacroiliac joint hypomobility.[21]

Movement analysis in the standing position also includes the observation of backward bending and side bending movements, which are commonly painful and restricted in the presence of lumbar spine dysfunction. Mellin[22] studied patients aged 35–55 years with chronic or recurrent low back pain and reported a stronger correlation for lateral flexion with low back pain than forward flexion and exten-

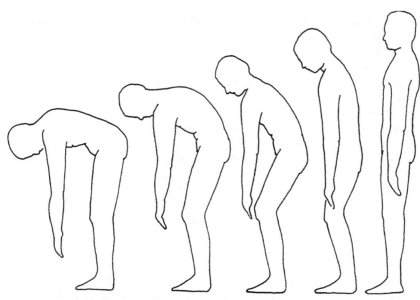

Figure 4.5 Reversal of spinal rhythm. On attempting to regain the erect position from forward flexion, the patient bends the knees and tucks the pelvis underneath the spine to stand erect. This type of movement is characteristic of segmental instability. (Reprinted with permission from I Macnab. Backache. Baltimore: Williams & Wilkins, 1977.)

sion. He also found thoracolumbar mobility had higher correlations with low back pain than mobility of the lumbar spine, which supports the clinical findings of Maigne[23] regarding the importance of the thoracolumbar junction in the evaluation and treatment of low back pain. Backward bending is assessed for range and recruitment of motion into the lumbar spine, particularly the lowest lumbar segments. Deviations from the midline on backward bending should also be noted. Restricted side bending to one side may be indicative of abnormal coupling (mobility) of the posterior lumbar facets or the loss of translation (side gliding), or both, secondary to a lateral lumbar shift.[8,24] Tenhula et al.[24] reported a significant relationship between the direction of a lateral lumbar shift (LLS) and pain provocation with lumbar spine side bending in patients with an obvious, observable LLS. They found that 71% of the patients reported reproduction or increase in symptoms with side bending contralateral to the side of the LLS, but no significant relationship between the side of symptoms and the direction of the LLS. Restrictions in side bending may also be the result of muscular shortening, particularly of the quadratus lumborum muscle, which Simon and Travell[25] believe is the most often overlooked source of myofascial low back pain. The hip drop test[20] (Figure 4.9) can indicate the patient's ability to symmetrically side bend at L5–S1, which is sometimes difficult to assess with the active side bending tests alone.

The final tests administered while the patient is standing include toe walking and heel walking to assess motor function of S1 and L4–L5, respectively. The patient's overall gait pattern with shoes off should be scrutinized for stride length, hip drop symmetry, arm swing, and head posture. A Trendelenburg gait may be indicative of gluteus medius weakness or hip pathology, which may be contributing to the patient's symptoms.

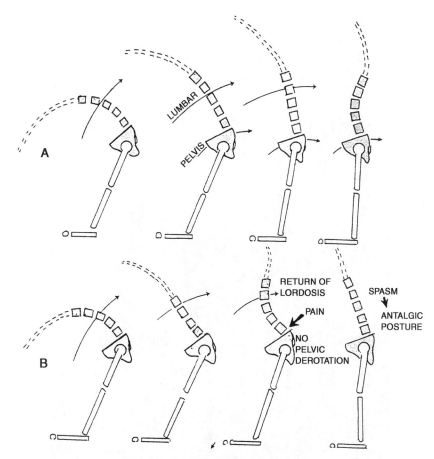

Figure 4.6 (A) Normal return to upright standing. **(B)** Late derotation of the pelvis. (Reprinted with permission from R Cailliet. Low Back Pain Syndrome [3rd ed]. Philadelphia: FA Davis, 1981.)

Sitting

One of the major objectives of postural and movement analysis of the patient in a sitting position is to observe the effect of removal of the lower quarter influences on the static posture and functional status of the lumbar spine. A functionally short leg is inferred when the iliac crest, trochanter, and posterior superior iliac spine are all lower on the same side in standing, but appear symmetric in the seated posture. A scoliosis noted in standing, but absent in sitting, indicates a compensatory scoliosis that occurs in response to the unleveling of the pelvis in the standing posture. Changes in the lumbar lordosis and thoracic kyphosis, as well as head and neck posture, should be noted.

Movement analysis in the sitting position also includes observation of forward bending mobility, but differs from forward bending in the standing position in that the influences of the lower extremities, particularly the hamstrings and hip flexor musculature, are eliminated. Deviations from the midline seen with forward bending in the standing position may not be apparent with forward bending in a sitting position, possibly due to reduction in nerve root tension or elimination of the lower extremity influences, or both. A sacroiliac joint screening test (Figure 4.10)

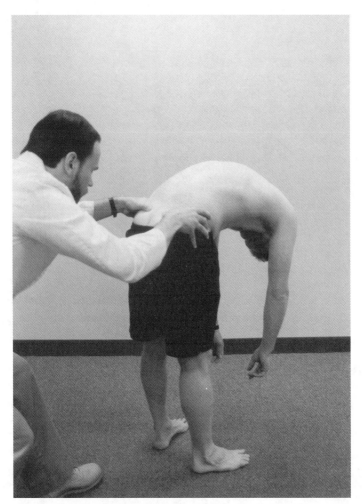

Figure 4.7 Standing forward flexion test. The examiner's thumbs are placed on the inferior slope of the posterior superior iliac spine, and the relative excursion of each thumb is noted while the patient bends forward fully.

is also done in this position, with the examiner's thumb contact again on the inferior slope of the posterior superior iliac spines. The relative excursion of both thumbs is noted when the patient is asked to forward bend fully. As with the standing test, the thumb that moves further indicates the side of restricted sacroiliac joint mobility.[19,20] A forward bending test that appears more positive in the standing than in the sitting position indicates imbalances in the lower extremity musculature or asymmetric movement of the ilium and pubis, or both, whereas a forward bending test that is more positive in the seated posture indicates dysfunction (hypomobility) involving the sacrum itself, as influences of the lower extremity have largely been removed.[19,20]

Active range of motion for rotation of the spine is best examined with the patient seated and the examiner looking for symmetric recruitment of motion from cephalad to caudal. Particular attention should be paid to the thoracolumbar junction, as restricted motion here is often ignored but has been found to have a high correlation with low back pain.[22,23]

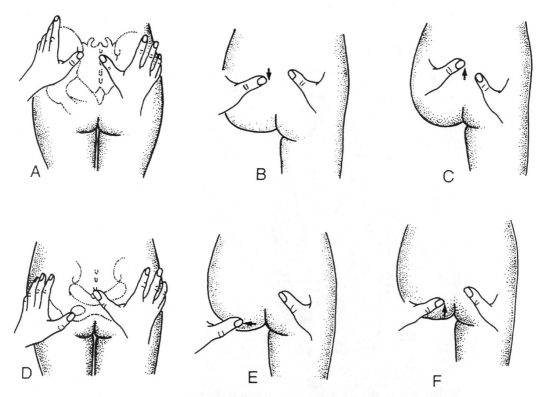

Figure 4.8 Standing hip flexion tests to demonstrate left sacroiliac joint fixation. Tests for the upper part of the joint in **A**, **B**, and **C**, and for the lower part in **D**, **E**, and **F**. **(A)** The examiner places the left thumb on the posterior superior iliac spine and the right thumb over one of the sacral spinous processes. **(B)** When movement is normal, the examiner's left thumb moves downward as the patient raises the left leg. **(C)** When the joint is fixed, the examiner's left thumb moves upward as the patient raises the left leg. **(D)** The examiner places the left thumb over the ischial tuberosity and the right thumb over the apex of the sacrum. **(E)** When movement is normal, the examiner's left thumb moves laterally as the patient raises the left leg. **(F)** When the joint is fixed, the examiner's left thumb moves slightly upward as the patient raises the left leg. (Reprinted with permission from WH Kirkaldy-Willis. Managing Low Back Pain [2nd ed]. New York: Churchill Livingstone, 1988.)

Neurologic testing in the sitting position includes segmental muscle tests and deep tendon reflexes (i.e., knee-jerk reflex for L4 and ankle-jerk reflex for S1). Even in the presence of neurologic findings, physical therapy should be considered. A patient with neurologic findings often has associated biomechanical dysfunctions that can be addressed by a physical therapist. Therapeutic procedures, such as traction, may in some cases effectively relieve nerve root tension signs and reverse neurologic findings. A study by Saal and Saal[26] supports the use of conservative therapy measures, even in the presence of confirmed lumbar disk herniations with radiculopathy.

Supine

When the patient is in the supine posture, direct observation of spinal movements is obviously impeded. Supine movement tests are primarily pain provocation tests to determine which types of movements and which tissues may be the source of the

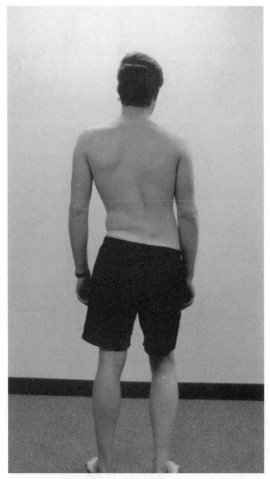

Figure 4.9 Hip drop test. The patient is asked to bend the right knee to allow the right side of the pelvis to drop. In this photograph, right hip drop provides information regarding the patient's ability to side bend to the left in the lower lumbar spine.

patient's pain. Laslett and Williams[27] reported on the interrater reliability of selected pain provocation tests for sacroiliac joint pathology. They found reliability for pain provocation with the anterior superior iliac spine gapping or compression tests, the posterior shear test, and the pelvic torsion or Gaenslen's test, but their diagnostic specificity is yet to be determined. Straight leg raising is the classic test to assess for sciatic nerve root irritation.[28] The straight leg raising test can be made more sensitive for adverse neural tension by the addition of hip adduction and internal rotation, ankle dorsiflexion, and neck flexion.[29] Butler[30] has pointed out the importance of sequencing when testing for adverse neural tension, noting that the best reproduction of symptoms occurs if the source of the symptoms is placed on tension first (i.e., straight leg raising, then hip adduction and internal rotation, then ankle dorsiflexion versus ankle dorsiflexion, hip flexion, and knee extension). Occasionally, a patient has a positive cross straight leg raising test, in which pain in the contralateral leg or hip is increased when the asymptomatic leg is raised.[31] Khuffash and Porter[32] found that a positive cross straight leg raising test, coupled

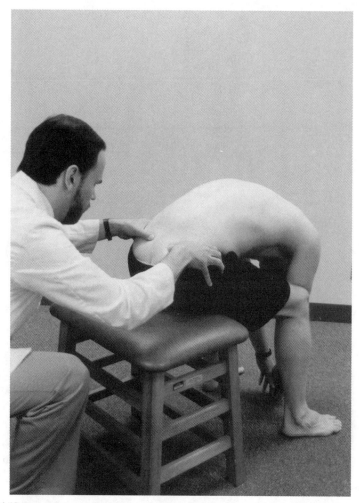

Figure 4.10 Seated forward flexion test. In this example, the examiner's left thumb traveled further, indicating a restriction in the left sacroiliac joint.

with a trunk list (lateral shift), indicates a poor prognosis for nonoperative management, as the majority of patients with this presentation are found to have a sequestrated or extruded disk fragment when taken to surgery. In addition to straight leg raising, McKenzie[8] uses bilateral pulling of knees to chest, especially repetitively, to provoke pain, especially peripheralization of symptoms, in patients he suspects have a disk herniation. If repeated pulling of knees to chest increases the patient's symptoms and results in peripheralization of pain, flexion activities should be temporarily avoided in the treatment program. If centralization of symptoms occurs with repeated pulling of knees to chest, flexion of the lumbar spine should be included in the treatment program.

The hip joint is assessed in the supine posture for both passive range of motion and provocation of pain. Faber's test (flexion, abduction, and external rotation) is a classic test for osteoarthritic changes in the hip and should not be overlooked, as the hip can refer pain into the buttocks and leg. In my experience, more commonly, the combined movements of hip flexion, adduction, and internal rotation are restricted

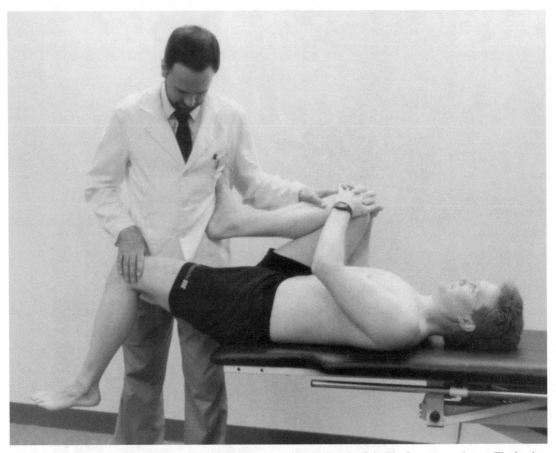

Figure 4.11 Thomas test. This test provides information regarding the length of the hip flexor musculature. The lumbar spine is kept in neutral position by fully flexing the right knee to the chest. The left hip should be able to extend to neutral (0 degrees). Tightness of the left iliopsoas is illustrated.

and cause a pinching sensation in the groin, usually indicative of posterior hip capsule tightness. Posterior hip capsule tightness is usually associated with a tight piriformis muscle. The piriformis muscle, because of its close anatomic relationship to the sciatic nerve, has been described as a source of sciatic-like referred pain.[33] Stretching of the piriformis by the application of flexion, internal rotation, and adduction of the hip, provides information regarding length and irritability of the piriformis muscle. The Thomas test (Figure 4.11) provides information regarding the length of the hip flexor musculature. The iliopsoas is one of several muscles that tends to shorten with low back dysfunction and seems to have an inhibitory effect on gluteal muscle strength through some type of reciprocal inhibitory loop.[34]

Although the role of muscle as a primary source of low back pain remains controversial,[35] length and strength of the musculature supporting and moving the low back should be considered in the assessment and treatment plan, as muscle imbalances contribute to faulty mechanics of the lumbar spine, pelvis, and hips. Strengthening of the abdominal muscles has long been advocated as a preventive measure to avoid low back pain. Weakness of the abdominal musculature has traditionally been

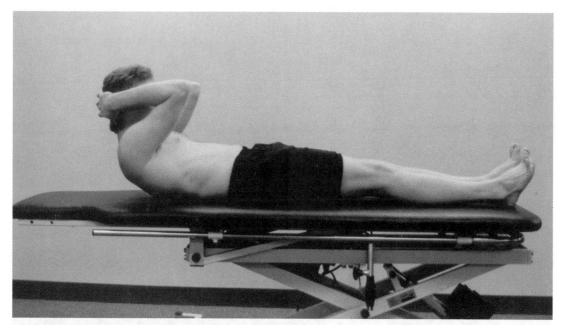

Figure 4.12 Abdominal curl-up. Normal strength is present if the patient is able to flex the vertebral column, bringing the scapula off the table with the hands clasped behind the head.

assessed in the supine posture primarily by two tests, both described by Kendall and McCreary.[36] The abdominal curl-up (Figure 4.12) assesses the ability to flex the trunk on a relatively fixed pelvis, whereas the leg lowering test (Figure 4.13) assesses abdominal strength with a relatively fixed thorax. Recently, the role of the transversus abdominis in contributing to spinal stability has been discovered.[37] The transversus abdominis has been shown to be the first trunk muscle normally activated before movement of the lower extremity in any direction.[38] In patients with low back pain, there is a delay in firing of the transversus abdominis, indicating a change in postural control of the low back.[39]

Hides et al.[40] have used real-time ultrasound imaging in patients with first-time acute unilateral low back pain, showing wasting of the multifidus muscle at a single segmental level ipsilateral to the side of pain. Subsequently, Hides et al.[41] found that multifidus recovery, as measured by cross-sectional area, is not automatic after symptomatic relief of low back pain, implying that inhibition of the multifidus after the first episode of low back pain may predispose patients for recurrent symptoms.

Prone

When the patient is in the prone position, passive extension of the lumbar spine (Figure 4.14) may be used as a test of both mobility and pain provocation, and should include assessment of range of motion and recording of the patient's subjective responses to repetitive movements. As previously mentioned in the section Standing, centralization of symptoms is a desired response to repetitive test movements and dictates the direction of spinal movement to be incorporated in the patient's home exercise program. A comparison is made between the patient's

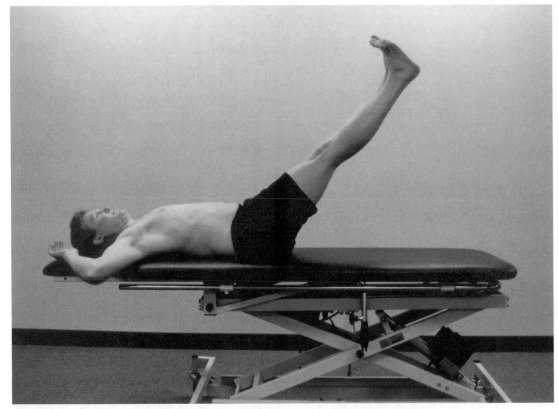

Figure 4.13 Leg lowering test. The legs are brought up to a right angle by the examiner. The patient is asked to slowly lower the legs while keeping the lower back flat on the table by posteriorly tilting the pelvis. This test is thought to be more specific than the abdominal curl-up for weakness of the external oblique musculature. Normal strength is present if the legs can be fully lowered to the table while the patient maintains a posteriorly rotated pelvis and a flat lower back.

response to repeated knees-to-chest motions in the supine position (flexion) and repeated press-ups (extension) of the lumbar spine in prone lying. In my experience, repeated knees-to-chest motions in the supine posture aggravate and peripheralize a patient's symptoms when a herniated disk or annular tear is the source of pain, whereas repeated prone press-ups performed after lateral shift correction, if a list is present, often centralize (improve) the patient's symptoms. Kopp et al.[42] have shown that patients with acute herniated disks who are unable to achieve normal lumbar extension within 3–5 days of initiation of treatment have a poor prognosis for improvement with conservative therapy.

Mechanical dysfunction in one of the posterior facet joints is often associated with a herniated disk at either the same level or neighboring levels above and below, and, therefore, makes a differential diagnosis difficult. Dysfunction in mobility of one of the posterior facets at a segmental spinal level can be assessed with the patient in the prone position through the use of manually applied pressures to the spinous process or transverse processes of the lumbar vertebrae. Central posterior to anterior, unilateral posterior to anterior (Figure 4.15), and transverse pressures (Figure 4.16) can be used to evoke pain and to detect restriction in accessory movements of a specific segmental level. Accessory movements are defined as

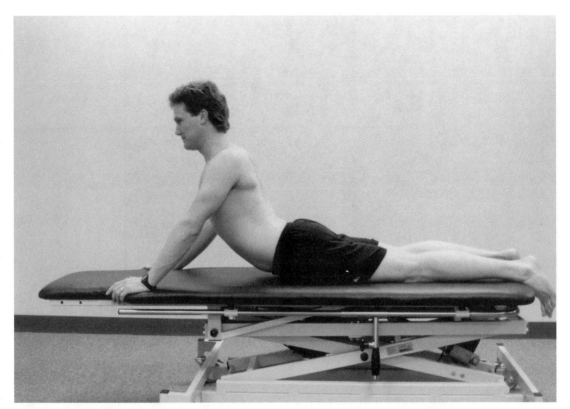

Figure 4.14 Passive prone press-up. The patent is asked to push up through the arms and to relax the lower back musculature during the motion.

those joint movements that cannot be performed voluntarily or in isolation by a patient but are necessary components for normal joint function.[43] Loss of accessory movements of a spinal segment is the most sensitive indicator of abnormality of movement (dysfunction) in a joint.[44]

Hip range of motion can be further assessed in the prone posture by examining bilateral internal rotation and external rotation. Range of motion for hip extension should also be assessed in the prone posture, as a restriction in hip extension is a common clinical finding in patients with low back pain. The relative strength of hip extension should be tested after assessment of passive range of motion. Frequently, active hip extension is limited, and gluteus maximus strength is notably weakened on manual muscle testing. Janda[34] has noted a characteristic pattern of tight postural muscles (i.e., hip flexors and hamstrings, and weak dynamic muscles, especially the gluteus maximus and medius) in patients with low back pain. Frequently, when hip extension is impaired, the lumbar erector spinae musculature compensates for gluteus maximus weakness, resulting in hyperextension and possibly hypermobility of the lumbar spine.[45]

Palpation concludes the assessment in the prone position, including palpation for myofascial trigger points as described by Simon and Travell.[46] Reproduction of the patient's symptoms is sought. Skin rolling is useful for assessing tissue texture changes associated with dysfunction at a segmental spinal level and can be helpful in localizing the area of dysfunction.[19,20,23] Palpation along the sides of the spinous

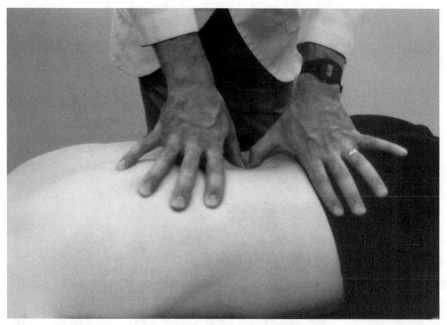

Figure 4.15 Application of unilateral posterior to anterior pressures. Thumb pressure is applied to the transverse processes of the lumbar spine in a posterior to anterior direction to detect a loss of mobility or to provoke symptoms, or both.

processes may reveal hypertonicity in the deeper multifidus and sacrospinalis musculature at the level of segmental dysfunction.

SUMMARY

On completion of the biomechanical examination, the following questions should be answered: (1) Does the patient have a musculoskeletal problem? (2) In which of the three pathophysiologic stages defined by Kirkaldy-Willis[2] does the patient fit? (3) If dysfunction is present, where is the area of greatest dysfunction (i.e., hip, lumbar spine, sacroiliac joint), and where are the associated dysfunctions? (4) What tissue(s) are at fault?

Musculoskeletal problems typically respond to biomechanical stresses, with certain positions or activities exacerbating the patient's pain and other positions giving some relief of symptoms. The treatment plan is guided by the patient's response to the test movements during the biomechanical assessment. If a patient states that his or her pain is constant, unchanged by any position or activity, the evaluation process is obviously more difficult. This situation should cause the examiner to suspect a nonmusculoskeletal cause.

Kirkaldy-Willis[2] described three phases in the degenerative process of the lumbar spine: dysfunction, instability, and restabilization. Dysfunction characterizes by far the greatest number of patients seen for low back pain. Loss of symmetry with active movements, especially backward bending and side bending, is characteristic of patients with lumbar spine dysfunction. Whether an intervertebral disk, one of the posterior facet joints, or other soft tissue structures are at fault remains a point

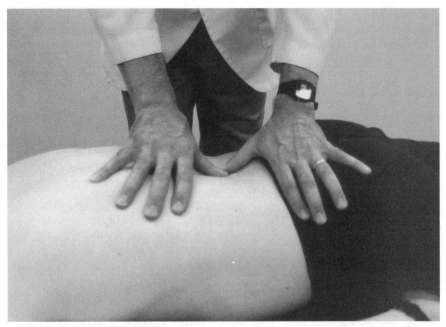

Figure 4.16 Application of transverse pressures. The examiner's thumbs are placed on the lateral aspect of the spinous process and pressure is applied transversely to the spinous process of each lumbar spinal segment to detect loss of mobility or to provoke symptoms, or both.

of controversy. The role of muscle in lumbar spine dysfunction is a subject for study to determine whether abnormal muscle function leads to abnormal movement and strain of the three-joint complex, or whether muscle hypertonicity is a result of faulty spinal mechanics.

The second phase of the pathophysiologic model, instability, is characterized by spinal dysrhythmia observed as the patient bends forward and returns to an upright standing position. The treatment program for the patient with instability differs significantly from that for the patient with lumbar spine dysfunction. Frequently, however, the patient with instability also has neighboring areas of dysfunction (hypomobility) near the unstable segment. Theoretically, treatment addressing the hypomobile segments can diminish the strain placed on the unstable segment, and reduction of symptoms may occur.

The third phase, restabilization, is, by nature, age related and therefore more common among older patients with low back pain. The patient characteristically has a generalized loss of mobility and complains of stiffness, and back pain complaints are minimal compared to leg pain complaints, which may be severe when central or lateral stenosis is present.[47]

In most patients presenting with low back pain in the dysfunction phase, the dysfunction involves the lumbar spine, the sacroiliac joints, the hips and lower extremities, or the thoracolumbar junction. Determining the area of greatest dysfunction and the tissue(s) at fault can often be a challenge. Production of the patient's symptoms by the placement of selective tension on different tissues during the biomechanical examination can help to define the source of pain. The treatment plan should emphasize the restoration of normal biomechanics of the spine, pelvis, and lower quarter, with consideration given to the tissues at fault (i.e., the intervertebral disk, the posterior facet joints, the nerve roots, and the myofascial soft tissues). Only by the constant reassessment of the patient after treatment intervention can we confirm our suspicions and learn from our mistakes.

REFERENCES

1. Mooney V. The syndromes of low back disease. Orthop Clin North Am 1983;14:505–515.
2. Kirkaldy-Willis WH. The Pathology and Pathogenesis of Low Back Pain. In WH Kirkaldy-Willis (ed), Managing Low Back Pain. New York: Churchill Livingstone, 1983;23–43.
3. Wedge JH. The Natural History of Spinal Degeneration. In WH Kirkaldy-Willis (ed), Managing Low Back Pain. New York: Churchill Livingstone, 1983;3–8.
4. Paris SV. The Spine Course Notes. Atlanta: Institute Press, 1979;12.
5. Finneson BE. Low Back Pain (2nd ed). Philadelphia: JB Lippincott, 1980;302.
6. Porter RW, Miller CG. Back pain and trunk list. Spine 1986;11:596–600.
7. Matsui H, Ohmori K, Kanamori M, et al. Significance of sciatic scoliotic list in operated patients with lumbar disc herniation. Spine 1998;23:338–342.
8. McKenzie RA. The Lumbar Spine: Mechanical Diagnosis and Therapy. Waikanae, New Zealand: Spinal Publications, 1981.
9. Farfan HF, Kirkaldy-Willis WH. The present status of spinal fusion in the treatment of lumbar intervertebral joint disorders. Clin Orthop 1981;158:198–214.
10. Donelson R, Silva G, Murphy K. Centralization phenomenon—its usefulness in evaluating and treating referred pain. Spine 1990;15:211–213.
11. Long, AL. The centralization phenomenon. Its usefulness as a predictor of outcome in conservative treatment of chronic low back pain (a pilot study). Spine 1995;20:2513–2521.
12. Sufka A, Hauger B, Trenary M, et al. Centralization of low back pain and perceived functional outcome. J Orthop Sports Phys Ther 1998;27:205–212.
13. Nachemson AL. Disc pressure measurements. Spine 1981;6:93–97.
14. Stoddard A. Manual of Osteopathic Technique. London: Hutchinson Medical Publications, 1959;212–213.
15. Giles LG, Taylor JR. Low back pain associated with leg length inequality. Spine 1981;6:510–521.
16. Macnab I. Backache. Baltimore: Williams & Wilkins, 1977.
17. Cailliet R. Low Back Pain Syndrome. Philadelphia: FA Davis, 1981.
18. Rask M. Knee flexion test and sciatica. Clin Orthop 1978;134:221.
19. Greenman PE. Principles of Manual Medicine (2nd ed). Baltimore: Williams & Wilkins, 1996.
20. Bourdillon JF, Day EA, Bookhout MR. Spinal Manipulation (5th ed). Oxford, U.K.: Butterworth–Heinemann, 1992.
21. Kirkaldy-Willis WH. The site and nature of the lesion. In WH Kirkaldy-Willis (ed), Managing Low Back Pain. New York: Churchill Livingstone, 1983;91–107.
22. Mellin G. Correlations of spinal mobility with degree of chronic low back pain after correction for age and anthropometric factors. Spine 1987;12:464–468.
23. Maigne R. Low back pain of thoracolumbar origin. Arch Phys Med Rehabil 1980;61:389–395.
24. Tenhula JA, Rose SJ, Delitto A. Association between direction of lateral lumbar shift, movement tests, and side of symptoms in patients with low back pain syndrome. Phys Ther 1990;70:480–486.
25. Simon DG, Travell JG. Myofascial origins of low back pain. Part 3: torso muscles. Postgrad Med 1983;73:81–92.
26. Saal JA, Saal JS. Nonoperative treatment of herniated lumbar intervertebral disc with radiculopathy: an outcome study. Spine 1989:14:431–437.
27. Laslett M, Williams M. The reliability of selected pain provocation tests for sacroiliac joint pathology. Spine 1994;19:1243–1249.
28. Laseque C. Considerations sur la sciatique. Arch Gen de Med Paris 1864;2:558–580.
29. Breij A, Troup JD. Biomechanical considerations in the straight leg raising test. Spine 1979;4:242–250.

30. Butler DJ. Mobilization of the Nervous System. Melbourne: Churchill Livingstone, 1991.

31. Hudgins WR. The crossed straight leg raising test: a diagnostic sign of herniated disc. J Occup Med 1979;21:407–408.

32. Khuffash B, Porter RW. Cross leg pain and trunk list. Spine 1989;14:602–603.

33. Retzlaff EW, Berry AH, Haight AS, et al. The piriformis muscle syndrome. J Am Osteopath Assoc 1974;73:799–807.

34. Janda V. Muscles, Central Nervous Motor Regulation and Back Problems. In IM Korr (ed), The Neurobiological Mechanism in Manipulative Therapy. New York: Plenum, 1978;27–41.

35. Jull GA. Examination of the Lumbar Spine. In GP Grieve (ed), Modern Manual Therapy of the Vertebral Column. Edinburgh: Churchill Livingstone, 1986;547–560.

36. Kendall FP, McCreary EK. Muscle Testing and Function. Baltimore: Williams & Wilkins, 1983.

37. Cresswell AG, Oddsson L, Thorstensson A. The influence of sudden perturbations on trunk muscle activity and intra-abdominal pressure while standing. Exp Brain Res 1994;98:336–341.

38. Hodges PW, Richardson CA. Contraction of the abdominal muscles associated with movement of the lower limb. Phys Ther 1997;77:132–142.

39. Hodges PW, Richardson CA. Delayed postural contraction of transversus abdominis in low back pain associated with movement of the lower limb. J Spinal Disord 1998;11:46–56.

40. Hides JA, Stokes MJ, Saide M, et al. Evidence of lumbar multifidus muscle wasting ipsilateral to symptoms in patients with acute/subacute low back pain. Spine 1994;19:165–172.

41. Hides JA, Richardson CA, Jull GA. Multifidus muscle recovery is not automatic after resolution of acute, first-episode low back pain. Spine 1996;21:2763–2769.

42. Kopp JR, Alexander AH, Turocy RH, et al. The use of lumbar extension in the evaluation and treatment of patients with acute herniated nucleus pulposus. Clin Orthop 1986;202:211–218.

43. Corrigan B, Maitland GD. Practical Orthopaedic Medicine. London: Butterworth–Heinemann, 1983.

44. Magarey ME. Examination and Assessment of Spinal Joint Dysfunction. In GP Grieve (ed), Modern Manual Therapy of the Vertebral Column. Edinburgh: Churchill Livingstone, 1986; 481–497.

45. Lewit K. Manipulative Therapy in Rehabilitation of the Locomotor System (2nd ed). Oxford, U.K.: Butterworth–Heinemann, 1991.

46. Simon DG, Travell JG. Myofascial origins of low back pain. Part 1: principles of diagnosis and treatment. Postgrad Med 1983;73:66–77.

47. Kirkaldy-Willis WH. The Three Phases of the Spectrum of Degenerative Disease. In: WH Kirkaldy-Willis (ed), Managing Low Back Pain. New York: Churchill Livingstone, 1983;75–89.

Chapter 5

Radiographic Evaluation of the Lumbar Spine

Fred J. Laine and A. John Kuta

With the advent of modern technologies, the clinician has never had a more complete armamentarium of imaging studies to aid in the diagnosis and treatment of disorders of the spine. Although newer studies can be invaluable, they also increase the complexity of deciding which of these studies to order. In some cases, older procedures may provide equivalent or even better data than the newer procedures. The cost of the various studies also becomes an issue. In an ideal world, we might hope for the ability to order all tests at minimal cost. But even this approach brings with it problems of patient compliance and an increasing detection of false-positive or confounding results. This chapter attempts to shed some light on when imaging studies may be most helpful.

TESTING TECHNIQUES

Conventional Radiographs

Technique

Conventional plain films of the lumbar spine should include an anteroposterior (AP) view, a large port lateral view of the whole lumbar spine, and a small port lateral view of the sacrum and coccyx. These films are performed to evaluate the number, general appearance, and alignment of the vertebral bodies and the posterior elements. Bilateral oblique examinations, obtained 45 degrees off lateral, are often added and are helpful in evaluating the pars interarticularis and the lamina.

Normal Plain Film Examination

There are typically five lumbar vertebral bodies, although there can occasionally be four or six. Each vertebra is composed of three sections: the body, the pedicles and lamina, and the spinous process. The vertebral bodies are separated by intervertebral disks. The primary weightbearing column is composed of the vertebral bodies and the disks. The posterior elements provide some weightbearing and control the motion of the spine. The vertebral body, pedicles, and laminae form the ring of the spinal canal. The dural sac and spinal cord lie within the canal.

The pedicles and lamina are jointed to the adjacent superior and inferior vertebra by the facet or zygapophyseal joints (z-joints). These are synovial joints and are subject to the inflammatory and degenerative diseases common to synovial joints. They allow bending and rotation of the spinal column to occur. Each joint level has a superior and an inferior articulating facet where there is connection to the facet of the ring above and to the ring below. The bony strut between the superior and inferior facets of each side is called the *pars interarticularis*. The laminae fuse in the posterior midline to form a large bulbous posterior protuberance called the *spinous process*. This is the attachment site for the paraspinous musculature and ligaments.

The intervertebral disk height is approximately one-fourth that of the adjacent body; the L5–S1 disk is significantly narrower in height. On the lateral view, the anterior and posterior border of the bodies normally form a smooth lordotic curve. On the oblique examination, the pedicle, lamina, and facet complex has the appearance of a "Scottie dog." The normal anatomy of the lateral, AP, and oblique views is shown in Figure 5.1.

Indications

Plain films remain an excellent modality for the evaluation of bony anatomy. They are relatively inexpensive, rapid, and widely available. For these reasons, they remain an important study in the initial evaluation of pathology involving the spine. Plain films are accurate in evaluating the bony alignment by visualizing the posterior and anterior margins of the vertebral bodies. They are therefore frequently the first modality used in acute trauma and spinal degenerative disease. Oblique views are extremely useful in the evaluation of disruption of the pars interarticularis and any associated spondylolysis. Pathology that affects primarily the bone marrow (tumor, endocrine abnormality, infection, and hematologic disorders) is also evaluated by plain films. However, as explained in the sections Computed Tomography: Indications and Magnetic Resonance: Indications, other examinations have an increased sensitivity to marrow changes and have replaced plain films as the modality of choice. The results of the plain film examination can help to establish the appropriate secondary imaging study.

One shortcoming of plain films is an inability to discern soft tissue anatomy directly; only indirect conclusions can be drawn based on the effects of the bone involvement. In addition, they do not allow adequate evaluation of spinal canal contents or spinal ligaments. Therefore, plain films are infrequently indicated when evaluating an acute radiculopathy or a specific soft tissue abnormality.

One variant of radiography is the tomogram. Although it largely has been replaced by newer imaging studies, the x-ray tomogram may occasionally be useful. It is performed by synchronously moving the x-ray source and the film in opposite directions, with the slice of interest placed at the fulcrum of motion. The plane of interest is represented clearly, whereas the surrounding structures are blurred. This can be used to detect some fractures not otherwise seen on plain films. Another variant of radiography is fluoroscopy, a continuous x-ray image. This is often used to aid in injections (for localization). It is also used along with myelography to view the spine under motion.

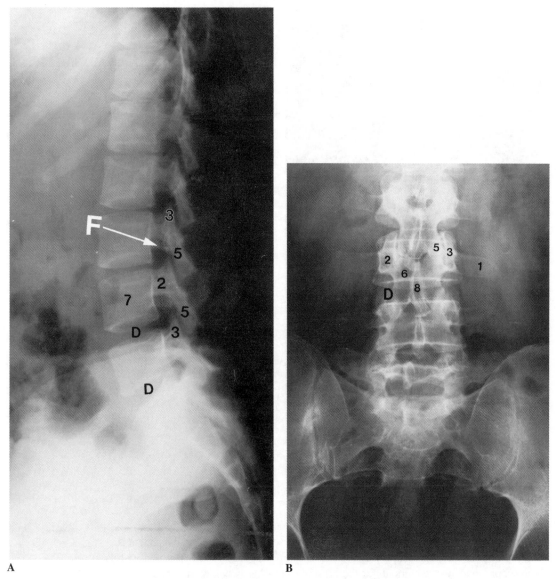

Figure 5.1 Normal plain films. (**A**) Lateral view shows the normal lordotic curvature with the anterior and posterior margins of the bodies describing a smooth curve. The intervertebral disk height is approximately one-fourth the height of the vertebral body. (**B**) Anteroposterior view demonstrates the pedicles and spinous processes and assists in evaluating any scoliotic curves. The number of nonrib-bearing vertebral bodies can be counted. Vertebral body anomalies are also most notable on this view. *Continued on page 98.*

Myelography

Technique

Myelography is the imaging of the spine with conventional radiographs after the intrathecal administration of contrast material. This should always be followed immediately

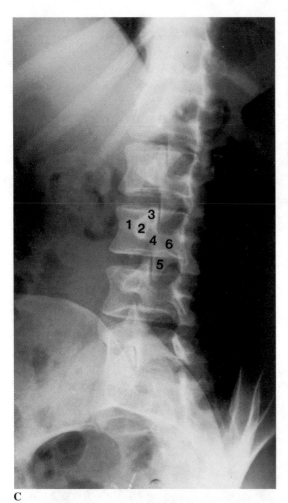

C

Figure 5.1 (*continued*)
(C) Oblique view helps in evaluation of the pars interarticularis. The image of a "Scottie dog" is demonstrated. The transverse process (1) forms the nose, the pedicle (2) forms the eye, the superior articulating facet (3) forms the ear. The pars interarticularis (4) forms the neck of the dog, the inferior articulating facet (5) forms the front leg, and the lamina (6) forms the body of the dog. (7 = body; 8 = spinous process; D = disk space; F = neuroforamen.)

by a computed tomography (CT) study. Informed consent is obtained, and the patient is placed prone on the fluoroscopy table. A routine lumbar puncture is performed with fluoroscopic guidance, commonly at the L2–L3 level (this is below the conus medullaris and above most degenerative disk disease). The skin is prepared sterilely and anesthetized. A spinal needle with trocar in place is introduced into the thecal sac. Proper placement is confirmed by the return of clear cerebrospinal fluid (CSF) after the removal of the trocar. A small amount of water-soluble iodinated intrathecal contrast material is injected. The needle is removed, and radiographs are obtained in multiple projections, including AP, lateral, oblique, and upright weightbearing. Flexion and extension upright weightbearing views can also be obtained to evaluate spinal stability. The patient is then imaged by CT. The contrast mixes with the CSF and is absorbed into the blood by the arachnoid granulations and within hours is excreted by the kidneys.

Normal and Abnormal Examination

The normal lumbar myelogram shows a contrast-filled thecal sac that gradually narrows to a point at the sacral level (Figure 5.2). The nerve roots are seen as

Figure 5.2 Normal lumbar myelogram. Oblique view from a lumbar myelogram demonstrating the high density contrast material within the thecal sac. The nerve roots (*arrows*) are represented as linear defects within the contrast column. Their course can be followed beneath the corresponding pedicle (P).

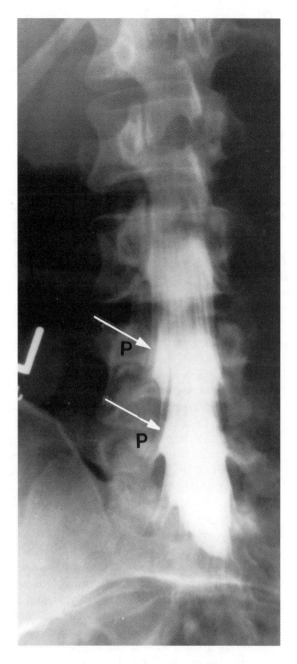

thin linear filling defects in the midst of the contrast. The nerve roots gradually veer laterally and gently curve under the appropriate lumbar pedicle. Each root is surrounded by a narrow nerve root sleeve, which is filled with contrast. The sleeve fills to approximately the mid-pedicle and then disappears. The anterior border of the contrast column on the lateral film should be smooth. Anterior indentations of the column are typically due to disk disease. Posterior indentations are due to facet and ligamentous disease. Oblique images best display the infrapedicle course of the nerve roots. A narrowing and rewidening of the contrast column is seen with extradural disease and is most prominent with spinal stenosis. Nerve roots widen and become serpiginous with a spinal canal stenosis or block.

Indications

The advent of magnetic resonance imaging (MRI) of the spine has decreased the frequency of myelography. Myelography should be performed if the patient is unable or unwilling to have MRI of the spine or has a contraindication (such as a pacemaker). Myelography has the advantage of giving a global view of the lumbar spine and allows easy comparison between levels and sides. This is often useful for spine surgeons. The diagnostic accuracy of myelography alone is approximately 80%, compared to 85% when used with CT, and 95% with MRI. The advantage of myelography is the demonstration of nerve root compression and the global evaluation of anatomy. Weightbearing views can provide evidence of abnormality that is in some cases missed on other imaging studies.

Complications

Myelography is an invasive procedure and can cause complications in up to 10% of patients.[1,2] Postprocedural headache is the most common complication. This is thought to be related to CSF leak or to meningeal irritation from the contrast material. The incidence of headache can be reduced by adequate patient hydration and by using small-diameter spinal needles (22–25 gauge). After the procedure, the patient is placed at bed rest in a slightly head-up position to decrease the "dumping" of contrast into the head. Treatment of postmyelogram headaches includes pain medications, bed rest, and continued hydration. If the headache persists for longer than 2 days, a CSF leak may be present. If this is the case, an epidural blood patch, the epidural injection of a small amount of autologous blood clot at the level of the puncture, may be required.

Seizures are another potential complication of myelography and are more common in patients who have a prior history of seizure. Patients on tricyclic antidepressants may have a lower seizure threshold. Therefore, such medications should be avoided for at least 2 days before the myelogram and 1 day afterwards.

Bleeding or epidural hematoma can occur after myelography because of the rich vascular supply of the spinal canal and the trauma that the myelographic needle can produce. Patients should be off anticoagulants and should have normal coagulation tests before the examination. The use of aspirin is unlikely to cause problems.

Patients with a history of allergic reactions to contrast material have a higher incidence of myelographic contrast reactions and should avoid the procedure. If the myelogram is necessary, the patient should be adequately premedicated with steroids to prevent a reaction. Antihistamines are also used occasionally.

Infection is a rare complication of myelography, and the incidence of meningeal infection is low and most commonly found in patients with skin infections of the lower back. Myelography should be avoided in these patients, or the contrast material should be administered in the cervical canal.

Diskography

Technique

Diskography is an invasive procedure that requires the insertion of a small-gauge needle into a disk space followed by the injection of a small amount of contrast material. The procedural technique of performing diskography varies widely. In essence, after informed consent, the disk space is localized under fluoroscopic guidance. After sterile preparation and local anesthesia, a needle is inserted into the individual disks. Some advocate that the needle be placed transdurally at the midline. However, a lateral approach is now generally the preferred method.[3] This allows easier needle placement with fluoroscopy and earlier patient mobilization by avoiding a transdural puncture. No more than 3 cc of contrast is injected. A note is made of the amount of contrast that is actually injected and the degree of resistance that is encountered to this injection. In addition, a note is made of any pain that is provoked by the injection, especially if this reproduces the patient's main pain complaint. After the fluoroscopic observation of disk injection, plain films are obtained in AP and lateral projections. Some centers obtain CT after the plain film examination.

Normal and Abnormal Examination

Normal and abnormal diskogram findings are illustrated in Figure 5.3. Interpreting a diskogram requires knowledge of the amount of contrast injected, the degree of resistance encountered, the production (reproduction) of pain, and the radiographic appearance of the study.[4] The normal lumbar disk holds up to 1.5 cc of contrast, has a firm end point of injection, and is painless. An abnormal disk allows greater than 1.5 cc of contrast to be injected, and the injection does not have a distinct end point. An abnormal disk may result in a painful study. The imaging characteristics of a normal disk shows a fairly concentric collection of contrast that remains within the central disk. An abnormal study is nonspecific, but shows diffusion of contrast throughout the disk.

Indications

The value of diskography has been controversial since its original description.[4] Advocates of this technique suggest that diskography is indicated in diagnosing internal disk derangement and in evaluating patients with back pain in which other standard imaging procedures have been normal or equivocal.[5] The test is also considered useful in determining which disk is symptomatic when multilevel disk degeneration is present.[6]

The sensitivity of CT and MRI has continued to fuel the controversy concerning diskography. Earlier comparative studies between MRI and diskography had variable results ranging from poor correlation[7] to high correlation.[6] Some studies have found diskography to be superior to CT alone or to myelography in identifying disk degeneration and tears in the annulus fibrosus.[8,9] Diskography may also be superior to MRI in identifying tears in the annulus fibrosus.[10] More recent studies have demonstrated that the presence of a high-signal intensity zone in the posterior annulus on MRI is extremely specific for a symptomatic annular tear.[11] A

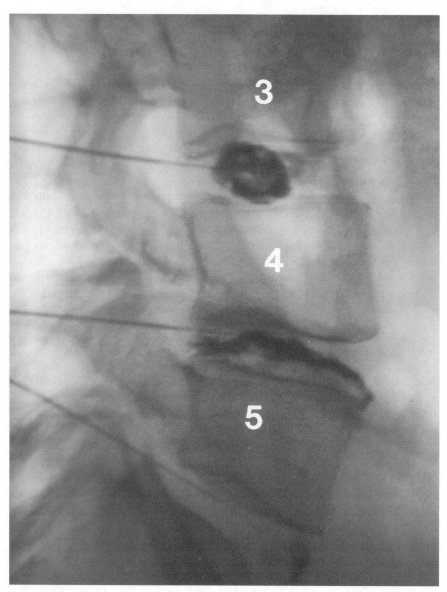

Figure 5.3 The normal and abnormal diskogram. Lateral view of the lumbar spine demonstrates needle placement at the L3–L4, L4–L5, and L5–S1 disk levels. Injection of contrast at the L3–L4 level reveals a normal collection of contrast remaining within the central disk. At the L4–L5 level, there is abnormal diffusion of the contrast throughout the disk. For appropriate evaluation, the radiographic abnormalities should be correlated with the patient's pain during the examination. (3 = L3; 4 = L4; 5 = L5.)

prospective randomized study, however, is not yet available, and the use of diskography will most likely continue to be controversial and dependent on individual preferences.[4,12]

Complications

Diskitis occurs in 1–4% of patients who have had diskograms and can usually be avoided by meticulous attention to sterile technique and prophylactic antibiotic treatment.[13] Although pain is an expected outcome of an abnormal diskogram, the postprocedural continuance of pain can be lessened by the injection of 1% lidocaine into the disk after the diagnostic procedure.

Computed Tomography

Technique

High resolution CT scanners provide cross-sectional images to identify and evaluate spinal structures and pathology. The CT scanner measures the difference between radiation emitted and the amount detected when an x-ray beam is passed through a body part. This difference is known as the *attenuation coefficient* and can be converted to a gray scale value. A cross-sectional layer of the body is divided into many tiny blocks or volume elements (voxels), and each block is assigned a number proportional to the degree in which it attenuates the x-ray beam. Attenuation values (Hounsfield numbers) are converted to a gray scale of density readings, with the values ranging from +1,000 for cortical bone to –1,000 for air, with 0 representing water. The projected image, therefore, is composed of various shades of gray. The lighter (white) areas are produced by structures with high attenuation, such as bone. The darker (black) areas are produced by structures with low attenuation, such as fat.

Standard CT requires multiple axial slices through the spine. Slice thickness usually varies from 3 mm to 5 mm in thickness, depending on the area of the spine that must be evaluated and the need for detailed imaging. Thinner sections as low as 1 mm are reserved for specific locations that require detailed high resolution. Overlapping axial slices should be obtained when reconstructed images are necessary. The technique may also vary in the angle of axial orientation. Axial slices may be obtained that are parallel to the orientation of each disk or obtained contiguously from the top of the scanning volume to the bottom. The use of intravenous contrast administration is useful in evaluating vascular abnormalities, the enhancement characteristics of pathology, and in the postoperative state.

A significant advantage of CT lies in the postprocessing techniques that are available on most standard CT machines. Varying the window levels permits evaluation of both osseous and soft tissue structures. Wide (bone) windows optimally display osseous structures, and narrow (soft tissue) windows are best suited for evaluation of soft tissue structures. Another postprocessing technique allows the spinal column to be viewed in multiple additional planes within minutes after the axial study. Axial multislice images can be "stacked up" and reconstructed into coronal and sagittal planes or any obliquity that helps evaluate bony relationships and pathology.

One advancement, spiral (helical) CT, is now widely available. The principles of CT remain the same, but the method of acquiring the CT data has significantly changed. Data can now be obtained at a fraction of the time of previous studies, with minimal motion artifact and without significant loss of spatial resolution. Imaging time is significantly reduced, which allows more rapid patient turnover and the ability to accommodate uncooperative patients more easily.

Normal Examination

A normal CT examination is illustrated in Figure 5.4. Cortical bone, which includes the vertebral body end plates, is composed of compact bone and appears dense (white) on standard CT images because of its densely packed calcium. The central aspect of the vertebral body is composed of cancellous bone with fatty marrow, which decreases the density of the bone. Thicker trabeculations can usually be seen appearing as dots on cross-sectional images. The articular facets are separated by a true synovial joint lined by hyaline cartilage. Disk material, ligaments, and other soft tissue structures appear gray, being isodense to adjacent muscle. The dural or thecal sac normally is slightly darker than disk material due to the presence of CSF. Individual nerve roots within the sac usually are not identified. Epidural fat fills the space around the dural sac. The ligamentum flavum arises from the capsule of the articular joint and the lamina and can be seen as a band of soft tissue density along the posterior epidural space. The nerve root sheath originates from the dural sac close to the posterior disk border and exits the canal below the pedicle of the next inferior vertebra. Nerve roots and ganglia can be identified as soft tissue densities within the lateral recess and neural foramen. Differentiation between all of these structures is assisted by the contrast between epidural and paraspinal fat, which usually is the darkest area on the study.

One limitation of the CT scan is volume averaging artifact. This occurs because of intrinsic limitations of slice thickness. Each CT slice represents the average signal intensity of that slice. Tissue that extends only partially through a slice is averaged with the rest of that slice. Obviously, thinner slices result in less volume averaging artifact, but at the cost of a longer, more cumbersome study with higher radiation dosage. CT scans also demonstrate artifacts around metal implants.

Indications

Since the advent of MRI, the use of CT for evaluation of low back pain has declined. However, because of its ability to accurately demonstrate cortical bone, marrow, and spinal soft tissues, it remains an important modality.[14] The indications for CT include degenerative facet and disk disease and spinal stenosis. In particular, spondylolysis can be more clearly delineated on CT than MRI.[15] Marrow infiltrative disorders, as seen with some hematologic and systemic diseases, and bony destructive processes, as seen with primary and metastatic tumors, can also be adequately evaluated with CT. However, CT usually remains a complementary study to MRI in these cases.

Spinal trauma is an additional indication for CT. In fact, CT remains superior to plain films and MRI for the direct evaluation of bone injury.[14] CT can demonstrate fractures, fragment displacement, and, with the additional use of reconstructions, alignment abnormalities. Soft tissue structures can be evaluated directly (disk herniations and hematomas) or indirectly (by the position of bony structures).

Figure 5.4 Normal computed tomography (CT) examination. **(A)** Axial CT obtained at the level of the pedicles and body and filmed with bone window technique. **(B)** Axial CT obtained at the level of the disk and filmed with bone window technique.

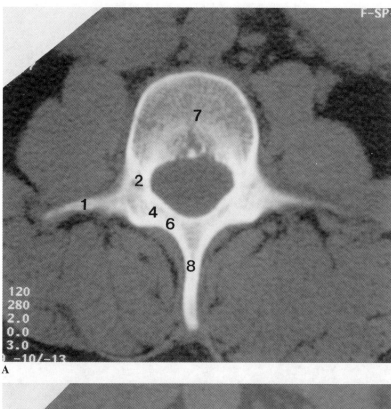

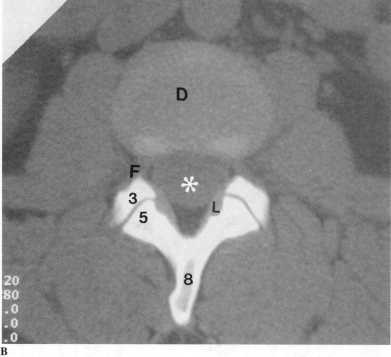

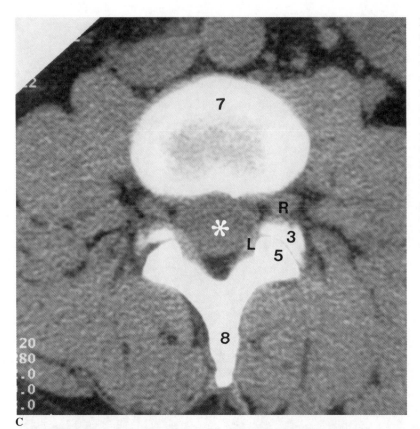

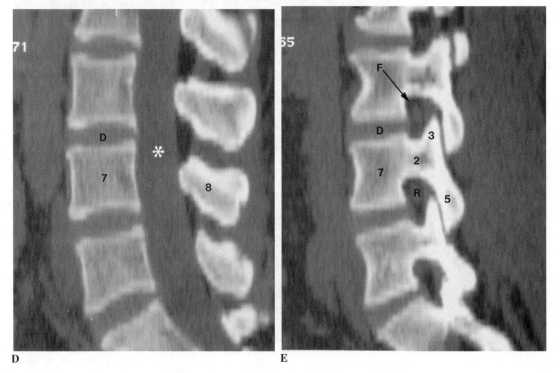

Figure 5.4 *(continued)* **(C)** Axial CT obtained at the level of the disk and filmed with soft tissue technique. **(D)** Sagittal and **(E)** parasagittal reconstructed CT views filmed with bone window technique. (1 = transverse process; 2 = pedicle; 3 = superior articulating facet; 4 = pars interarticularis; 5 = inferior articulating facet; 6 = lamina; 7 = body; 8 = spinous process; D = disk space; F = neuroforamen; L = ligamentum flava; R = nerve root; * = thecal sac.)

Myelography-Computed Tomography

Technique

CT can be performed after a routine myelogram (myelo-CT). Alternatively, a myelo-CT study can be performed as a low-dose method. In this case, the study requires a lumbar puncture but with the instillation of only a few milliliters of contrast material. This reduction in contrast material reduces the risk of some side effects. Similar to routine CT, coronal and sagittal reconstructed views can be performed following myelography.

Normal Examination

A normal myelo-CT scan is illustrated in Figure 5.5. Intrathecal contrast material has a higher attenuation value than CSF, which allows a greater degree of tissue contrast. The gray density of the normal CSF is replaced by bright density from the contrast material. Spinal cord, individual nerve roots, and the surrounding extradu-

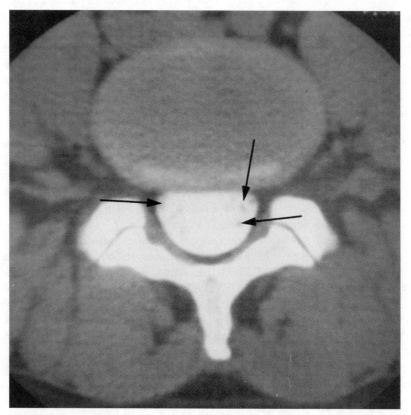

Figure 5.5 Normal myelography-computed tomography scan. Axial postmyelogram computed tomography image obtained at the disk level demonstrates individual nerve roots (*arrows*) surrounded by the bright contrast.

ral compartments can be assessed with a higher degree of accuracy. Intradural and extradural pathology can also be readily identified.

Indications

The indications for myelo-CT are essentially the same as those for CT (see previous section). However, because of the added tissue contrast, this procedure is also valuable in detecting soft tissue abnormalities such as disk herniation and intradural tumor, especially for those patients who are unable to undergo an MRI. The limitations and contraindications are similar to those of routine myelography and routine CT. If the low dose technique is performed, the risks are similar, but the risk of side effects may be reduced slightly.

Magnetic Resonance Imaging

Technique

MRI has made a significant impact in the diagnosis and treatment of spinal disease. The physics involved is beyond the scope of this chapter, but it should be emphasized that images are produced by magnetic-field effects and radiofrequency waves rather than by the ionizing radiation used in previously described procedures. When placed in a magnetic field, a small percentage of hydrogen protons align with the main magnetic field. Specific radiofrequency waves are used to displace the protons off alignment. As the protons realign with the field, they generate a radio wave that can be measured and converted to a gray scale value. The MRI is a gray scale map that reflects the percentage of protons characteristic for the hydrogen density of a tissue. The protons realign (relax) by two mechanisms, which are specific for each tissue type. These mechanisms are termed *T1 decay* and *T2 decay* and are based on inherent tissue characteristics. By altering operator-dependent imaging times, one can take advantage of these different decay mechanisms and change the contrast between the soft tissues. T1-weighted images emphasize T1 decay and T2-weighted images emphasize T2 decay. The relative signals (degree of brightness) from each tissue can, therefore, be altered to produce different contrasts between tissues. Intravenous administration of a heavy metal chelate, gadolinium, can be used to increase conspicuity of pathologic lesions.

MRI is consistently evolving. Newer, faster, and more disease-specific sequences are constantly being developed.[16] Many of these techniques are still under evaluation for usefulness. Gradient-recalled echo (GRE) sequences require less time to acquire and have replaced routine spin-echo T2-weighted sequences in evaluating most diseases of the spine. GRE sequences are available that can obtain data as a three-dimensional volume and allow reformation of images in any plane. Fast spin-echo sequences are available on most scanners. These sequences significantly reduce imaging times, increase resolution, and can improve signal-to-noise ratios on T2-weighted images.

High signal from fat on T1-weighted sequences can make it difficult to detect and define pathologic processes.[17] Fat-suppression sequences remove the bright fat signal on T1-weighted images. The use of contrast enhancement of pathologic processes has the disadvantage of occasionally masking pathology by making lesions isointense to fat. Fat-suppression sequences used in conjunction with intravenous gadolinium contrast injection improves the contrast between enhancing tissues and background tissues. Fluid attenuated fat-saturation sequences suppress CSF and fat signal and allow certain pathologic processes to be more conspicuous.

By combining heavily T2-weighted fast spin-echo sequences and fat-suppression techniques, an MR-myelogram can be created.[18] Individual slices are reformatted into a composite image resembling an intrathecal contrasted myelogram. This technique can create high-quality images of the thecal sac, thecal margins, nerve roots, and nerve root sheaths. A variation of this is the sequence, the neurogram, allowing the depiction of individual nerves coursing within the soft tissues.[19]

Standard imaging uses both T1- and T2-weighted sequences, usually in sagittal planes. In addition, at least one sequence should be performed in the axial direction. Specific sequences sensitive to certain pathologic changes can also be added. Gadolinium-based intravenous contrast can be injected to better delineate vascular abnormalities, tumor, and epidural scar. Because of the numerous sequences available to image the spine, clinical information is now mandatory. To optimize imaging time, only appropriate sequences should be performed and can be customized to varying clinical circumstances. The radiologist should be informed by the clinician as to what pathology is suspected on clinical evaluation.

Normal Lumbar Examination

The normal MRI appearance of the spine is complex because of the numerous sequences (Figure 5.6). Many imaging parameter combinations are available, and there is no one correct method to perform an individual study. Each MRI center should optimize the sequences available to provide the most useful information.

Bone.   With MRI, cortical bone does not emit a signal due to the presence of calcium and relative lack of hydrogen. Cortical bone, therefore, appears on all MRIs as a black line outlining the bony element. The central aspect of the vertebral bodies and other bony elements is composed of marrow. MRI signal in these areas is produced by both water and fat protons of the marrow. The high-fat content of normal adult marrow results in high signal on T1-weighted images and low signal on T2-weighted images. Normal trabecular bone is usually not apparent because of the dominant signal produced by the marrow. Focal fatty deposits are commonly seen and appear as high signal intensity on T1-weighted and intermediate signal intensity on T2-weighted images. On T2-weighted images, the synovial joint between the articular facets appears as an area of high signal intensity outlined by the dark signal void of the adjacent cortical bone.

Intervertebral Disk.   The intervertebral disk is composed of two major components, the central gelatinous nucleus pulposus and the peripheral fibrous annulus fibrosus. The central portion of the annulus is composed of fibrocartilaginous fibers (type II collagen), whereas the peripheral portion is composed of collagenous fibers (type I collagen).[20] On T1-weighted images, the distinction between the regions is not pronounced. Peripherally, there is a gray-black band that corresponds to the outer fibers of the annulus and its confluence with the longitudinal ligaments. Centrally, there is an area of low signal intensity, slightly brighter than the peripheral component, that corresponds to the inner annulus fibers and the nucleus pulposus. On T2-weighted images and GRE images, the peripheral region retains its low signal intensity, but the central

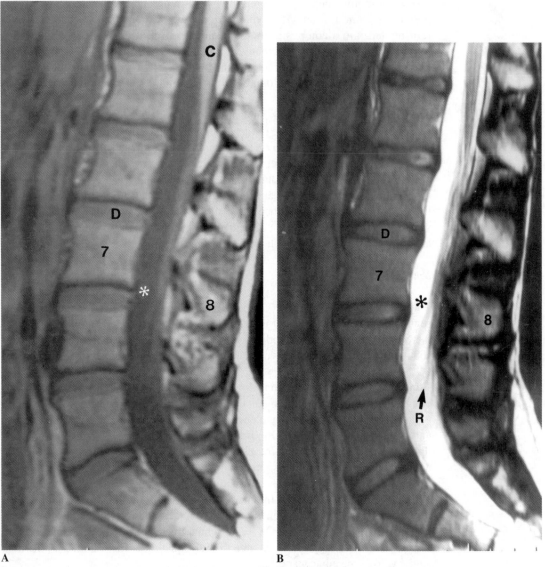

A   B

Figure 5.6 Normal magnetic resonance imaging (MRI) scan. Sagittal **(A)** T1-weighted and **(B)** T2-weighted MRI demonstrate the normal signal characteristics of the vertebral body marrow, disks, conus, and cerebrospinal fluid (CSF). **(C)** Parasagittal T1-weighted MRI shows the nerve root (*arrow*) surrounded by fat as it exits beneath the pedicle (p). Axial T1-weighted MRI.

region becomes bright. It is important to note that the normal intervertebral disk is slightly hypointense relative to the signal of the vertebral body bone marrow on T1-weighted images.

Associated Structures. The spinal cord normally terminates at the L1–L2 level, and the dural sac, containing CSF and nerve roots, continues to the middle of the

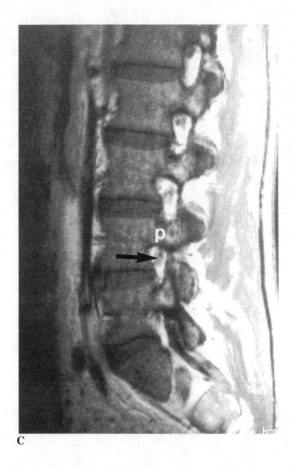

C

sacrum. On T1-weighted images, CSF is low in signal intensity, with the cord and nerve roots slightly brighter. On T2-weighted and GRE images, a myelographic effect is produced, with the CSF being bright and the cord and nerve roots being hypointense.

The epidural space primarily contains fat, which is bright on T1-weighted images and dark on T2-weighted images. The thickness of the fat typically increases progressively from L1 to L5. Within the fat are epidural veins and nerve roots that bud off the dural sac and enter the neural foramen. The epidural fat surrounds many soft tissue structures that are in contrast to the signal of fat. The dorsal root ganglion is an oval enlargement of the exiting nerve root and lies in the neural foramen. The ligamentum flavum covers the capsule of the facet joint and extends from one lamina to another. The anterior and posterior longitudinal ligaments cover the anterior and posterior aspects of the vertebral bodies, respectively. These ligaments adhere firmly to the vertebral bodies and the interposed annulus fibrosus of the disk.

The lateral recess is that portion of the spinal canal that is bound anteriorly by the vertebral body and disk, laterally by the pedicle, and posteriorly by the supe-

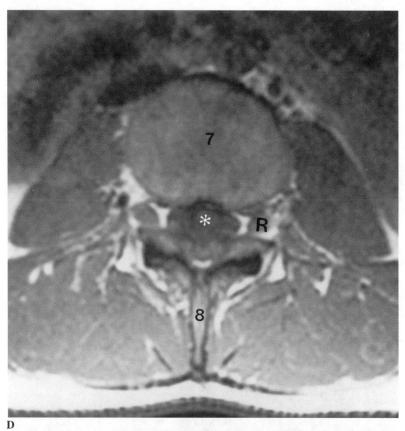

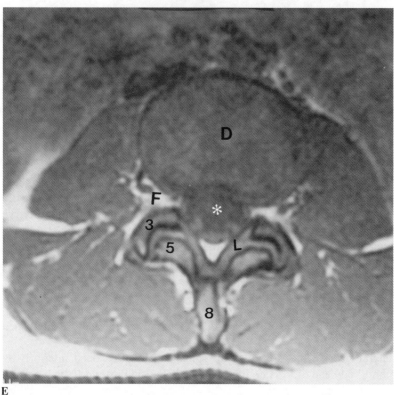

Figure 5.6 (*continued*) (**D**) at the level of the body inferior to the pedicle and (**E**) at the level of the disk. (**F**) MR-myelogram showing the ability of MR to mimic a myelographic picture. The nerve roots are well seen within the bright CSF signal. (3 = superior articulating facet; 5 = inferior articulating facet; 7 = body; 8 = spinous process; C = conus; D = disk space; F = neuroforamen; L = ligamentum flava; R = nerve root; * = thecal sac.)

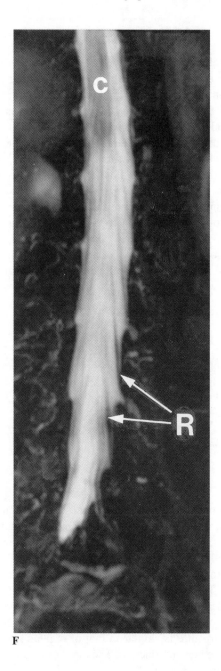

F

rior articular facet. The descending nerve root lies in the lateral recess along with surrounding fat. The neural foramen is a fibro-osseus canal that is the continuation of the lateral recess. On sagittal MRI, it is shaped like an hourglass with a wider superior portion that contains the nerve roots, dorsal root ganglion, arteries and veins, and the smaller inferior portion that contains primarily fat and intervertebral veins.

Indications

Excluding acute spinal trauma, MRI is the imaging modality of choice for evaluating most spinal pathology. In comparison to other imaging modalities, MRI has various advantages in imaging of the lumbar spine. Included are its noninvasive nature, the absence of ionizing radiation, direct multiplanar imaging, complete coverage of the spine, and the high-contrast resolution.[21] High tissue contrast has made MRI the primary modality when evaluating low back pain and radiculopathy when a herniated disk is suspected. MRI is also the modality of choice when a spinal infection is considered. For evaluation of any spinal neoplastic process, MRI is also the modality of choice, when marrow infiltrative processes, intramedullary neoplasms, and cord compressive lesions are suspected. In the evaluation of traumatic injury, MRI plays a role complementary to CT and plain films. CT better delineates fractures and bony displacement, but MRI better defines soft tissue injuries such as ligamentous injury, post-traumatic disk herniation, cord contusion, and hematoma, as well as the secondary effects of fractures such as epidural hematoma and cord compressive lesions.

Complications

Like CT, MRI is also limited by the volume averaging artifact. Metallic implant artifact can be a problem as well. MRI is contraindicated in persons with cardiac pacemakers and metallic aneurism clips. Claustrophobia is frequently a problem but can be minimized with open-sided magnets or sedation.

Nuclear Medicine Scanning

Technique

Nuclear medicine bone scanning uses a radioactive compound to evaluate metabolic activity or turnover of bone.[22] The most commonly used radioactive agent is the technetium (Tc) tracer, Tc–99m, in which 99 is the atomic weight and "m" stands for metastable, a descriptor of its radioactive state. Technetium 99m has a half-life of 6 hours and emits gamma radiation that can be detected by a gamma-scintillation camera. The number of radioactive emissions from each area of the body is counted, and an image is compiled. The tracer is chelated to an inorganic phosphate molecule or an organic phosphonate molecule before administration. The diphosphonate structure is similar to that of organic phosphorus and calcium and is taken into active bone production. The diphosphonate molecules bind avidly to amorphous hydroxyapatite crystals in areas of increased osteogenic activity. More tracer is delivered to areas with increased blood flow. In areas with no bone matrix or absent blood flow, there is no tracer uptake. Technetium can also be attached to pertechnetate, which binds to serum albumin, and can be used for angiographic studies of bone.

Gallium-67 citrate is a radiopharmaceutical that has been used to complement technetium studies. This agent binds to polymorphonuclear leukocytes and has been used in the evaluation of vertebral osteomyelitis and septic arthritis.

The patient having a bone scan should be well hydrated and void immediately before the examination. Approximately 20 milliCuries of Tc–99m diphosphonate is injected intravenously. Imaging begins 2–4 hours after injection. If a dynamic angiographic scan is necessary, images are taken 5–15 minutes after injection. Single photon emission computed tomography (SPECT) is useful for both more detailed localization of a pathologic finding, including the creation of a three-dimensional appearance, and also for increased sensitivity of identifying pathology.[23,24]

Normal and Abnormal Examination

The nuclear medicine bone scan creates an image of bone with osteoblastic and osteoclastic activity. The normal scan shows near uniform uptake in the whole skeletal system (Figure 5.7). There is usually greater conspicuity of the axial skeleton (spine and pelvis). There is light background activity of the soft tissues. The kidneys, ureters, and bladder are also visible in patients with normal renal function. The kidneys usually are not as intense as the spine. If the kidneys are not visible, there is either renal failure or severe widespread metastatic disease to the bone (as is commonly seen with prostate carcinoma). The phenomenon of extreme bone activity that outshines renal activity is called a *superscan*.

Three general abnormal bone scan patterns are seen.

1. High tracer activity is seen in areas of rapid bone turnover. This is commonly seen with metastatic or primary neoplasm, infection, or healing trauma. Metastatic disease causes remodeling of the bone through osteoclastic and osteoblastic processes and is detected as increased activity on the bone scan. The nuclear study is not as sensitive to small metastases as MRI is, but is used to localize areas of disease to determine what other imaging studies may be necessary. Marrow changes can often be first seen on MRI before there is enough remodeling to be seen on the nuclear scan. Severe diffuse osteoblastic metastatic disease is seen as a superscan.
2. A mild to moderate increase in tracer activity is commonly seen with degenerative joint disease. In the spine, this is usually seen in the facet joints or diskovertebral joints. A small amount of remodeling of the joint or end plate can cause a change in tracer uptake. This is most often seen in degenerative joint disease of the spine. Occasionally, an intense abnormality may be present on SPECT bone scan due to severe degenerative changes.
3. The least common pattern and most difficult to discern is low activity. This pattern is seen with diseases of extremely high osteoclastic activity with little osteoblastic activity, such as multiple myeloma. Bone infarction or severe sclerosis can also give this picture.

With healing of metastatic disease as a result of therapy, the bone scan can revert to normal, whereas the conventional radiographs may remain abnormal. If a process is indolent or diffusely lytic and widespread, the bone scan may also appear normal. This is often the case with multiple myeloma. Other diseases can cause abnormal uptake, including infection, trauma, degenerative disease, Paget's disease, and multiple infarctions.

Indications

Nuclear bone imaging is useful as a screening test to identify active areas of bone turnover. The level and distribution of activity can help in suggesting an underlying cause of the disorder. The entire skeletal system can be screened. Common reasons

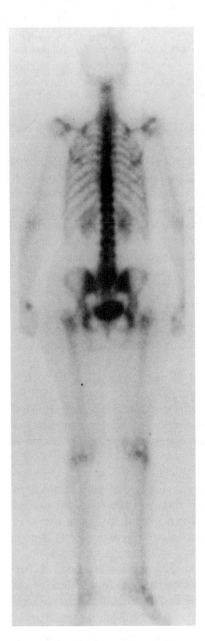

Figure 5.7 Normal nuclear bone scan. Posterior view of a technetium bone scan shows that the axial skeleton is slightly more pronounced than the appendicular skeleton. The kidneys and soft tissues of the body are barely visible.

for obtaining a nuclear bone scan are to assess for degenerative changes of the z-joints or diskovertebral joints, post-traumatically to assess for stress fracture, or to evaluate the presence and extent of metastatic disease.

IMAGING APPEARANCES OF LOW BACK DISORDERS

Mechanical Low Back Pain Syndromes

When evaluating mechanical low back pain syndromes, a convenient categorization that assists with obtaining the most reasonable imaging study first, is axial or radicular pain.

Axial pain can be further subdivided into pathology of the anterior or posterior column structures, or both, each either traumatically or nontraumatically induced. Radicular syndromes typically have a diskogenic origin or are secondary to spinal stenosis.

Axial Pain Syndromes

Axial pain syndromes include pain that is primarily in the low back region—central, unilateral, or bilateral—possibly with referred pain to the hip girdle or proximal lower extremity. Potential pain generators within the anterior column are the vertebral body and intervertebral disk and in the posterior column are the facet joint and pars interarticularis. The history and physical examination determines when and what type of advanced imaging study is ordered. Generally, disk disease is better demonstrated by MRI and facet disease is better demonstrated by CT.

The intervertebral disk may be the source of the majority of axial low back pain syndromes. There exists a continuum of disk pathology that may present with axial pain without radiculopathy, including internal disk disruption, annular tear, and central disk herniation—any of which can become symptomatic with or without trauma. Degenerative disk changes are universal in humans. Although the exact etiology of disk degeneration is not known, repetitive trauma coupled with immunologic, metabolic, or genetic factors may all play a role.[25] As the intervertebral disk degenerates, the primary changes are loss of water, fibrous tissue accumulation, and collapse. MRI is clearly the test of choice when evaluating these disk abnormalities. This imaging modality is the only noninvasive method to assess the internal architecture of the intervertebral disk. With MRI, the loss of disk hydration can be readily seen by the loss of water signal and the loss of disk height (Figure 5.8). The degenerative disk is lower than normal in signal intensity on T1- and T2-weighted images. The gas from vacuum phenomenon does not produce a signal and may simulate calcification. CT scanning, with or without contrast enhancement, does not demonstrate the internal aspect of the disk. On CT and myelo-CT, desiccation of the disk may be appreciated by the loss of disk height and occasionally by demonstration of the vacuum phenomena, in which normal disk material is replaced by gas, primarily nitrogen (Figure 5.9).

The presence of areas of high signal intensity on MRI in the posterior or posterolateral annulus fibrosis suggest a radial annular tear and is usually visualized on both sagittal and axial T2-weighted images. This high signal intensity zone may be as sensitive and specific in regard to predicting a clinically painful disk as diskography. MRI is also an ideal test for evaluating central disk pathology and disk bulges (i.e., a nonfocal or circumferential symmetric extension of disk beyond the margin of the vertebra end plate due to annular laxity). The benefits of MRI versus noncontrast CT for this specific pathologic entity is that it provides a much clearer distinction between the posterior disk margin and the thecal sac and a clearer differentiation between the thecal sac and the epidural venous plexus. The addition of intrathecal contrast, however, narrows this difference. On myelography, a disk bulge is seen as a diffuse anterior extradural defect that narrows the contrast column to a variable degree (Figure 5.10). On cross-sectional imaging studies, a bulging disk is demonstrated by disk material extending beyond the vertebral body margins (see Figure 5.9).

Abnormalities of the bony elements of the anterior and posterior columns can either develop acutely from a traumatic injury or result from chronic overload, result-

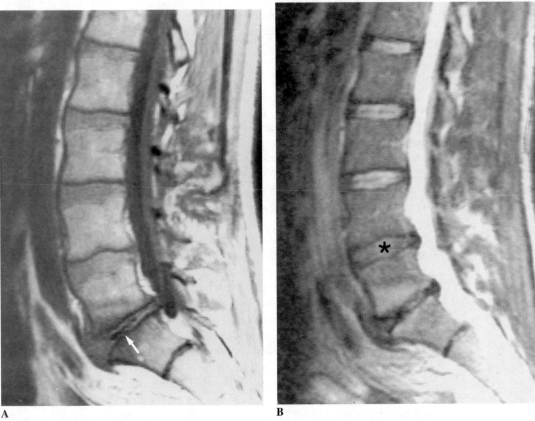

A   B

Figure 5.8 Degenerative disk disease. Sagittal (**A**) T1-weighted and (**B**) T2-weighted magnetic resonance images of the lumbar spine. The study demonstrates severe degenerative disk disease at the L5–S1 level as noted by a decrease in disk height and hydration. There are also type I end plate sclerotic changes at the L5–S1 level. The hypointense cleft within the L5–S1 disk on T1 image (*arrow*) represents calcification or vacuum phenomenon. Note that although the L4–L5 level (*asterisk*) appears normal on the T1-weighted image, the T2-weighted image shows loss of hydration when compared with the upper most lumbar disk levels.

ing in degenerative changes. Fractures of the vertebral body usually result from sudden axial and flexion overloads. Plain radiographs are always required if a significant axial load injury has occurred and should evaluate for loss of vertebral body height, displacement of the superoposterior portion of the vertebral body in the lateral plane, and splaying of the pedicles in the AP plane. These findings suggest a burst component. If any question arises regarding a vertebral body fracture, then an advanced imaging test is required, which can be a CT or MRI. CT is more easily obtained on an emergent basis and clearly demonstrates the presence of spinal canal compromise due to bony encroachment. T2-weighted MRI can also identify an acute fracture (including microfractures) by demonstrating edema in the bone marrow. It has the additional advantage over CT of assessing the neurologic components of the spinal canal and the presence of a soft tissue disk injury, including an acute Schmorl's node. Although MRI may be able to determine the acuity of the bony injury, nuclear bone scan imaging may also be helpful. A negative, or cold, bone scan essentially rules out an acute fracture, whereas an abnormal bone scan does not necessarily indicate acuity as bone scans can remain abnormal for months after an injury.

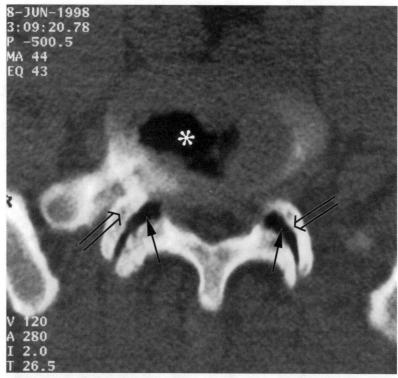

Figure 5.9 Degenerative disk disease. Axial computed tomography scan through a disk with significant degeneration. There is concentric disk bulge with vacuum phenomenon (*asterisk*). There is also significant bilateral facet joint degeneration (*open arrows*) with vacuum phenomenon (*arrows*).

Vertebral body marrow and end plate changes frequently accompany degenerative disk changes. These changes are referred to as *diskogenic sclerosis* and can be seen on plain radiographs and CT scans as regions of increased density in the vertebral end plate adjacent to a degenerative disk. The MRI appearance of these marrow changes is variable and is dependent on the underlying pathologic response. Modic et al. have classified these changes into three groups (see Figures 5.8 and 5.11).[26,27] Type I end plate sclerosis represents vascularized fibrous tissue with an increase in intracellular water. On MRI, these changes are seen as low signal on T1-weighted images and increased signal on T2-weighted images with respect to normal marrow. With type II end plate sclerosis, the marrow converts to fat. On MRI, this is seen as an increase in signal on T1-weighted images and an isointense to slightly hyperintense signal on T2-weighted images. Type III end plate changes represent dense bone sclerosis without fibrous or vascularized tissue. On MRI, these changes are seen as areas of low signal on both T1- and T2-weighted images. Although this classification seems trivial, they should be reported because they are thought to be clinically relevant. Type II and type III changes indicate a chronic process, whereas type I changes represent an acute or subacute inflammatory process that may explain acute pain.[28]

The lumbar facet joints are susceptible to mechanical wear and tear, resulting in arthropathic changes. Both an acute overload injury and chronic or repetitive extension and rotation overload injury can cause breakdown of the articular cartilage and subchondral bone. These synovial joints respond to repetitive mechanical stress

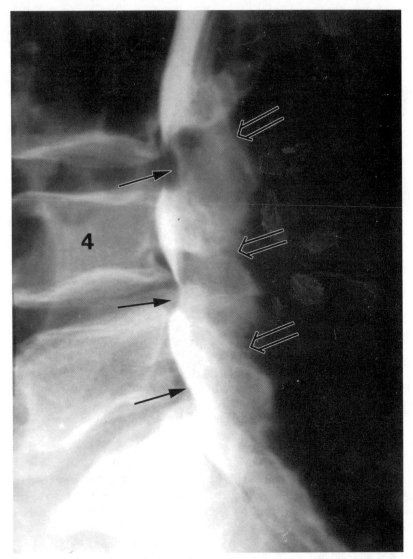

Figure 5.10 Disk bulge and spinal stenosis. Lateral myelogram shows "waisting" and near complete obliteration of the contrast column at the L3–L4 level. The L4–L5 level shows a disk bulge. The anterior defects are due to disk pathology (*arrows*); the posterior defects (*open arrows*) are due to facet and ligament pathology.

with the formation of osteophytes, bony sclerosis, and subchondral cyst formation (Figure 5.12). Because facet joint degenerative changes are common, determining whether an abnormal joint is a pain generator requires the combination of a high clinical index of suspicion and results from appropriate imaging studies as well as response to selective spinal injection (see Chapter 9). Plain radiographs frequently demonstrate facet joint degenerative changes, but these are typically nonspecific. However, after an acute injury in which a significant injury is suspected, including a facet fracture, radiographs should be obtained. Advanced imaging studies, such as SPECT bone scan, may identify a substantial bony injury such as a fracture of a facet joint process or subchondral bone by demonstrating an intense focal uptake in

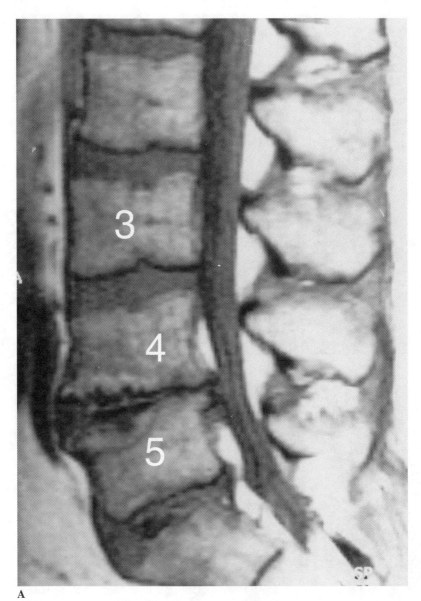

Figure 5.11 Degenerative disk disease with type II and type III end plate sclerosis. (**A**) Sagittal T1-weighted.

the posterior column. SPECT scanning may also be useful for evaluating a patient with chronic low back pain in whom plain radiographs reveal severe facet joint arthritis to determine whether a single level can be implicated as a source of pain. If a SPECT scan is abnormal, then a limited CT (with bone algorithm and thin slices) through the suspected region is appropriate to evaluate for a specific fracture, the degree of joint space narrowing, periarticular hypertrophy, subchondral cysts, and possible vacuum phenomena. A further benefit of CT is that the anatomy of the

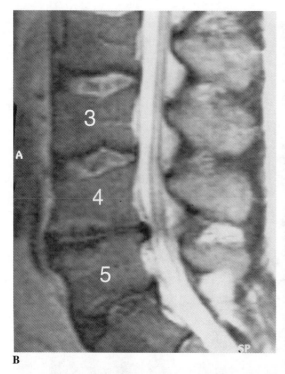

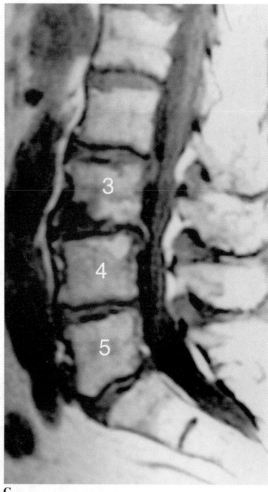

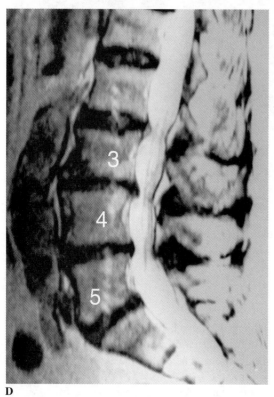

Figure 5.11 (*continued*) (**B**) T2-weighted magnetic resonance images demonstrate type II end plate changes at L4–L5. The end plates are hyperintense on the T1-weighted image and hypointense on the T2-weighted image with respect to the vertebral body. (**C**) Sagittal T1-weighted and (**D**) T2-weighted images demonstrate type III end plate changes at L3–L4. The signal characteristics are hypointense on both images.

Figure 5.12 Facet joint (z-joint) disease. Axial **(A)** computed tomography image and **(B)** T1-weighted magnetic resonance imaging (MRI) demonstrate bony degenerative changes of the facet joints. Bony hypertrophy and the associated effect on the neural foramen can be seen. Subchondral cysts (*straight arrows*) and associated ligamentum flavum thickening (*curved arrows*) can also be seen.

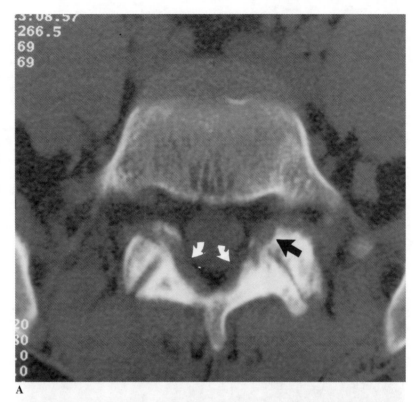

A

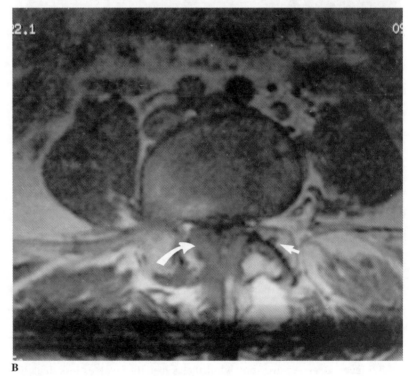

B

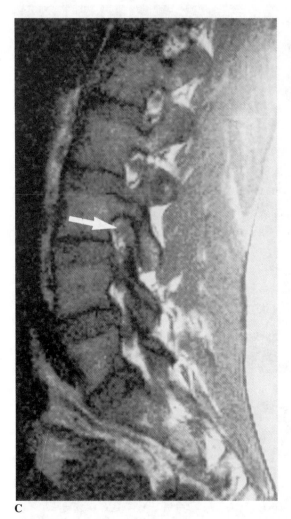

Figure 5.12 (*continued*)
(**C**) Parasagittal T1-weighted MRI demonstrates the foraminal narrowing and nerve root compression (*arrow*) associated with facet hypertrophic changes. There is loss of foraminal fat.

C

facet joint can determine whether an intra-articular facet joint injection is technically feasible. MRI can also depict some of these bony changes, although not with the same degree of detail as CT. However, MRI may demonstrate asymmetrically increased signal within the facet joint on T2-weighted imaging, suggesting an inflammatory reaction.

Spondylolisthesis is the subluxation of a vertebral body on the underlying body. This is usually anterior, but can be posterior. The grade of spondylolisthesis is based on the percentage of movement over the underlying vertebral body. Grade I is a displacement of less than 25% of the vertebral body width; grade II is 25–49%; grade III is 50–74%; and grade IV is greater than 75% of displacement. The most common cause of spondylolisthesis is degenerative, and this is most common at the L4–L5 level. Degenerative spondylolisthesis usually involves less than 30% vertebral body width subluxation. Spondylolisthesis can also be iatrogenic after surgical laminectomy with resultant destabilization of the spine, or post-traumatic.

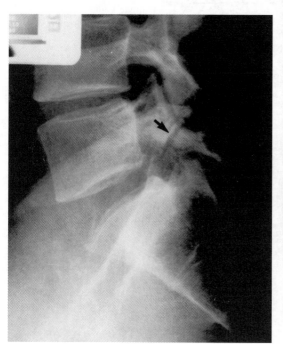

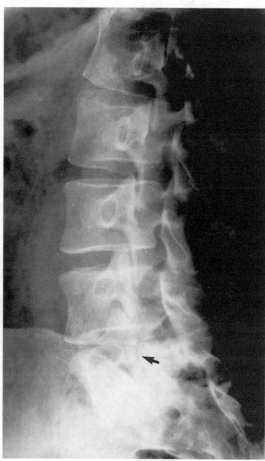

A   B

Figure 5.13 Spondylolysis and spondylolisthesis. **(A)** Lateral and **(B)** oblique plain films demonstrate the presence of a pars defect (*arrows*). Note the classic appearance of the collar (or broken neck) on the Scottie dog on the oblique view.

Spondylolysis is another common cause of spondylolisthesis (Figure 5.13). This is a disruption of the pars interarticularis between the superior and inferior facets of a vertebral level. This is thought to be due to repeated mild trauma and is unlikely to be congenital. The classic radiographic finding is the "collar on the Scottie dog" on oblique conventional radiographs. Flexion and extension plain films or myelographic films help to identify areas of instability.[29]

SPECT imaging has been reported as a method of distinguishing symptomatic from asymptomatic spondylolysis.[23,24] If the SPECT is abnormal, a CT should be done to evaluate in more detail the extent of the pars interarticularis abnormality. A limited CT with thin slice thickness is usually sensitive in evaluating stress fractures or pars stress reaction. Computer generated sagittal reformats may be required to identify more subtle fractures. Sagittal MRIs can also help identify the defect as well as establish the degree of subluxation. There is also evidence that MRI may

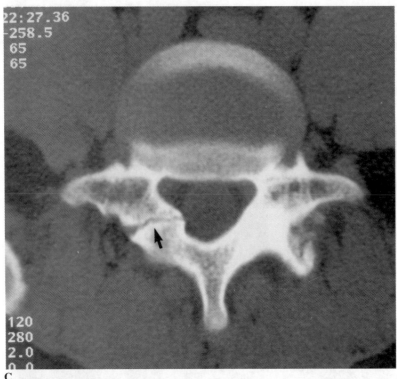

C

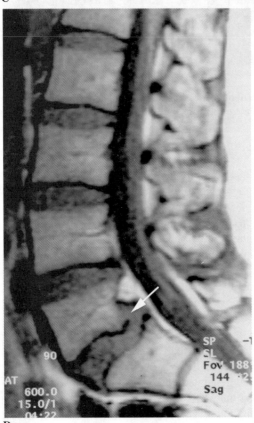

D

Figure 5.13 (*continued*) (**C**) Axial computed tomography scan reveals the presence of an incomplete ring due to a unilateral pars defect (*arrow*). (**D**) Sagittal T1-weighted magnetic resonance imaging demonstrates grade I anterior subluxation of L5 on S1 (*arrow*).

detect associated abnormalities in the pars (changes similar to end plate sclerosis) before they are seen on CT and plain films.[30]

Radicular Pain Syndromes

Lumbar radicular syndromes are usually related to disk pathology, although in the older population, spinal stenosis becomes the more typical etiology. The test of choice when evaluating for a disk herniation as the cause of a radicular syndrome is MRI. This includes evaluation for central, posterolateral, and lateral disk herniations. Most often, lumbar disks herniate posterolaterally where the posterior longitudinal ligament is thinnest. Central disk herniations do occur, but radicular pain secondary to these is not common unless the spinal canal is small. Lateral (i.e., foraminal or extraforaminal) disk herniations are least common, but are seen in the senior population.

A key issue in the imaging of disk herniation is the terminology used to describe such herniations.[25,28,31,32] A widely accepted anatomic classification system to describe disk herniations has been proposed to provide accurate and consistent imaging information. This system includes the terms *disk protrusion*, *disk extrusion*, and *free* (or *sequestered*) *disk fragment*. The distinction between a disk protrusion and disk extrusion may be difficult with any imaging modality. A protruding disk indicates the presence of a focal disk herniation through the annulus with a variable amount of the outer annular fibers remaining intact. An extruded disk is a true herniated disk that has extended through all layers of the annulus. The herniated disk material may remain beneath or extend through the posterior longitudinal ligament (subligamentous), but typically remains in continuity with the parent disk material. Many authors combine the terms *protrusion* and *extrusion* and use the term *herniated disk* to encompass both.[33] A free disk fragment may lie at the disk level or migrate superiorly or inferiorly.

On MRI, protruded or extruded herniated disks are identified by a focal contour abnormality of the disk margin (Figures 5.14 and 5.15). The herniated disk fragment has a variable intensity, depending on the sequence used and the presence of calcification or gas. Obliteration of epidural fat planes, displaced nerve roots, and thecal sac contour deformities all contribute to the diagnosis. In most cases, the disk material appears to remain connected to the parent disk by a thin strand of disk material. With a free fragment, this bridge is not seen (see Figure 5.15). A far lateral disk herniation is seen on MRI as a soft tissue mass extending from the disk into the foramen or paraspinal space. The normally visualized fat plane between the disk and nerve root is lost and the nerve root is displaced (see Figure 5.14C).

Focal disk protrusions and extrusions can be identified on myelography as filling defects, which are seen as double-density changes in the contrast column (Figure 5.16). Trumpeting, or enlargement, of the adjacent nerve root indicates nerve root compression. On CT (Figure 5.17), disk protrusions, extrusions, and free fragments may be identified by noting focal deformity of the posterior disk border, soft tissue material with disk density in the extradural space, displacement of epidural fat, deformity of the dural sac, or compression and displacement of the nerve root sheath, or a combination of these elements. However, nonenhanced CT has substantial limitations, as indicated in the section Computed Tomography. Myelo-CT can demonstrate these findings to greater degree due to the ability to outline the thecal sac and nerve root sleeves. Myelography alone is ineffective in identifying a lateral

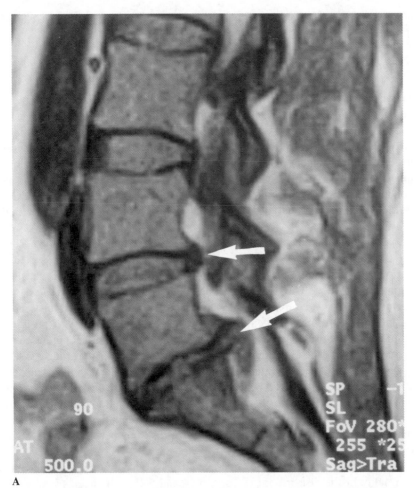

A

Figure 5.14 Herniated disk. **(A)** Parasagittal T1-weighted magnetic resonance imaging (MRI) demonstrates herniated disk material at the L5–S1 level (*arrow*) and disk bulge at L4–L5 (*arrowhead*). **(B)** Axial T1-weighted image demonstrates a right paracentral herniated disk (*arrow*). The herniated disk material is isointense to the parent disk. The effacement of epidural fat and the herniated disk's relation to nerve roots and fat (*asterisks*) is nicely demonstrated.

disk herniation because the dural sleeve does not typically extend beyond the foramen and, therefore, lateral nerve root compression is not seen.

Spinal stenosis is the narrowing of specific areas of the spinal canal with resultant pressure on the nerves. There are three main categories of spinal stenosis based on the region of the spinal canal that is narrowed: central canal stenosis, lateral recess stenosis, and foraminal stenosis (Figure 5.18; see Figure 5.10). Central stenosis is narrowing of the central oval portion of the canal with symptoms typically occurring when the AP diameter is 11 mm or smaller. This is commonly due to a disk herniation or bulge and posterior ligamentous thickening. Subluxation of a vertebral body (spondylolisthesis) also can cause central stenosis. Lateral recess stenosis is most often due to facet osteophyte formation, disk herniation, and ligamentous thickening. Foraminal stenosis can occur from a lateral disk herniation,

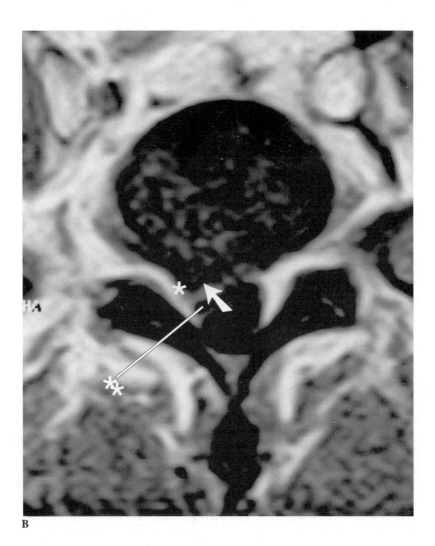

B

vertebral osteophyte encroachment, or collapse of the disk due to degenerative change. A lumbar myelogram and postmyelo-CT may be the test of choice if spinal stenosis is suspected, because the bony detail is better defined than with MRI. Myelography and nonenhanced CT alone are typically ineffective in properly evaluating for spinal stenosis. MRI can also identify spinal stenosis, and the sagittal image is particularly valuable in demonstrating foraminal stenosis with the finding of diminished epidural fat within the foramen (see Figure 5.12C).[34] Occasionally, synovial cysts can arise from the facet joint lining. These are typically associated with osteoarthritis, trauma, and rheumatoid arthritis.[35] These cysts appear as posterior extradural lesions and may be asymptomatic or cause compressive radicular symptoms. The CT appearance is that of a cystic mass extending from the facet joint medially into the spinal canal (Figure 5.19A). The MRI appearance is variable due to the variable concentration of protein and the presence or absence of hemor-

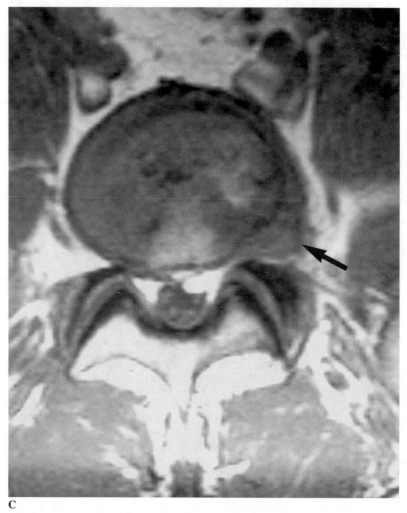

C

Figure 5.14 (*continued*) **(C)** Axial T1-weighted MRI demonstrating a far lateral disk herniation (*arrow*).

rhage or calcification, but frequently a high signal mass is visualized on T2-weighted images (Figure 5.19B and C).

Postoperative Findings

Postoperative studies are commonly necessary, both to assess bony healing after fusion and to evaluate patients with persistent and recurrent symptoms. Plain radiographs with flexion and extension views can be particularly useful in assessing general alignment and stability of the spine, as well as any hardware implants. CT with sagittal and coronal reformats is often necessary to more clearly evaluate incorporation of the fusion graft and to assess stability. Soft tissue abnormalities, such as epi-

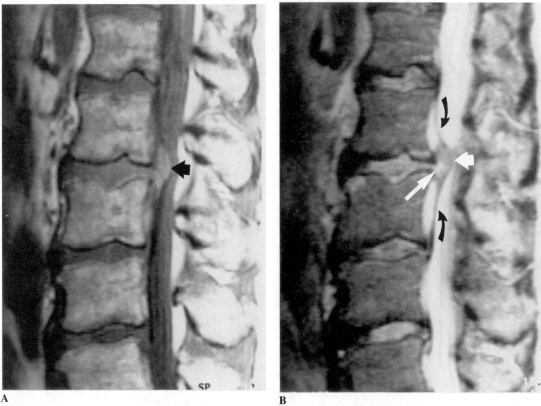

Figure 5.15 Herniated disk. Sagittal (**A**) T1-weighted and (**B**) T2-weighted images of the lumbar spine demonstrate a large herniated disk (*short arrow*) at the L2–L3 level. The T2-weighted image demonstrates that the herniated disk (*short arrow*) is subligamentous, beneath the posterior longitudinal ligament (*curved arrows*). The ligament is pulled away from the adjacent vertebral bodies. Note that the loss of connection of the disk material to the parent disk (*long arrow*) suggests a free fragment.

dural scarring or persistent or recurring disk herniation, are best evaluated with pre- and postcontrast MRI.

Rheumatologic Disorders

Rheumatologic disorders are a group of inflammatory diseases that affect joints, ligaments, tendons, and muscles, as well as bones. They are frequent causes of back pain.[36]

Rheumatoid Arthritis

Rheumatoid arthritis is a chronic systemic inflammatory disease that affects synovial joints. The cervical spine is frequently involved, whereas the lumbar spine is rarely involved. Low back pain associated with rheumatoid arthritis is typically seen in patients with long-standing disease. Imaging studies of the lumbar spine are usually performed to rule out other disease processes. Radiographic studies

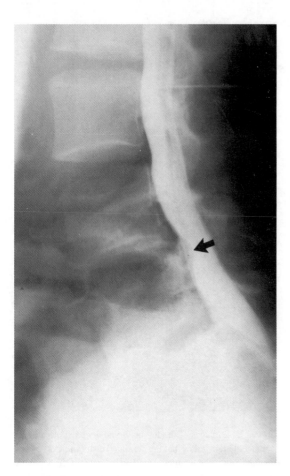

Figure 5.16 Herniated disk. Lateral view of a myelogram demonstrates a double density of the contrast column, suggesting a herniated disk (*arrow*).

demonstrate z-joint erosion without sclerosis and secondary disk space narrowing without osteophytosis.[37] Sacroiliac joint involvement may be unilateral or bilateral. The fibrous part of this joint is not affected. The sacroiliac joint is best viewed on angulated or oblique radiographic views. CT can also be used to image the sacroiliac joints.

Ankylosing Spondylitis

Ankylosing spondylitis (AS) is a seronegative spondyloarthropathy that involves the sacroiliac and axial skeletal joints (Figure 5.20). Plain film radiographic changes in the sacroiliac joints and spine are classic and help establish the diagnosis. However, early changes may be difficult to identify. Bone scan, CT, and MRI studies have been used in the evaluation of the early stages but are usually reserved for unusual cases.[36] Sacroiliitis is usually bilateral and symmetric; it progresses through various stages, ranging from pseudowidening with sclerosis or erosion and progressing to total obliteration of the joint.[38] Ligamentous structures surrounding the joint may also calcify. In the lumbar spine, osteitis affects the anterior corners of the vertebral bodies, resulting in loss of the normal concavity of the anterior vertebral body or "squaring" of the

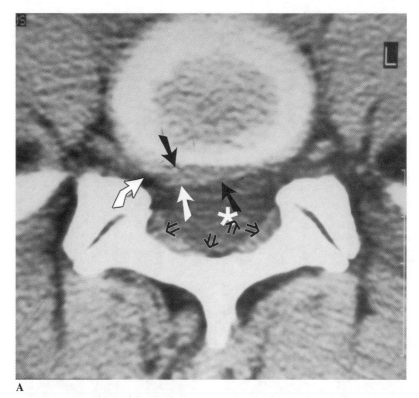

A

Figure 5.17 Herniated disk. **(A)** Axial computed tomography scan demonstrates a right paracentral disk herniation (*arrows*). The soft tissue disk (*open arrows*) is outlined by the surrounding epidural fat (*curved arrow*) and slightly lower density thecal sac (*asterisk*).

body. Syndesmophytes, vertical calcifications of the annulus fibrosis and anterior and posterior longitudinal ligaments, appear in association with osteopenia. Extensive continuous syndesmophytes can encase the axial skeleton and have been described as "bamboo spine" (see Figure 5.20). Z-joints are also affected and can lead to fusion.

Reiter's Syndrome

Reiter's syndrome consists of a clinical triad of urethritis, arthritis, and conjunctivitis. It is the most common cause of arthritis in young men and primarily affects the low back and lower extremity joints.[36] Radiographic changes are helpful to confirm the diagnosis in patients who do not manifest the complete triad. Sacroiliitis may be symmetric or asymmetric and may mimic AS. Sacroiliac joint and z-joint fusion occurs, but less frequently than in AS. Involvement of the spine is discontinuous (skip lesions) and is characterized by nonmarginal bony bridging of the vertebral bodies.[39]

Psoriatic Arthritis

Psoriatic arthritis is a characteristic pattern of joint disease that develops in patients with psoriasis. Classically, psoriatic arthritis is described as involving the distal

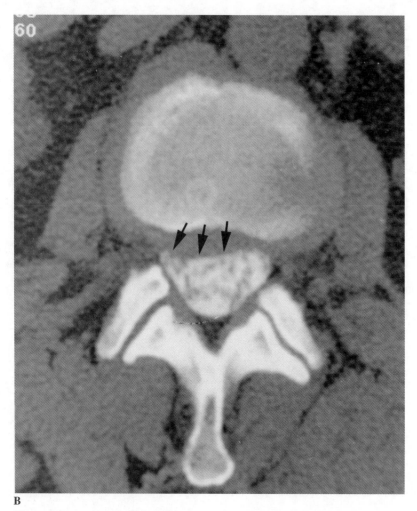

B

Figure 5.17 (*continued*) (**B**) Axial myelo-computed tomography demonstrates a right herniated disk. The contrast helps identify the location of the nerve roots and thecal sac (*arrows*).

interphalangeal joint and is associated with nail disease. Involvement of the spine occurs in 5% of patients, and sacroiliac involvement is seen in 25%.[36,40] Radiographic findings of psoriatic sacroiliitis are nonspecific. Erosions and sclerosis occur primarily on the ilium, and there is joint widening. Ankylosis occurs, but less commonly than in AS. Spine involvement is characterized by asymmetric involvement of the vertebral bodies and nonmarginal syndesmophytes.

Enteropathic Arthritis

Enteropathic arthritis is an inflammatory arthritis of the peripheral and axial joints that is associated with ulcerative colitis and Crohn disease. Axial skeletal disease resembles AS and follows a course that is independent from the activity of the

Figure 5.18 Spinal stenosis. (A) Axial myelogram-computed tomography demonstrates marked spinal stenosis (*arrows*) and lateral recess stenosis (*open arrow*) due to ligamentous thickening and facet hypertrophy. (B) Axial gradient-echo magnetic resonance imaging demonstrates central canal stenosis (*arrows*) and lateral recess stenosis (*open arrows*) secondary to concentric disk bulge, facet hypertrophy (*two asterisks*), and ligamentous thickening.

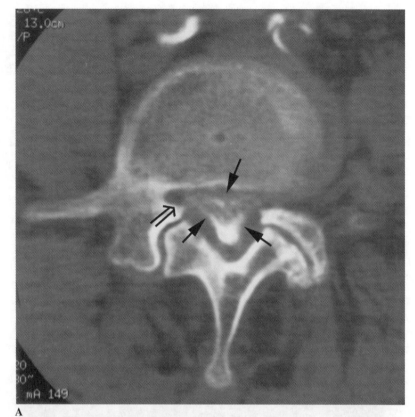

A

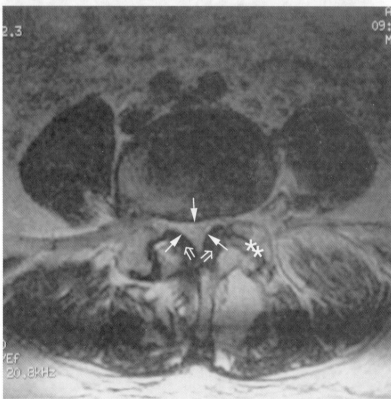

B

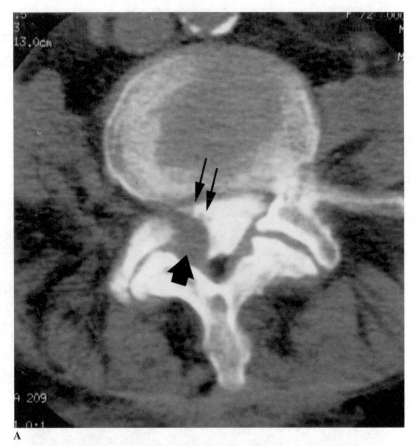

A

Figure 5.19 Synovial cysts. **(A)** Axial myelogram-computed tomography demonstrates a rounded soft tissue mass *(arrowhead),* which communicates with the right facet joint. The displacement of the nerve roots *(arrows)* is well seen with the intrathecal contrast. **(B)** Axial T1-weighted image of a second patient demonstrates a slightly hypointense mass *(arrows),* with respect to the thecal sac, adjacent to the left facet joint.

bowel inflammation.[36] The radiographic changes of the spine and sacroiliac joint are indistinguishable from changes seen with AS.

Diffuse Idiopathic Skeletal Hyperostosis (Forestier's Disease)

Diffuse idiopathic skeletal hyperostosis is a relatively common disorder of the spine (thoracic, then lumbar) associated with diabetes. It involves a "flowing" calcification of the anterolateral vertebrae due to a proliferative enthesopathy. It is often found as an incidental finding on conventional radiographs.

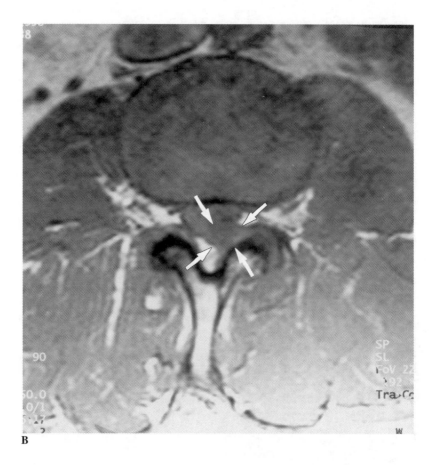

B

Infection

Clinical symptoms of spinal infections may be nonspecific and produce a diagnostic problem. Typical clinical presentation includes fever, back pain, and focal tenderness, but symptoms vary greatly. The nonspecific presentation may delay the diagnosis and increase morbidity and mortality.[41] Early radiologic evaluation to help establish the diagnosis is therefore critical.

Pyogenic Diskitis and Vertebral Osteomyelitis

Conventional plain films may be normal in the first 2–8 weeks of evolution of pyogenic diskitis.[42] Radionuclide studies have been effective, but are unreliable in differentiating cellulitis from frank osteomyelitis. There are also false-negatives secondary to impairment of blood supply to the infected region. Technetium bone scan coupled with a gallium scan has increased the sensitivity and specificity in identifying spinal infection (Figure 5.21). CT can detect bone destruction associated with osteomyelitis earlier than plain films, but is limited in depicting interspi-

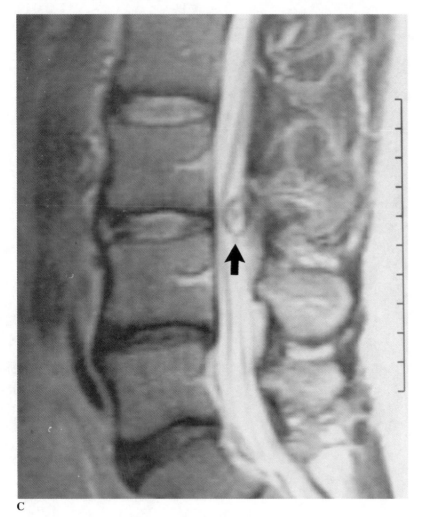

C

Figure 5.19 (*continued*) **(C)** Sagittal T2-weighted image confirms the cystic appearance of this mass (*arrow*).

nal soft tissue structures. MRI is now considered the study of choice.[41] Not only can MRI offer direct visualization of the disk, cord, and nerve roots, but it can also detect changes earlier and thereby affect patient management at an earlier stage.

Conventional film and CT findings in the early stages demonstrate disk space narrowing. Changes become more noticeable as the bony end plates begin to erode. On MRI, diskitis is usually seen as narrowing of the disk space with loss of the relative signal intensity of the disk on T1-weighted images and high intensity signal in the disk on T2-weighted images. Vertebral body involvement can be recognized by replacement of marrow with inflammatory tissue. This is seen as abnormal low intensity within the vertebral body on T1-weighted images and increased signal on T2-weighted images. The normal low signal of the cortical margins becomes difficult to delineate as end plate erosion progresses (see Figure 5.21).

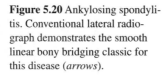

Figure 5.20 Ankylosing spondylitis. Conventional lateral radiograph demonstrates the smooth linear bony bridging classic for this disease (*arrows*).

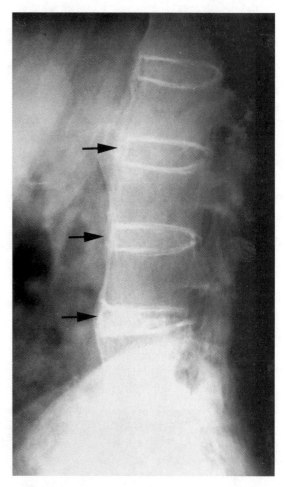

An epidural abscess is uncommon without osteomyelitis or diskitis. The abscess appears as a well-defined mass that is usually isointense to the spinal cord on T1-weighted images and hyperintense on T2-weighted images. With contrast enhancement, the extent of the abscess can be clearly delineated. Most epidural abscesses enhance homogeneously, although nonhomogeneous enhancement can also occur.

Nonpyogenic Infection

Tuberculous (TB) spondylitis is a more insidious process than pyogenic infections. Bone destruction is more extensive with TB, and disk space narrowing occurs secondarily and is relatively limited. Involvement of noncontiguous vertebral bodies can occur as infection spreads beneath the anterior ligament. Involvement of the posterior bony elements also appears more commonly with TB than with other infections. Paraspinal infection and gibbus deformity are common in TB spondylitis.

Involvement of the spine with other granulomatous and fungal lesions is still frequent in many parts of the world.[43] These infections may mimic other infectious lesions, but may have some distinguishing characteristics. With brucellosis infections, the vertebral body remains intact despite evidence of osteomyelitis. Coccid-

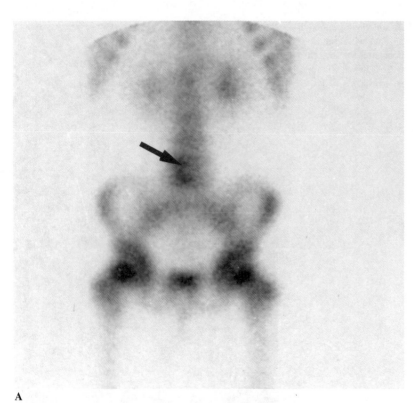

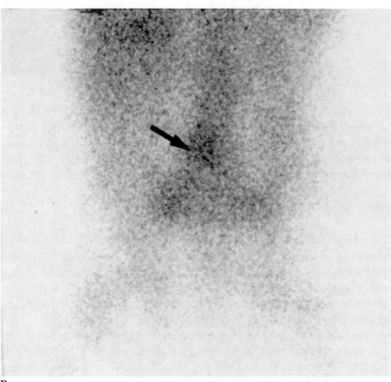

Figure 5.21 Diskitis. **(A)** Nuclear medicine technetium scan shows diffuse increased uptake in the lower lumbar level (*arrow*) indicating increased bone turnover. **(B)** Nuclear medicine gallium scan shows increased activity at the same level consistent with infection. **(C)** Sagittal T1-weighted magnetic resonance image shows loss of normal hypointense signal from the inferior end plate of L4 and the superior end plate of L5. The marrow and disk signals are hypointense to the normal vertebral bodies as well. **(D)** Sagittal T2-weighted magnetic resonance image shows the disc and adjacent vertebral bodies become hyperintense.

A

B

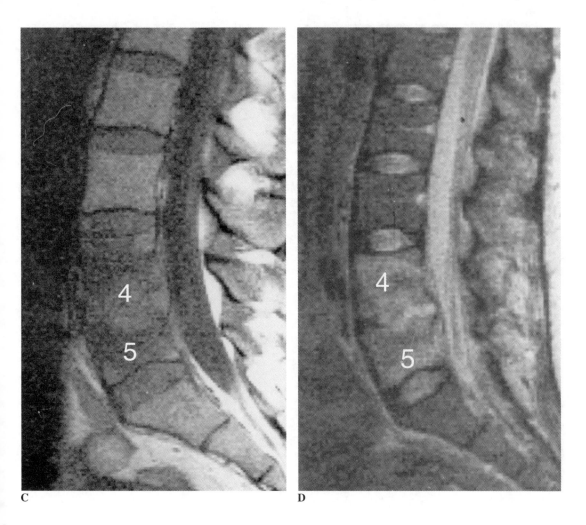

ioidomycoses involves multiple spinal foci with preservation of the disk space. Blastomycosis produces lytic lesions with surrounding sclerosis.

Leptomeningeal Infection and Arachnoiditis

Leptomeningeal infections of the spine are often seen in conjunction with cranial leptomeningeal infection. Infections of the lumbar region are often an extension of the inflammation and arachnoiditis seen in the basal cisterns. Granulomatous processes, such as TB and sarcoid, cysticercosis, bacterial, and viral etiologies, have also been implicated. On both T1- and T2-weighted images, the normal CSF spaces are obscured, and the spinal cord may have irregular margins.[43]

Arachnoiditis is an inflammatory process that involves all three meningeal layers. Multiple causes have been cited, including spinal surgery, infection, intrathecal steroid or anesthetic injection, subarachnoid hemorrhage, and ionic myelographic contrast material injection. The pathogenesis is a natural repair process that involves a fibrinous exudate and collagen deposition, which create

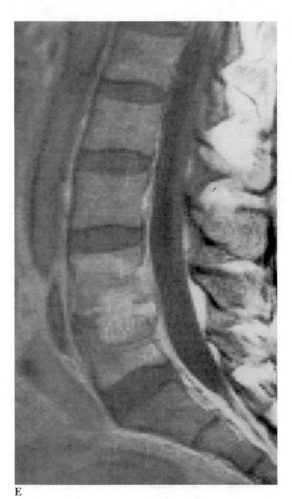

Figure 5.21 (*continued*) (**E**) Sagittal postcontrast T1-weighted magnetic resonance image shows enhancement of the disk and adjacent vertebral bodies and epidural involvement.

E

bands and adhesions between nerve roots or the thecal sac, or both. The myelographic picture of arachnoiditis can have two appearances.[44] In type I, the featureless sac, contrast fills the thecal sac with an absence of nerve defects within the contrast column (Figure 5.22A and B). In type II, there are localized or diffuse filling defects within the contrast column representing clumping and adhesions (Figure 5.22C and D). Myelo-CT and MRI demonstrate both types relatively accurately. Adhesion of the roots to the thecal sac wall results in the empty sac appearance. As the nerve root clumping progresses, the appearance changes to a variable number of soft tissue masses within the thecal space. These changes exist along a continuum, and overlap occurs.

Trauma

Trauma involving the spine can cause an interruption of the osseous structures and of the associated soft tissues. Often, the importance of osseous damage is not due to the fracture itself, but rather to the potential instability of the spine. For this reason,

Figure 5.22 Arachnoiditis.
(**A**) Anteroposterior (AP) view
of a myelogram demonstrates
type I arachnoiditis. The lower
portion of the thecal sac is
smooth and featureless (*arrows*).

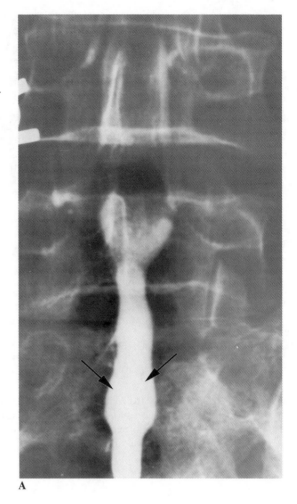

A

conventional films continue to be the modality of choice in the evaluation of acute spinal injury. Fractures, alignment abnormalities, and, occasionally, soft tissue injury can be identified. Screening of the spine can be performed rapidly and accurately and allows greater freedom of patient movement while other injuries are being addressed.

The difficult question in evaluating a traumatic injury is in choosing the follow-up study (if any). As a general guideline, indications for CT include: further evaluation of fractures detected or suspected on plain films, further evaluation of confusing plain film findings, and further evaluation of areas not well seen on plain films.[45] Indications for MRI include the evaluation of spinal cord involvement (intramedullary hematoma or edema), traumatic disk herniation, and ligamentous injuries. Epidural hematoma and its effect on the cord, thecal sac, or nerve roots, is also readily identified with MRI. MRI is also valuable in differentiating benign compression fractures from malignant compression fractures (see the section Compression Fracture Differentiation). Myelo-CT can be valuable when a dural tear is suspected, as it can demonstrate extravasation of contrast material.

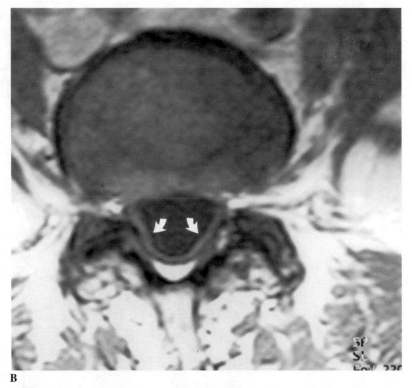

B

Figure 5.22 *(continued)* **(B)** Axial T1-weighted magnetic resonance imaging (MRI) confirms the adhesion of the nerve roots along the lateral margin of the thecal sac *(curved arrows)*. **(C)** AP view of a myelogram demonstrates type II arachnoiditis. The nerve roots are clumped together and give the appearance of a thick filling defect *(arrow)* within the contrast column.

Compression (wedge) and comminuted (burst) fractures are the most common injuries in the lumbar spine. Retropulsed fragments and the degree of canal compromise can be evaluated with CT and MRI (Figure 5.23). Transverse process fractures also occur in the lumbar spine and appear as vertical lucencies on CT. These fractures may be associated with renal or retroperitoneal injury. CT and MRI can be used to evaluate these associated injuries. Distraction injuries (Chance fracture) may occur in motor vehicle accidents with passengers wearing seatbelts (Figure 5.24). These horizontal fractures involve the vertebral body, pedicles, laminae, and spinous process, as well as disruption of the intervertebral disk, facet joint, and interspinous ligaments. CT demonstrates the fractured bony elements, and reconstructed sagittal views provide information on the degree of subluxation and instability.

Soft tissue injuries of the lumbar spine include traumatic disk herniation, ligamentous injuries, epidural hematomas, and pseudomeningoceles. Demonstration of cord or nerve root compression secondary to herniated disk material or the presence of an epidural hematoma may significantly alter management of the injured patient. On MRI, disruption of the ligaments can be seen as a discontinuity in the normally low signal intensity ligament. Edematous changes within the ligament may be seen as

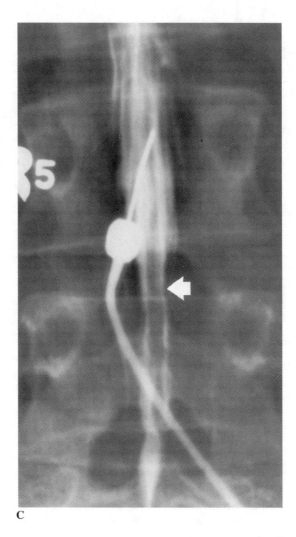

C

hyperintense signal change within the ligament on T2-weighted images. Early detection of ligamentous injury may identify patients who are at risk for delayed instability.

Neoplasms

Tumors of the spine are classified according to the space in which they arise. They can be extradural (outside the thecal sac, such as in the subdural space, epidural space, or the vertebral column), intradural extramedullary (in the thecal sac but outside the cord), or intramedullary (within the cord). The differential diagnosis can often be shortened if a tumor can be placed in a certain compartment, because most tumors arise within a specific space. Most tumors are extradural.[46]

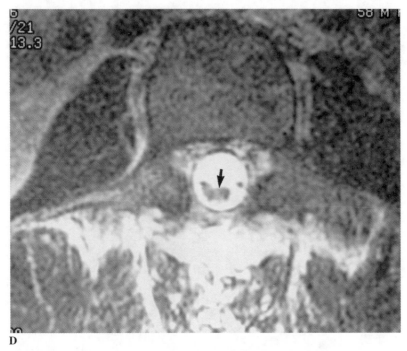

D

Figure 5.22 (*continued*) (**D**) Axial T2-weighted MRI demonstrates the clumped nerve roots (*arrow*) within the thecal sac.

Extradural Tumors

A complete list of extradural tumors is beyond the scope of this chapter. This includes myeloma, chordoma, aneurysmal bone cysts, osteoid osteoma, giant cell tumor, and osteoblastoma. The more common extradural tumors are metastatic lesions and hemangiomas.

Metastasis.   The most common lumbar spine neoplasm is metastatic disease. Any primary neoplasm can metastasize to the spine. The most common types of metastases are lung, breast, prostate carcinoma, and lymphoma. Most metastases are osteolytic, but prostate and breast cancer can be osteoblastic. The metastases most commonly spread hematogenously. The vertebral body is the most common site of metastasis due to its larger proportional size. Involvement of just the lamina or pedicle without involvement of the body is atypical for metastatic disease. The tumor fills and weakens the vertebral body. This increases the chance of structural failure and pathologic compression fracture. The metastases replace the fatty marrow in the vertebral body and destroy the trabeculae. The replacement of the fat causes a change in the MRI signal of the vertebral marrow and makes MRI the most sensitive imaging test for metastatic disease, especially early in the process (Figure 5.25). Metastases have irregular edges, are often multiple, and enhance with contrast. They can be small or can replace and expand the vertebral body and all its elements. The metastasis can also leave the

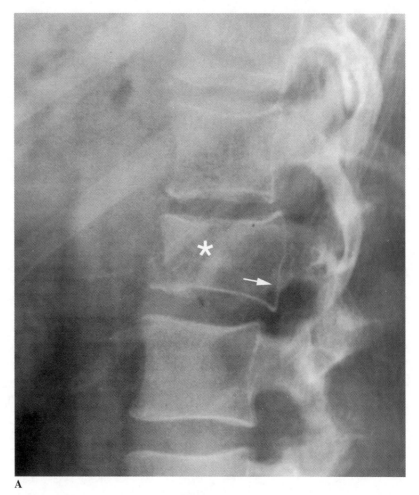

A

Figure 5.23 Burst fracture. **(A)** Lateral plain film view of the lumbar spine reveals the presence of a burst fracture involving the L1 vertebral body (*asterisk*). There is retropulsion of the posterior aspect of the vertebral body into the spinal canal (*arrow*).

bony confines and extend into the epidural space with resultant spinal canal stenosis. Nuclear imaging becomes sensitive after bony remodeling occurs. CT imaging is positive after destruction of bone. Conventional radiographs are the least sensitive and require approximately 50% of bone mass loss before the lesion can be seen. When metastatic disease is extensive, a diffuse infiltrative marrow process may be seen. This pattern of disease is discussed in the section on Compression Fracture Differentiation.

Hemangioma.   Hemangiomas are common benign tumors of the vertebral bodies. They are usually asymptomatic, but can occasionally be the site of pathologic fracture or can cause bony expansion with resultant spinal canal compression. These tumors are a mix of cavernous, capillary, and venous channels with thickened bony trabeculae. With MRI, they are typically bright on T1- and T2-weighted images and

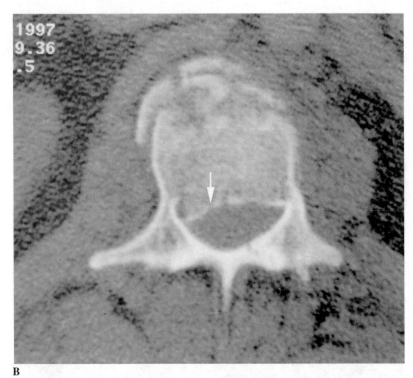

B

Figure 5.23 (*continued*) (**B**) Axial computed tomography image demonstrates the degree of retropulsion and can provide an accurate measurement of the degree of spinal canal narrowing (*arrow*). (**C**) Sagittal T2-weighted magnetic resonance image demonstrates the burst fracture of the vertebral body. This image also helps evaluate the effect on the compressed conus (*arrow*). The edema and hemorrhage within the conus are best evaluated on magnetic resonance.

can enhance (Figure 5.26B and C). On CT examination, hemangiomas are identified by the thickened trabeculae (see Figure 5.26A).

Intradural Extramedullary Tumors

Nerve Sheath Tumors.   Nerve sheath tumors include schwannomas and neurofibromas. These are benign overgrowths of elements of the nerve root and peripheral nerve. They are typically solitary lesions.

Meningiomas.   Meningiomas are the second most common intraspinal tumor. Approximately 5% of all meningiomas are within the lumbar spine.[46] Osseous changes can be seen in 10% of meningioma cases. This includes tumoral calcification, hyperostosis, pedicle erosion, and foraminal enlargement. With MRI, these tumors are typically similar in signal intensity to the spinal cord (Figure 5.27). Enhancement is usually strong and homogeneous.

Congenital Tumors.   The most common of congenital tumors are epidermoids and dermoids. These are usually congenital but can be post-traumatic. The CT and

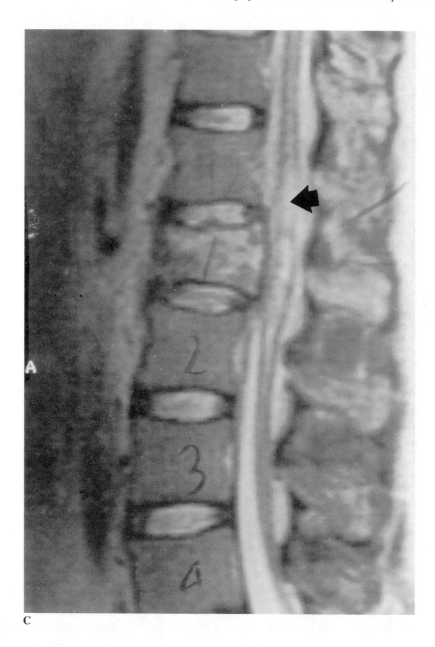

MRI characteristics are variable depending on the parenchymal elements. The parenchymal elements can be squamous and fatty elements and usually do not enhance. These are often large and fill the thecal sac.

Intradural Metastases.   Intradural metastases are metastases that adhere to the nerve roots. They typically are transported with the CSF from intrathecal primary tumors such as medulloblastomas, ependymomas, or glioblastoma multiforme. They can also occur with systemic metastatic disease and are most common with breast carcinoma, lymphoma, malignant melanoma, and lung cancer. Intradural

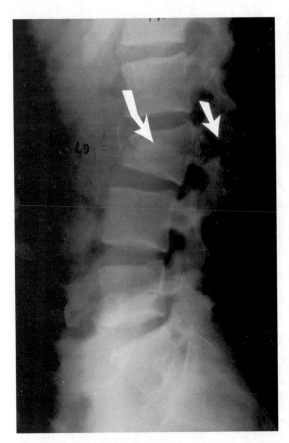

Figure 5.24 Chance fracture. Lateral plain film of the lumbar spine demonstrates a fracture involving the vertebral body (*curved arrow*) and posterior elements (*arrow*).

metastases, or drop metastases, are typically multiple, small, and brightly enhancing lesions. These are often seen as multiple excrescences of the nerve roots.

Intramedullary Tumors

Intramedullary tumors arise within the lowermost extent of the cord, the conus medullaris, or in the ligamentous extent of the cord, the filum terminale. The spinal cord typically does not extend below the L1–L2 interspace. Intramedullary lesions below this point are difficult to differentiate from intradural-extramedullary tumors. The most common tumor is the ependymoma. Astrocytomas can also arise in the lower cord, but are uncommon in this location. On MRI, ependymomas are rounded masses that are isointense to the cord on T1-weighted images and hyperintense on T2-weighted images. These enhance strongly and fairly uniformly. Astrocytomas appear similar to ependymomas but are less sharply defined and less often contain areas of hemorrhage. Otherwise, there is no specific pattern that permits their distinction.

Figure 5.25 Metastatic disease. Sagittal T1-weighted magnetic resonance imaging demonstrates multiple foci of abnormal signal within several vertebral bodies replacing the normal marrow (*arrows*).

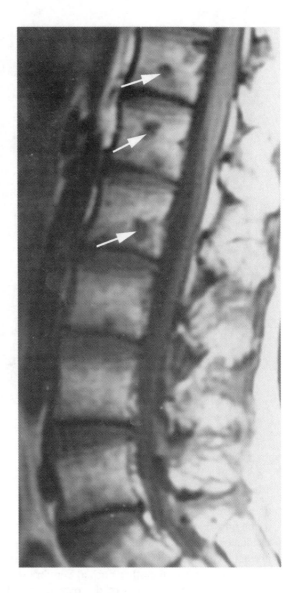

Miscellaneous Pathology

Compression Fracture Differentiation

A great clinical concern is the evaluation of the cause of a vertebral body compression fracture (Figure 5.28). The main differential concerns are metastatic disease versus osteoporosis. MRI examination before and after contrast is the most helpful diagnostic test. In osteoporotic fractures, the unaffected portion of the vertebral body has a normal bright T1 marrow signal. The T2 images have marrow signal similar to that of the adjacent normal bodies. Acutely, there may be marrow edema with low T1 signal. The acute marrow edema seen with osteoporotic frac-

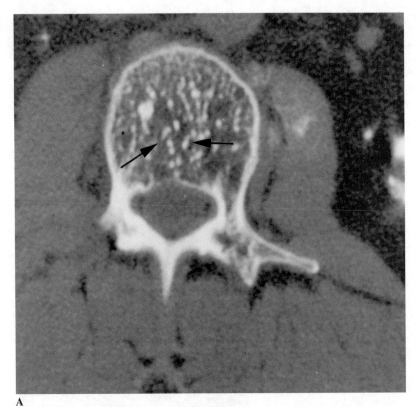

A

Figure 5.26 Hemangioma. **(A)** Axial computed tomography scan reveals the presence of a hemangioma (*arrows*) as noted by the thickened bony trabeculae. **(B)** Sagittal T1-weighted magnetic resonance imaging demonstrates a focal mass within the vertebral body which is hyperintense (*asterisk*).

tures regresses in approximately 1–3 months. There is no epidural mass. The posterior border of the vertebral body is typically concave. There is usually some residua of normal fatty marrow within the vertebral body. The pedicles are usually normal. After contrast administration, the T1 signal of the fractured vertebral body equals that of the other normal vertebral bodies and is homogenous. Occasionally, the central portion of the osteoporotic fracture does not enhance. The fractured body can have bands of low signal, which are parallel to the vertebral end plate.

Metastatic lesions in vertebral bodies show low T1 signal and increased T2 signal. The areas of abnormal signal are often patchy and poorly defined. There commonly are other abnormal vertebral bodies. Metastases often have at least one abnormal pedicle with low T1 signal. The metastases enhance nonhomogeneously, but are usually brighter than the normal fat signal. Myeloma often enhances markedly so that the signal is much higher than the normal vertebral bodies. Epidural masses and extension beyond the confines of the vertebral body are often seen. The posterior border of the vertebral body is often expanded and convex.[47]

Although these criteria may not absolutely make the diagnosis, the more characteristics filled, the more clear the diagnosis. A new MRI technique, diffusion-weighted MRI, which was originally developed for the evaluation of brain stroke,

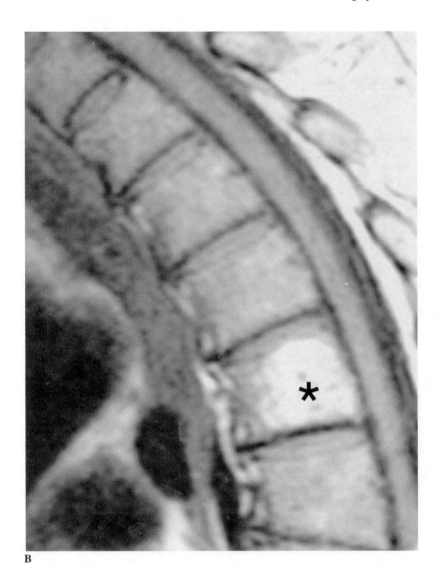

B

has been shown to be helpful in the differential.[48] If the clinical situation is still unclear, CT guided biopsy of the affected vertebral body can be performed.

Infiltrative Marrow Disease

A number of disease processes directly affect the marrow. These include disease processes that convert yellow marrow to red marrow (anemia, metastatic disease, myeloma, myelofibrosis), diseases that infiltrate or replace marrow (leukemia, lymphoma, metastases, and primary bone tumors), and diseases that cause myeloid depletion (aplastic anemia, radiation therapy, and chemotherapy).[49] The imaging of bone marrow is complex and dependent on patient age. At birth, the entire fetal skeleton is composed of red marrow. Conversion to yellow marrow takes place in

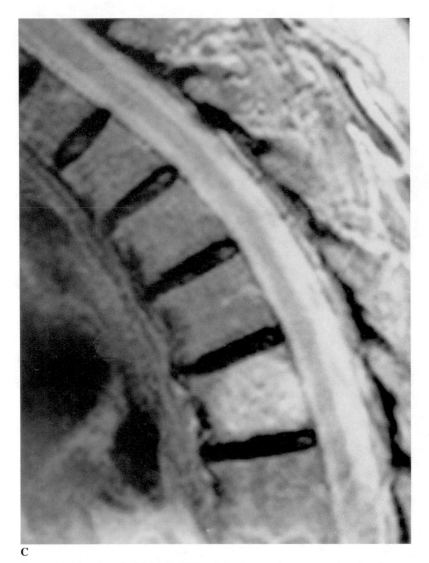

C

Figure 5.26 (*continued*) **(C)** Sagittal T2-weighted magnetic resonance imaging demonstrates a focal mass within the vertebral body, which is hyperintense on both images. These features are characteristic for a hemangioma.

an orderly and predictable pattern. Marrow conversion to the adult pattern usually is complete by the age of 25 years.

Considerable loss of trabecular bone is required before a marrow abnormality becomes evident on conventional films. Nuclear medicine studies provide a sensitive survey of the entire skeleton, but lack anatomic detail and specificity, especially when there is a diffuse infiltrative process. The so-called superscan may appear normal, but actually represents increased uptake throughout the skeleton. CT findings can be variable, and the appearance of infiltrative diseases is dependent on the different combinations of red and yellow marrow and cancellous bone. On MRI, the major contributor to adult marrow signal is fat. Therefore,

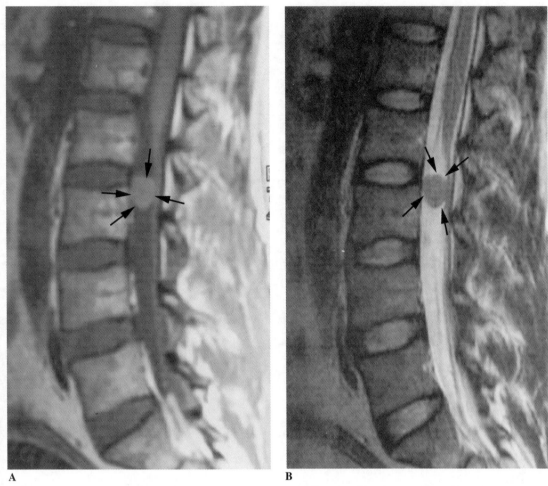

A   B

Figure 5.27 Intradural meningioma. Sagittal **(A)** T1-weighted and **(B)** T2-weighted magnetic resonance images demonstrate a nodular mass within the thecal sac at the L2–L3 level. The mass is isointense to the spinal cord on both sequences (*arrows*).

replacement of the fat signal by an infiltrative process alters the signal characteristics. When the process is diffuse, the changes may be subtle and may be recognized only by comparing bone and disk signal differences. Normally, the marrow signal is higher than disk material on T1-weighted images and lower than disk material on T2-weighted images. In diffuse infiltrative processes, the signal from bone approaches that of disk on both sequences (i.e., the bone decreases in intensity on T1-weighted images and increases in intensity on T2-weighted images). This change can be subtle and easily overlooked when the process is homogeneous and diffuse.

Paget's Disease

Paget's disease is a relatively common bone disease that is marked by increased osteoclastic activity followed by increased osteoblastic activity. It often affects the

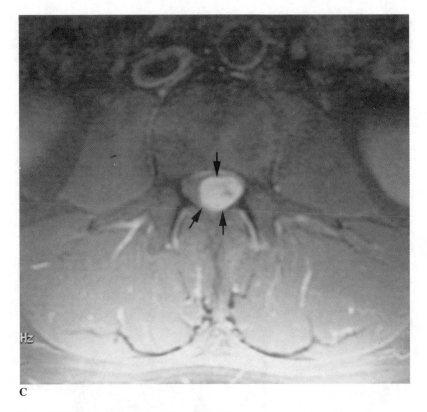

C

Figure 5.27 (*continued*) (**C**) Axial T1-weighted image after contrast administration reveals the diffuse enhancement of the mass (*arrows*).

vertebrae. It is usually asymptomatic or mildly symptomatic. It can be seen on plain films, often as an incidental finding.

Variations That May Produce Back Pain

Epidural Lipomatosis

Epidural lipomatosis is an abnormal accumulation of normal adipose tissue in the epidural space. This is seen most often in patients who receive exogenous corticosteroids and in endogenous hypercortisolemia.[50,51] Imaging studies help to demonstrate the accumulation of fat and the resultant spinal canal narrowing (Figure 5.29).

Tarlov (Perineurial) Cysts

Tarlov cysts are diverticula of spinal root sleeves that may become symptomatic. They are most often seen in the lumbar and sacral regions and are often multiple. These cysts usually fill with contrast on myelography and are identified on imaging

Figure 5.28 Compression fractures. (**A**) Lateral plain film shows a nonspecific compression fracture of L5. Sagittal (**B**) T1- and (**C**) (next page) T2-weighted magnetic resonance imaging (MRI) of the same patient shows the posterior portion of the L5 body to have normal marrow signal. There is a horizontal band of T2 hyperintensity. Arrows indicate collapsed bodies.

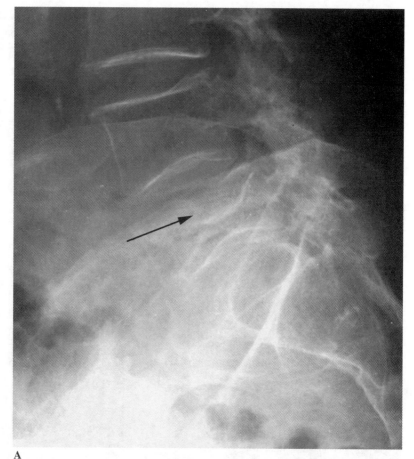

A

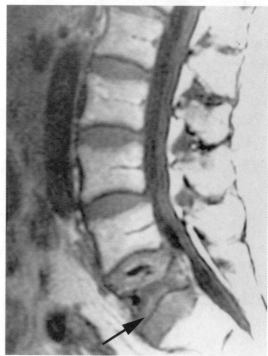

B

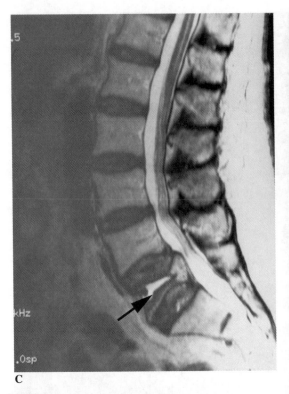

C

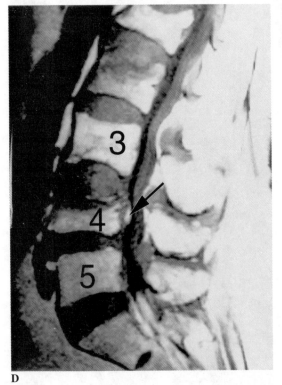

D

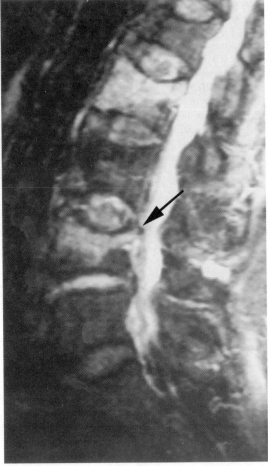

E

Figure 5.28 (*continued*) Sagittal (**D**) T1- and (**E**) T2-weighted MRI of a patient with known metastatic disease at L3–4 shows abnormal signal in the marrow of several vertebral bodies and the retropulsion (*arrows*) of the abnormal signal bone. Adjacent pedicles (not shown) were also abnormal in signal.

Figure 5.29 Epidural lipomatosis. Sagittal T1-weighted image of the lumbar spine demonstrates an abnormal accumulation of bright epidural fat producing spinal canal stenosis (*asterisks*).

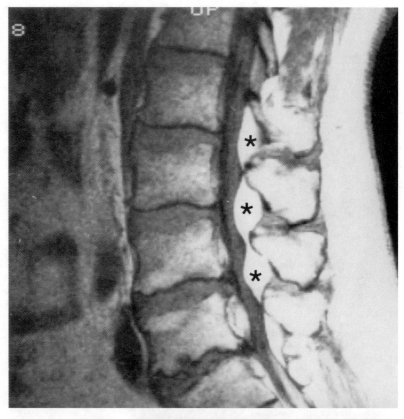

Figure 5.30 Tarlov (perineurial) cysts. (**A**) Parasagittal T2-weighted magnetic resonance imaging (MRI) demonstrates cystic masses (*arrow*) within the sacral region, which is slightly higher in intensity than cerebrospinal fluid.

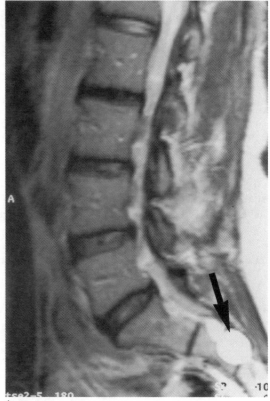

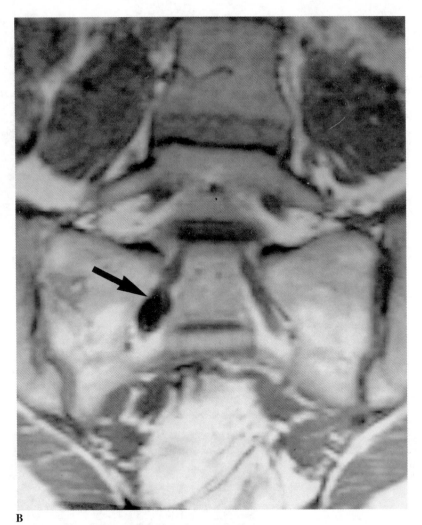

B

Figure 5.30 (*continued*) (**B**) Coronal T1-weighted MRI demonstrates this region to represent dilated nerve root sleeves (*arrow*).

studies as focal enlargements of nerve root sleeves (Figure 5.30). On MRI, the signal characteristics resemble CSF. However, changes in protein concentration secondary to altered CSF flow may produce a variable appearance.

Conjoined Root

Conjoined root is an anomaly consisting of a common origin of two root sheaths. Conjoined root is usually unilateral and most frequently involves the fifth lumbar and first sacral roots. Myelography demonstrates the common sheath and the presence of two roots (Figure 5.31). On cross-sectional imaging studies, there is enlargement of the sheath that may resemble a soft tissue mass in the lateral recess.[52]

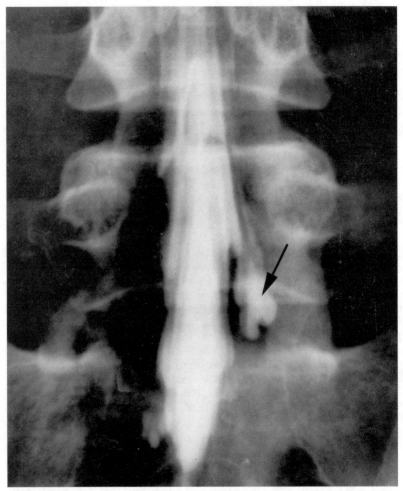

Figure 5.31 Conjoined root. Anteroposterior view of a myelogram demonstrates a common nerve root sleeve on the left (*arrow*).

SUMMARY

The timing and choice of imaging studies vary according to the diagnosis and patient-related factors and should be used to confirm the information gathered from a thorough history and physical examination. There is a high prevalence of abnormal findings on images of asymptomatic individuals, and excessive reliance on diagnostic studies without clinical correlation can lead to erroneous or unindicated treatment.[53] The ideal time to image a patient with back pain is when the information that is obtained affects the treatment plan.[12] With acute low back pain, imaging is often not necessary during the first 6 weeks unless there are neurologic findings, constitutional symptoms, a history of trauma, symptoms of a tumor, or patient age older than 50 years or younger than 18 years. After 6 weeks, if there is no clinical improvement, imaging the spine may prove useful. The choice of study is dependent on the suspected disease. Familiarity with each test's sensitivity, specificity, and predictive values is helpful.

REFERENCES

1. Sykes RH, Wasenaar W, Clark P. Incidence of adverse effects following metrizamide mye-lography in nonambulatory and ambulatory patients. Radiology 1981;138:625–627.
2. Peterman SB. Post-myelography headache rates with Whitacre versus Quincke 22-gauge spi-nal needles. Radiology 1996;200:771–778.
3. Sachs BL, Spivey MA, Vanharanta H, et al. Techniques for lumbar discography and com-puted tomography/discography in clinical practice. Appl Radiol 1989;18:28–30.
4. el-Khoury GY, Renfew DL. Percutaneous procedures for the diagnosis and treatment of lower back pain: diskography, facet-joint injection, and epidural injection. AJR Am J Roent-genol 1991;157:685–691.
5. Crock HV. Internal disc disruption: a challenge to disc prolapse fifty years on. Spine 1986;11:650–653.
6. Bernard TN. Lumbar discography followed by computed tomography: refining the diagnosis of low-back pain. Spine 1990;15:690–707.
7. Zucherman J, Derby R, Hsu K, et al. Normal magnetic resonance imaging with abnormal discography. Spine 1988;13:1355–1359.
8. Antti-Poika I, Soini J, Tallroth K, et al. Clinical relevance of discography combined with CT scanning. A study of 100 patients. J Bone Joint Surg Br 1990;72:480–485.
9. Milette PC, Raymond J, Fontaine S. Comparison of high-resolution computed tomography with discography in the evaluation of lumbar disc herniations. Spine 1990;15:525–533.
10. Yu SW, Haughton VM, Sether LA, et al. Comparison of MR and diskography in detecting radial tears of the annulus: a postmortem study. AJNR Am J Neuroradiol 1989;10:1077–1081.
11. Schellhas KP, Pollei SR, Gundry CR, Heithoff KB. Lumbar disc high-intensity zone: corre-lation of magnetic resonance imaging and discography. Spine 1996;21:79–86.
12. Boden SD. The use of radiographic imaging studies in the evaluation of patients who have degenerative disorders of the lumbar spine. J Bone Joint Surg 1996;78A:114–124.
13. Osti OL, Fraser RD, Vernon-Roberts B. Discitis after discography: the role of prophylactic agents. J Bone Joint Surg Br 1990;72-B:271–274.
14. Johnson BA, Tanenbaum LN. Contemporary spinal CT applications. Neuroimaging Clin N Am 1998;8:559–576.
15. Grenier N, Kressel HY, Schiebler ML, et al. Isthmic spondylolysis of the lumbar spine: MR imaging at 1.5T. Radiology 1989;170:489–494.
16. Gregory BA, Hasselink JR. MR imaging of the spine: recent advances in pulse sequences and special techniques. AJR Am J Roentgenol 1994;162:923–934.
17. Tien RD, Olson EM, Zee CS. Diseases of the lumbar spine: findings on fat-suppression MR imaging. AJR Am J Roentgenol 1992;159:95–99.
18. Krudy AG. MR myelography using heavily T2-weighted fast spin-echo pulse sequences with fat presaturation. AJR Am J Roentgenol 1992;159:1315–1320.
19. Dailey AT, Tsuruda JS, Goodkin R, et al. Magnetic resonance neurography for cervical radic-ulopathy: a preliminary report. Neurosurgery 1996;38:488–492.
20. Firooznia H, Rausching W, Rafii M, et al. Normal correlative anatomy of the lumbosacral spine and its contents. Neuroimaging Clin N Am 1993;3:411–423.
21. Takahashi M, Shimomura O, Sakae T. Comparison of magnetic resonance imaging with myelography and computed tomography—myelography in the diagnosis of lumbar disk her-niation. Neuroimaging Clin N Am 1993;3:487–498.
22. Thrall JH, Ziessman HA. Nuclear Medicine: The Requisites. St. Louis: Mosby Year Book, Inc., 1993;93–98.
23. Bodner RJ, Heyman S, Drummond DS, Gregg JR. The use of single photon emission com-puted tomography (SPECT) in the diagnosis of low-back pain in young adults. Spine 1988;13:1155–1160.
24. Lusins JO, Elting JJ, Cicoria AD, Goldsmith SJ. SPECT evaluation of lumbar spondylolysis and spondylolisthesis. Spine 1994;19:608–612.
25. Czervionke L. Lumbar intervertebral disk disease. Neuroimaging Clin N Am 1993;3:465–485.

26. Modic MT, Masaryk TJ, Ross JS, et al. Imaging of degenerative disk disease. Radiology 1988;168:177–186.
27. Modic MT, Steinberg PM, Ross JS, et al. Degenerative disk disease: assessment of changes in vertebral body marrow with MR imaging. Radiology 1988;166:193–199.
28. Milette PC. The proper terminology for reporting lumbar intervertebral disk disorders. AJNR Am J Neuroradiol 1997;18:1859–1866.
29. Rauch RA, Jinkins JR. Lumbosacral spondylolisthesis associated with spondylolysis. Neuroimaging Clin N Am 1993;3:543–555.
30. Yamane T, Yoshida T, Mimatsu K. Early diagnosis of lumbar spondylolysis by MRI. J Bone Joint Surg Br 1993;75:764–768.
31. Milette PC, Melanson D, Dupuis PR, et al. A simplified terminology for abnormalities of the lumbar disk. Can Assoc Radiol J 1991;42:319–325.
32. Kim KY, Kim YT, Lee CS, et al. MRI classification of lumbar herniated intervertebral disc. Orthopedics 1992;15:493–497.
33. Enzmann DR. Degenerative disk disease. In: DR Enzmann, RL DeLaPaz, JB Rubin (eds), Magnetic Resonance Imaging of the Spine. St. Louis: Mosby, 1990;437–509.
34. Griffiths HJ, Parantainen H, Olson PN. Disease of the lumbosacral facet joints. Neuroimaging Clin N Am 1993;3:567–575.
35. Lemish W, Apsimon T, Chakera T. Lumbar intraspinal synovial cysts: recognition and CT diagnosis. Spine 1989;14:1378.
36. Borenstein DG, Wiesel SW, Boden SD. Rheumatologic Disorders of the Lumbosacral Spine. In Low Back Pain: Medical Diagnosis and Comprehensive Management (2nd ed). Philadelphia: Saunders, 1995;218–298.
37. Helliwell PS, Zebouni LNP, Porter G, et al. A clinical and radiological study of back pain in rheumatoid arthritis. Br J Rheumatol 1993;32:16.
38. Dale K. Radiographic grading of sacroiliitis in Bechterew's syndrome and allied disorders. Scand J Rheumatol 1979;[Suppl]32:92.
39. Sundaram M, Patton JT. Paravertebral ossification in psoriasis and Reiter's disease. Br J Radiol 1975;48:628.
40. Harvie JN, Lester RS, Little AH. Sacroiliitis in severe psoriasis. AJR Am J Roentengenol 976;127:579.
41. Post MJ, Quencer RM, Montalvo BM, et al. Spinal infection: evaluation with MR imaging and intraoperative US. Radiology 1988;169:765.
42. Digby JM, Kensley JB. Pyogenic non-tuberculous spinal infection: an analysis of thirty cases. J Bone Joint Surg Br 1979;61B:47.
43. Sklar EM, Donovan Post MJ, Lebwohl NH. Imaging of infection of the lumbosacral spine. Neuroimaging Clin N Am 1993;3:577–590.
44. Jorgensen J, Hansen PH, Steenskov V, et al. A clinical and radiological study of chronic lower spinal arachnoiditis. Neuroradiology 1975;9:139–144.
45. Cornelius RS, Leach JL. Imaging evaluation of cervical spine trauma. Neuroimaging Clin N Am 1995;5:451–464.
46. Bazan C. Imaging of lumbosacral spine neoplasm. Neuroimaging Clin N Am 1993;3:591–608.
47. Cuenod CA, Laaredo JD, Chevret S, et al. Acute vertebral collapse due to osteoporosis or malignancy: appearance on unenhanced and gadolinium-enhanced MR images. Radiology 1996;199:541–549.
48. Baur A, Stäbler A, Bruning R, et al. Diffusion-weighted MR imaging of bone marrow: differentiation of benign versus pathologic compression fractures. Radiology 1998;207:349–356.
49. Vogler JB 3rd, Murphy WA. Bone marrow imaging. Radiology 1988;168:679–693.
50. Quint DJ, Boulos RS, Sanders WP, et al. Epidural lipomatosis. Radiology 1988;169:485–490.
51. Doppman JL. Epidural lipomatosis. Radiology 1989;171:581–582.
52. Hoddick WK, Helms CA. Bony spinal canal changes that differentiate conjoined nerve roots from herniated nucleus pulposus. Radiology 1985;154:119–120.
53. Boden SD, Davis DO, Dina TS, et al. Abnormal magnetic-resonance scans of the lumbar spine in asymptomatic subjects: a prospective investigation. J Bone Joint Surg Am 1990;72:403–408.

Chapter 6
Electrodiagnosis of Lumbosacral Radiculopathy

Robert H. Perkins, Ernest W. Johnson, William S. Pease, and Michael Giovanniello

Patients whose major complaint is back pain with associated buttock, thigh, leg, or foot pain, that could include paresthesias, numbness, or weakness, are frequently referred for electromyographic evaluation. Electrodiagnostic (EDX) testing can be helpful. In addition, several imaging techniques are available for this clinical condition, including magnetic resonance imaging, computed tomography, and myelography. None, however, can verify the precise functional deficit. Only EDX evaluation gives information on nerve root physiology.[1–4] Needle electromyography (EMG) is an extraordinarily useful EDX method when evaluating radiculopathy.[5] In cases in which the history, physical examination findings, and imaging studies are equivocal or contradictory, EDX testing can often clarify the diagnosis, even if history and physical examination findings are suggestive of radiculopathy, as it can confirm functional or neurophysiologic deficit and objectify the prognosis.

The history and physical examination remain a critical part of evaluating a patient with a suspected radiculopathy, but EDX testing should be considered an extension of these rather than a laboratory procedure. Most of the diagnoses of radiculopathy are made from the history, with pain as the presenting complaint. It can be solely buttock pain, but also with referral to posterior thigh, calf, or foot. The pain is usually a deep, aching pain located deep in the limb at myotomal and sclerotomal sites. The pain is not dermatomal; this is the region of paresthesias. The pain location is not root specific because mesodermal pain (i.e., myotomal and sclerotomal pain) is longitudinal, placed deep in the limb. For example, both L5 and S1 can produce buttock and shin pain. Back pain can occur initially, and usually becomes less prominent as buttock and other referred pain becomes more severe. Tingling (paresthesias) can occur in a dermatomal pattern (Figure 6.1).[6] The dermatome of S1 is the sole and lateral two toes; the dermatome of L5 is the dorsum of foot and great toe; and the dermatome of L4 is the medial leg.

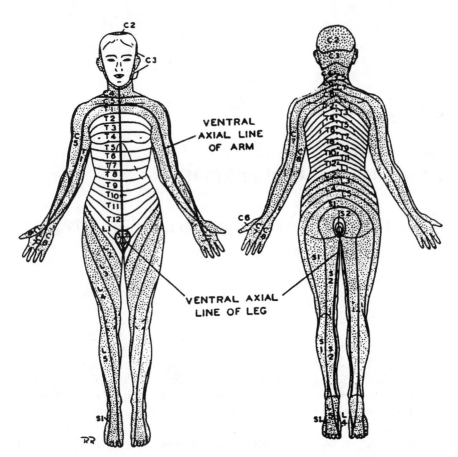

Figure 6.1 Dermatomal representation according to Keegan and Garret. Radicular pain is not referred in a dermatomal distribution. It refers to myotomes and sclerotomes. (Reprinted with permission from W Haymaker, B Woodhall. Peripheral Nerve Injuries. Philadelphia: Saunders, 1953;537.)

CLINICAL PEARL: MYTHS

1. Pain radiates down the leg. (Pain does not radiate. This means a continuous line from a point.) Pain refers to distal sites (e.g., buttocks, shin, calf, ankle, heel).
2. Pain refers to dermatomes. (Pain refers to myotomes or sclerotomes, not dermatomes.)
3. Skeletal muscle spasm is present and causes pain. (There is no such thing as skeletal muscle spasm.) Patients often use the term *spasm* as a synonym for pain. More accurately, the term *guarding* describes sudden contraction of paraspinal muscles to avoid pain. This contraction can be relaxed by slightly laterally flexing and extending the lumbar spine. If spasm is defined as *sustained involuntary skeletal muscle contraction*, it is nonexistent as shown by Harrell and Mead.[7]

On physical examination, muscle stretch reflexes (MSRs) can be reduced or absent (Table 6.1). For detecting muscle weakness, screening tests, such as walking on heels and toes, are too gross to pick up weakness of most radiculopathies. One should specifically check knee extensors for L4, toe extensors for L5, and 10 toe

Table 6.1 Physical Examination

Spinal Nerve Root	Muscle Stretch Reflex (Diminished or Absent)	Weakness	Paresthesias
L4	Knee jerk	Knee extensors	Medial leg
L5	Lateral hamstrings	Toe extensors	Dorsum of foot
S1	Ankle jerk	Ankle plantar flexors	Sole of foot; lateral two toes

rises on one foot with knee extended for S1, comparing with the normal side (see Table 6.1). Often, knee extensors are too strong to break, if even slightly weak; therefore, using a functional test like squatting can help detect weakness. Sensation is the least valuable sign because it goes through two nervous systems after a stimulus (patient and examiner). However, light touch or sharp-dull sensation can be reduced in a dermatomal pattern; therefore, it is still important to perform a good sensory examination. Straight leg raising (SLR) is the most reliable test for radiculopathy (especially if validated) and to follow the progress of the patient. To validate, repeat SLR in sitting position, then with neck flexion just below pain level. Pain, or an increase in pain, occurs with neck flexion, as well as with forced ankle dorsiflexion. Pain that occurs in the first 30 degrees of SLR usually is not radicular. Tight hamstrings can be a cause of pain. Check leg circumference for atrophy, which is greatest calf circumference compared with the opposite side. A difference of 2 cm or less is in the range of normal. Edema can often be the cause of measurement differences. Thigh circumference is measured at a given distance proximal to the superior pole of the patella. Differences less than one-half of an inch are not significant. Skeletal muscle atrophy can occur as early as 3 weeks after injury. Both hip and knee injuries and arthritis can result in significant thigh atrophy; therefore, circumference does not always reflect weakness.

Once a detailed history and physical examination are completed, EDX testing can be performed. The EDX testing should be planned based on the physical findings.

PRACTICAL ANATOMY

A thorough knowledge of anatomy is required to be a competent electromyographer. All muscles acting on the limbs are plurisegmentally innervated except for the rhomboids, which are innervated only by C5. All other limb muscles are innervated by at least two nerve roots. Generally, as one explores the muscle proximally to distally, medially to laterally, and anteriorly to posteriorly, the nerve roots are cephalad to caudad. The disk derangement is, in most instances, affecting the spinal nerve rather than being restricted to the root.

There is overlap in the root levels when exploring the paraspinals, but the specific spinal nerve level is more precisely identified by deep penetration of the paraspinal muscle bulk by the electrode. The distribution of the lumbosacral spinal nerve levels is more likely directly lateral to the spinous processes. By using proper technique, analysis of the multifidus muscles can be accurately performed.[8] The multifidus muscles are thought to be unisegmentally innervated.[9] There is no S2 representation in the paraspinal muscles. To access the S2 level, muscles innervated by the anterior primary rami S2 spinal nerve can be examined with the needle electrode. These muscles include the gluteus maximus, lateral head of the gastrocnemius, soleus, and foot intrinsics. To assess the S3–S4 spinal level, the external anal sphincter can be evaluated by needle EMG.

GUIDES TO SPINAL NERVE INNERVATION

1. Only L4 innervation below the knee is anterior tibial muscle.
2. Only L5 below the ankle is extensor digitorum brevis.
3. From medial to lateral in the foot, more S1 to more S2.

ELECTRODIAGNOSIS

Certain steps should be taken by the electromyographer to ensure a complete but concise examination when evaluating a patient with a suspected lumbosacral radiculopathy. The following sequence of steps should be followed by the electromyographer once the patient is on the examining table:

1. Perform a needle study of the paraspinals bilaterally, and record any spontaneous activity (Figure 6.2).
2. Perform a needle study of a proximal muscle innervated by suspected nerve root involved in radiculopathy.
3. Perform a needle study of a distal muscle innervated by suspected nerve root involved in radiculopathy.
4. Perform a needle study of muscles innervated by the affected root, but two different peripheral nerves.
5. Perform a needle study of muscles innervated by a root above and below the suspected root.
6. Perform a needle study of the muscle most involved (weakest), and perform a needle study on the same muscle on the contralateral limb.
7. Determine the H-reflex latency of both limbs.
8. Compare compound muscle action potential (CMAP) response of suspected spinal nerve to the normal contralateral limb (i.e., L4—anterior tibial or vastus lateralis; L5—extensor digitorum longus (EDL) or peroneus longus; S1—medial head of gastrocnemius or soleus).
9. If peripheral neuropathy is suspected, perform more detailed sensory and motor nerve conduction studies (NCSs), including the sural, peroneal, and tibial nerves, as well as upper limb NCSs.

Case 1

A 17-year-old high school football player presented with low back pain of 5 days' duration. He reported that he was jumping up to receive a pass when he was hit from behind, resulting in hyperextension of his back. Furthermore, as he landed, an opposing player took the patient's legs out from beneath him, causing him to jackknife at the waist. He indicated that after the injury he was able to walk off the field unassisted, but was unable to play due to moderate to severe low back pain and muscle spasms. On presentation, his primary symptoms were intense low back pain

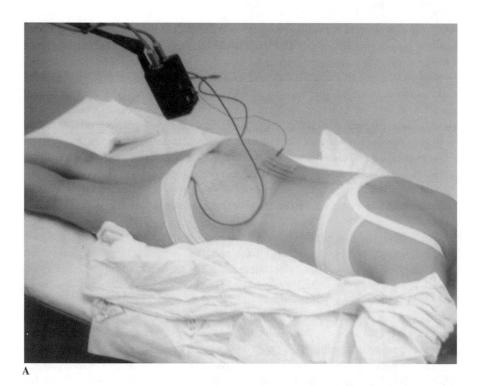

A

Figure 6.2 (A) Proper positioning of patient in prone position
for paraspinal needle examination. **(B)** L4, L5, and S1 spinous
processes are indicated. Distribution of the lumbosacral root levels occurs directly lateral to the
lumbar   spinous   processes.
Appropriate root level can usually be isolated by deep penetration of the paraspinal muscle by
the electrode.

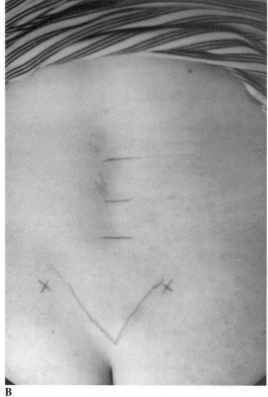

B

with some referred pain into the buttocks. He denied numbness and tingling in his lower limbs bilaterally, or referred pain down his legs. He reported no bowel or bladder dysfunction. His low back pain was aggravated with all physical activity, prolonged sitting, and standing. Physical examination revealed an antalgic gait with mild listing to the right. Inspection of the low back was remarkable for loss of lordotic curve with no other gross deformities. Tenderness to palpation was present over lumbar paraspinal muscles. Lumbar flexion and extension were decreased, with pain reported at extremes of range of motion. Manual muscle testing of bilateral lower limbs revealed no specific weaknesses. Sensory examination was within normal limits. SLR bilaterally provoked pain in his low back with no referred pain into the legs. Hip flexion with knees flexed at 90 degrees exacerbated low back pain bilaterally. MSRs were symmetric in lower limbs bilaterally.

The differential diagnosis included lumbar strain or sprain, pars interarticularis fracture, spondylolisthesis, fracture of the vertebral body, and lumbar radiculopathy. Lumbosacral spine films were obtained and were negative for spondylolysis, spondylolisthesis, or vertebral body fracture. Patient's history and physical were consistent with an acute lumbar strain.

To establish the diagnosis of a lumbar strain or sprain, there should be pain on palpation over the lumbar paraspinals, decreased lumbar range of motion, and pain at extreme range of motion. This type of injury is the result of heavy lifting, twisting movements, and flexion or extension injuries. Pain worsens as the day goes on because daily activities, such as bending, twisting, lifting, sitting, and standing for prolonged periods, aggravate pain. There should be no associated neurologic signs, and coughing or sneezing should not refer pain into lower limbs. Plain radiographs are usually not helpful in evaluating patients with an acute low back sprain, because they typically show changes appropriate for age with little or no disk space narrowing in adolescents. Spondylolysis is a likely consideration in a young athlete. Teenagers who engage in athletic activity with low back pain have a 45% likelihood of having spondylolysis.[10] Plain radiographs were indicated to rule out a pars fracture, with oblique films being the most helpful in seeing the pars interarticularis defect. EDX studies are not indicated in evaluating acute lumbar strain or sprain without clear radicular symptoms. They might be useful later, if the pain persists for an extended period, to rule out a neuropathic component as the cause of pain.

Case 2

A 43-year-old man was moving furniture 5 days before evaluation and developed stiffness in his back. The next morning, he was unable to get out of bed because of sharp pain in his low back. He developed an aching pain in his right buttock and calf, and noticed numbness at the top of his foot and complained that his foot did not work. Physical examination revealed weakness in his right ankle dorsiflexors (3/5) and right big toe extension (3/5). He had trouble walking on his right heel. There was a mild sensory deficit to light touch and pinprick on the dorsal aspect of the right foot. SLR was positive on the right at 70 degrees.

EMG of selected muscles in the right lower limb and bilateral lumbosacral paraspinal muscles revealed no evidence of membrane irritability. There was a decreased number of motor units in the muscles supplied by L5. Early polyphasics were seen in the right L5 paraspinal muscles.

Table 6.2 Results of Needle Electromyography in Case 2

Muscle (Right Lower Limb)	Root(s)	Insertional Activity	Spontaneous Activity	Number of MUAPs/Amplitude and Duration
Adductor longus	L2, L3, L4	Normal	None	nl/nl
Vastus medialis	L2, L3, L4	Normal	None	nl/nl
Tensor fascia lata	L4, L5	Normal	"Early polyphasics"	decr/nl
Anterior tibial	L4, L5	Normal	None	nl/nl
Peroneus longus	L5, S1	Normal	None	decr/nl
Extensor hallucis longus	L5, S1	Normal	None	decr/nl
Flexor digitorum longus	L5, S1	Normal	None	decr/nl
Lateral gastrocnemius	S1, S2	Normal	None	nl/nl
Abductor hallucis	S1, S2	Normal	None	nl/nl
Biceps femoris	L5, S1, S2	Normal	None	decr/nl
Gluteus medius	L4, L5, S1	Normal	"Early polyphasics"	decr/nl
Gluteus maximus	L5, S1, S2	Normal	"Early polyphasics"	decr/nl
Right Lumbosacral Paraspinals	**Posterior Primary Rami**			
L1–L4	L1–L4	Normal	None	—
L5	L5	Normal	"Early polyphasics"	—
S1	S1	Normal	None	—
Left Lumbosacral Paraspinals	**Posterior Primary Rami**			
L1–S1	L1–S1	Normal	None	—

decr/nl = decreased number of MUAPs with normal amplitude and duration; nl/nl = normal; MUAPs = motor unit action potentials.

Table 6.2 shows the results of needle EMG in Case 2. NCSs of the right lower limb revealed normal sensory and motor studies. H-reflex was normal bilaterally. Table 6.3 shows the results of NCSs in Case 2.

Sensory and motor NCSs were within normal limits. Needle EMG revealed decreased recruitment in right L5 innervated muscles, as well as early polyphasic motor units in the right L5 paraspinals. With normal H-reflexes, the lesion was

Table 6.3 Results of Nerve Conduction Studies in Case 2

Nerve	Peak Latency (ms)	SNAP (μV)	Distal Latency (ms)	CMAP (mV)
Right sural	3.3	18.0	—	—
Left peroneal (to EDL)	—	—	—	5.5
Right peroneal (to EDL)	—	—	—	6.0
Left H-reflex	—	—	28.8	—
Right H-reflex	—	—	29.0	—

CMAP = compound motor action potential amplitude; EDL = extensor digitorum longus; SNAP = sensory nerve action potential amplitude.

likely to be at L5 on the right. Furthermore, with normal CMAP amplitudes recorded over the EDL, the prognosis for full recovery in this patient was excellent because there was little, if any, axonal loss. EDX testing can be helpful regarding prognosis in a patient suspected of a radiculopathy after 5 days, even if one is confident of the diagnosis of radiculopathy based on physical examination and history. One cannot determine the severity based solely on the physical examination. A patient can have a foot drop on physical examination, but this may be only from a conduction block at the spinal nerve as contrasted to permanent axonal loss. EDX testing can provide early information on the severity of the lesion, providing reassurance to the patient. The management of the patient could be more aggressive if substantial axonal loss were present (e.g., pulse steroids, epidural blocks).

How would EDX studies have been different in Case 2 if they were performed 3 weeks after onset of symptoms? Findings on EMG would have been more remarkable at this time if significant axonal loss was present. Membrane irritability could have been seen in both proximal and distal muscles supplied by the L5 nerve root as well as in the L5 paraspinal muscles. One could have seen a diminished CMAP amplitude of an L5 muscle on NCSs if axonal loss was present.

"EARLY POLYPHASIC" MOTOR UNIT ACTION POTENTIAL

Within the first few days of an acute radiculopathy, on needle examination one can see what looks like polyphasic motor unit action potentials (MUAPs), but they are actually two or three MUAPs firing synchronously, but not simultaneously. Thus, the MUAPs are grouped closely together and appear to be polyphasic. Colachis et al.[11] reported 20 cases of cervical and lumbar radiculopathies in which they observed these polyphasics within 1–3 weeks of the onset of symptoms. They hypothesized when a nerve root is inflamed, ephaptic activation of neighboring axons occurs as the nerve impulse travels across the inflamed root. Thus, ephaptic activation of a second and third axon can occur from an active axon. The second axon is stimulated synchronously at the spinal level with the volitionally active axon. A variation of conduction occurs along the nerves, so the impulses reach the motor unit at different times, leading to synchronous, but not simultaneous, activation of the unit. This variation leads to the appearance of a polyphasic motor unit (Figures 6.3 and 6.4). Because these units can occur at the onset of inflammation and look like polyphasics, they are referred to as *early polyphasics*. Recognizing early polyphasics is helpful in diagnosing acute radiculopathies within the first 2–3 weeks when the radiculopathy is limited to a root distribution because fibrillation potentials and positive waves would not be seen yet in the peripheral muscles. Lumbosacral radiculopathies can be diagnosed early by recognizing these early polyphasics, and appropriate treatment can be directed toward the inflamed root.

CHRONOLOGY OF ELECTRODIAGNOSIS IN RADICULOPATHY

To use EDX to its fullest potential, one can start with the onset of radicular pain (inflamed spinal nerve). In most instances, the herniated nucleus pulposus does not mechanically compress the spinal nerve. Although in some instances of foraminal encroachment and narrow recesses, certain lumbar motion can cause some compression, most radiculopathies result from irritation and subsequent inflammation

Early Polyphasic M.U.P

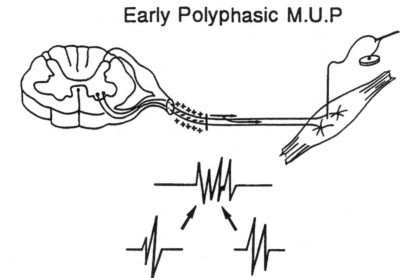

Figure 6.3 Hypothesis to explain early polyphasic motor unit potential in acute radiculopathy. Ephaptic transmission between adjacent nerve axons in the region of the inflamed root results in synchronous, but not simultaneous, firing of two or more motor units. (Reprinted with permission from SC Colachis, WS Pease, EW Johnson. Polyphasic motor unit action potentials in early radiculopathy: their presence and ephaptic transmission as a hypothesis. Electromyogr Clin Neurophysiol 1992;32:29.)

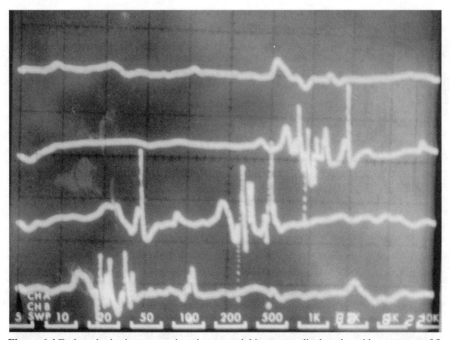

Figure 6.4 Early polyphasic motor unit action potential in acute radiculopathy with symptoms of 5 days' duration. Monopolar needle electrode in extensor digitorum longus muscle. (Line width = 10 ms/division; line height = 50 μV/division.)

of spinal nerves. The nucleus pulposus is highly irritating to nerve tissue. The usual good response to steroids is explained by the presence of inflammation. From the onset of S1 radiculopathy, the H-reflex latency is prolonged by 1 ms or more because of localized myelin dysfunction, thus slowing in the injured S1 nerve root segment is evident when compared to the normal limb (Figure 6.5).[12]

If significant weakness is present (e.g., less than four out of five on MRC system), then the recruitment pattern is reduced on maximum contraction. If there is only minimal weakness, it is difficult to recognize a pattern of decreased recruitment. However, with a minimal contraction, one can see an increase in recruitment frequency (or a reduction in recruitment interval). In early L5 radiculopathy, Pease et al.[13] showed a recruitment interval of 70–90 ms (recruitment frequency of 16 Hz) in the EDL, compared to a normal interval of 100–120 ms (recruitment frequency of 10 Hz) (Figure 6.6). After 4–5 days, CMAP of the weak muscle is reduced compared to the normal side if the weakness is permanent and the nerve is undergoing Wallerian degeneration (Figure 6.7). Conversely, if there is simply neurapraxia (conduction block), the CMAP will be near normal. The medial head of the gastrocnemius for S1 and the EDL for L5 are the usually used muscles. This can be helpful to determine the prognosis as early as possible.[14]

During the first few days of an acute radiculopathy, spontaneous activity in the form of "early polyphasics" can be seen; these are believed to be due to ephaptic transmission.[11] These "early polyphasics" are usually seen before other types of spontaneous activity are present and can be helpful in verifying a specific spinal nerve compromise. In cases of litigation involving reinjuries of the back, early polyphasic MUAPs add to the notion of acuteness. By 7–8 days, the paraspinal

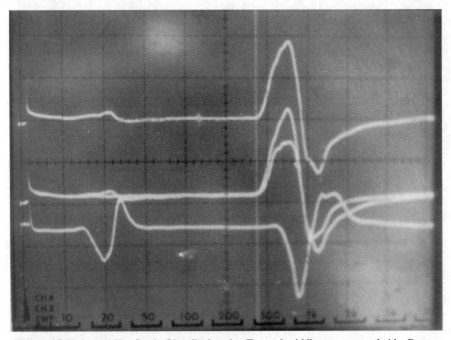

Figure 6.5 Prolonged H-reflex in S1 radiculopathy. Top and middle trace: normal side. Bottom trace: S1 radiculopathy. (Line width = 5 ms/division; line height = 500 μV/division.)

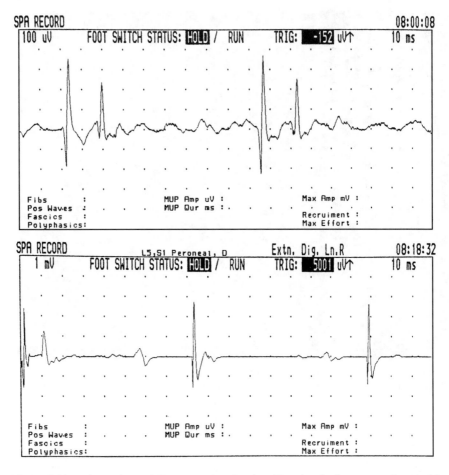

Figure 6.6 Recruitment interval. Top trace: normal patient. Note that the first motor unit potential is firing at 10 Hz when the second unit begins to activate. Recruitment interval = 100 ms; recruitment frequency = 10 Hz. (Each square = 10 ms, 500 μV.) Bottom trace: patient with L5 radiculopathy. Note that the first motor unit is firing at 12.5 Hz when the second unit begins to activate. Recruitment interval = 80 ms; recruitment frequency = 12.5 Hz. (Each square = 10 ms, 1 mV. Monopolar needle electrode in extensor digitorum longus.) (MUP = motor unit potential.) (Reprinted with permission from EW Johnson, WS Pease. Practical Electromyography [3rd ed]. Baltimore: Williams & Wilkins, 1997;127.)

muscles demonstrate positive sharp waves at the appropriate level. At this time, one can use H-reflex latency side-to-side difference to help to distinguish between an L5 and S1 radiculopathy. By 12–14 days, the proximal muscles supplied by the involved root show positive waves, and the paraspinals begin to have fibrillation potentials. At 18–21 days, the distal muscles begin to show the classic signs of denervation. As early as 4–5 weeks, collateral innervation begins, and polyphasic motor units begin to appear. By 2–3 months, reinnervation is established with some large amplitude MUAPs. The chronology of EDX changes suggests that the paraspinals are the most fruitful area to investigate, especially early in the course. In a study by Johnson and Fletcher,[15] fewer than 3% of the patients had abnormalities only in the limb muscles.

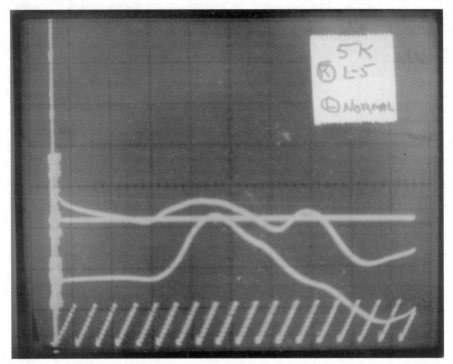

Figure 6.7 Reduced compound muscle action potential in radiculopathy. Top trace: right extensor digitorum longus compound muscle action potential in L5 radiculopathy. Bottom trace: normal left extensor digitorum longus compound muscle action potential. (Each square = 2 ms, 5 mV.)

Sensory nerve action potentials are usually unaffected, because the nerve root compromise can be proximal to the dorsal root ganglion, which is more likely in cervical radiculopathy. An extreme lateral compromise could decrease the sensory nerve action potential amplitude by involvement of the spinal nerve distal to the dorsal root ganglion. F waves are not of practical use in radiculopathy because all limb muscles have at least two, and usually three, nerve roots supplying them. Normal F waves can therefore traverse unaffected roots to the muscle evaluated. However, the number of F waves can be reduced if substantial weakness is present (thus, blocking at inflamed root). This reduction does not help with prognosis, however, and is only present if significant weakness is present and the clinical diagnosis is apparent.

The ability to recognize the different potentials seen during EMG is critical in arriving at the accurate diagnosis. Positive waves are artifactual recordings of a single muscle fiber discharge, and can be either a fibrillation potential from a spontaneous activation of a single muscle fiber, or from a single muscle discharge with the needle electrode in the end plate area and recording an end plate spike with the tip of the needle electrode in contact with the depolarized zone (Figure 6.8).[16] This part of the needle examination is the most commonly misinterpreted and has led to many misdiagnoses. Fibrillation potentials are spontaneous discharges of single muscle fibers, which can also be recorded as positive waves. These positive waves differ in their regularity and frequency of

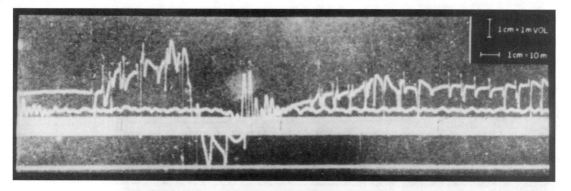

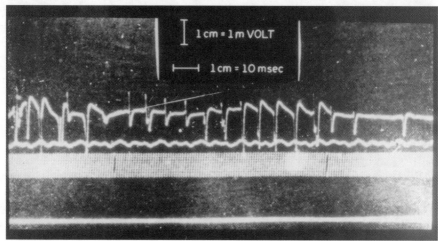

Figure 6.8 Example of end plate spikes, resulting from a single muscle fiber discharge with the needle electrode in the end plate area. The tip of the monopolar needle is in contact with the depolarized zone. (Each square = 10 ms, 1 mV.)

firing rate—2–20 Hz. Those positive waves associated with end plate spikes are usually irregular and faster in their discharge frequency. The fibrillation potential is usually initially positive and diphasic or triphasic. Occasionally, if the tip of the needle electrode is at the site of the beginning of the depolarization, the initial phase is negative (Figure 6.9). End plate spikes are always initially negative because the tip of the needle initiates the potential. Fibrillation potentials generally appear after 18–21 days of nerve injury (Figure 6.10). Complex repetitive discharges are hyperactive single muscle membranes that become generators of linked activated muscle cell membranes. They are considered high frequency if they fire at faster than the fastest motor unit fires—45 Hz. They are usually not seen until significant denervation occurs (Figure 6.11). Myokymic discharges are grouped discharges from ephaptic activation of injured axons with defective myelin. These discharges can occur at the inflamed area of the nerve root with activation either associated with volition or occurring spontaneously. These discharges are grouped MUAPs, not single muscle fiber potentials. Myokymic discharges can be seen as early as 2–3 weeks after acute radiculopathy. Paradoxically, these potentials can also be found in lumbar stenosis. They

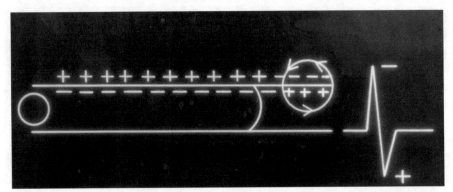

Figure 6.9 Fibrillation potential can be recorded as negative-to-positive potential if electrode is at the point where depolarization begins.

can be seen as group discharges when the sweep speed is reduced to 20–50 ms/cm (Figure 6.12).

SPINAL NERVE STIMULATION

Direct spinal nerve stimulation is another recognized test that is both objective and sensitive in the diagnosis of acute lumbosacral radiculopathy, and the results may change the treatment plan. It allows one to distinguish between true weakness versus conduction block, which affects management. With conduction block, one may

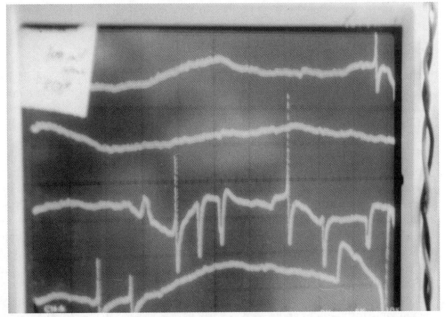

Figure 6.10 Fibrillation potentials and positive waves recorded from medial gastrocnemius in S1 radiculopathy. (Each square = 10 ms, 100 μV. Monopolar needle electrode in medial gastrocnemius.)

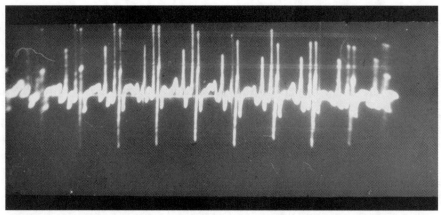

Figure 6.11 Complex repetitive discharge in lumbar paraspinal muscles in L5 radiculopathy. (Each square = 10 ms, 100 μV. Monopolar needle electrode in lumbar paraspinal at L5 level.)

choose to treat more conservatively with oral steroids. Chang[17] compared needle EMG with spinal nerve stimulation in patients suspected of having either an L5 or S1 radiculopathy. For L5 spinal nerve stimulation, the recording electrode was placed over the anterior tibial muscle. For S1 spinal nerve stimulation, the recording electrode was placed over the medial gastrocnemius. Side-to-side differences in CMAP amplitudes greater than 9.6% were considered abnormal. Their study showed that

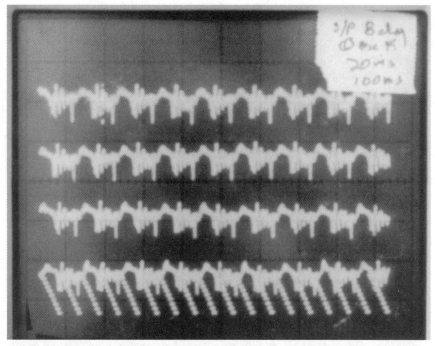

Figure 6.12 Myokymic discharges recorded from the biceps femoris in acute radiculopathy. (Each square = 20 ms, 100 μV. Monopolar needle electrode in biceps femoris.)

spinal nerve stimulation was highly sensitive in the diagnosis of lumbosacral radicul-opathy, and can be used when other EDX testing is equivocal in a patient suspicious of having a radiculopathy.

In a study by Colachis et al.,[18] they looked at the peak amplitude of the M response from the EDL in 26 healthy subjects. The mean amplitudes of the EDL were 6.5 mV on the right and 6.1 mV on the left. The side-to-side difference in amplitude of the M response was 0.4 mV (±1.1 mV). When using the amplitude of the EDL from the right lower limb as a reference, the left EDL was not over 2.8 mV, or 33% less than the right side. The amplitude of the right EDL was not over 1.8 mV, or 22% less than that of the left side when the EDL from the left lower limb was used as a reference. A criterion of greater than 50% reduction in amplitude of the CMAP compared to the normal side has often been used by oth-ers to indicate axonal degeneration has occurred.[2,5,19] The surface electrodes' placement can affect CMAP amplitude. Ideal site is E-1 over the motor point and E-2 over a silent area. The study by Colachis et al. indicates that the meaningful differences in the amplitude of the M response between the affected and unaf-fected limbs in focal nerve root lesions may not be detected by using a criterion of greater than 50% variation.

Case 3

A 33-year-old woman presented with a 6-month history of back and left lower limb pain. The pain was most intense in her left buttock and was referred to her calf, and she complained of occasional tingling in her sole. The pain was worse when driving her car and with prolonged sitting. She worked as an insurance sales representative and spent many hours driving her car. The onset of pain was insidious, but had been unremitting the past 12 weeks. She had increased difficulty climbing stairs. Physi-cal examination revealed moderate sensory deficit to light touch and pinprick on the lateral and plantar aspect of her left foot, and sensation was intact on the right. She was able to walk on her heels, but was unable to perform 10 toe rises on the left, and was noted to have some difficulty rising from a squatting position. SLR caused mild discomfort in her back and left posterior thigh. MSRs revealed 1+ ankle reflex on the left, and a 2+ on the right. Hamstring reflexes were 2+ bilaterally.

Needle EMG of selected muscles in the left lower limb and corresponding paraspinals revealed membrane irritability in S1 innervated muscles. Evaluation of the MUAPs revealed increased amplitude and duration in muscles supplied by S1, as well as decreased recruitment. EMG of right lumbosacral paraspinals was nor-mal (Table 6.4). Sensory nerve conduction study of the left sural nerve was within normal limits. Motor NCSs recording over the medial gastrocnemius revealed a 40% smaller CMAP amplitude on the left side compared to the right. H-reflex was also slowed on the left compared to the right by 2 ms. Table 6.5 shows the results of NCSs in Case 3.

EMG revealed evidence of an S1 radiculopathy with signs of ongoing degenera-tion and regeneration. NCSs revealed diminished CMAP of medial head of gastroc-nemius compared to the right side, but less than a 50% decrease, which indicated a good prognosis for recovery. H-reflex was prolonged on the left side. With large MUAPs and a good CMAP amplitude, collateral innervation could restore near nor-mal function in this patient.

Table 6.4 Results of Needle Electromyography in Case 3

Muscle (Left Lower Limb)	Root(s)	Insertional Activity	Spontaneous Activity	Number of MUAPs/ Amplitude and Duration
Adductor longus	L2, L3, L4	Normal	None	nl/nl
Vastus medialis	L2, L3, L4	Normal	None	nl/nl
Tensor fascia lata	L4, L5	Normal	None	nl/nl
Anterior tibial	L4, L5	Normal	None	nl/nl
Peroneus longus	L5, S1	Few positive waves	1+Fibs	decr/incr
Extensor digitorum longus	L5, S1	Few positive waves	1+Fibs	decr/incr
Flexor digitorum longus	L5, S1	Few positive waves	2+Fibs	decr/incr
Medial gastrocnemius	S1, S2	Many positive waves	3+Fibs	decr/incr
Abductor hallucis	S1, S2	Many positive waves	3+Fibs	decr/incr
Biceps femoris	L5, S1, S2	Few positive waves	2+Fibs	decr/incr
Left Lumbosacral Paraspinals	**Posterior Primary Rami**			
L1–L5	L1–L5	Normal	None	—
S1	S1	Many positive waves	3+Fibs	—
Right Lumbosacral Para-spinals	**Posterior Primary Rami**			
L1–S1	L1–S1	Normal	None	—

decr/incr = decreased number of MUAPs with increased amplitude and duration; MUAPs = motor unit action potentials; nl/nl = normal.

IMPORTANCE OF H-REFLEX IN S1 RADICULOPATHY

The H-reflex is a monosynaptic reflex that was first described by Hoffman in 1918 and was standardized by Braddom and Johnson.[12] It measures afferent and efferent conduction mainly along the S1 nerve root and is used in localizing nerve root compromise at that level.[12,20,21] To obtain the H-reflex, a recording electrode is applied over the medial aspect of the soleus, with a reference electrode over the Achilles' tendon. Percutaneous stimulator or needle stimulating electrode is inserted over the tibial nerve in the popliteal fossa (junction of middle and lateral 1/3) just lateral to

Table 6.5 Results of Nerve Conduction Studies in Case 3

Nerve	Peak latency (ms)	SNAP (μV)	Distal latency (ms)	CMAP (mV)
Left sural	3.2	18.0	—	—
Left tibial (medial gastrocnemius)	—	—	—	3.0
Right tibial (medial gastrocnemius)	—	—	—	5.0
Left H-reflex	—	—	31.0	—
Right H-reflex	—	—	29.0	—

CMAP = compound motor action potential amplitude; SNAP = sensory nerve action potential amplitude.

the popliteal artery (Figure 6.13). A low-intensity stimulus should be applied at a rate of 0.5 Hz and a duration of 0.5–1.0 ms. Sweep speed should be set at 5 ms/division and gain should be at 1 mV/division. The H-reflex appears after a latency from 28–35. As stimulus intensity is increased, the M wave appears at 5–8 ms, and the H-reflex becomes smaller. At maximum stimulating intensity, the H-reflex disappears and F wave (variable and low amplitude) appears after approximately the same latency. The latency of the H wave is constant. Side-to-side latency difference should be less than 1 ms (SD = 0.4 ms).[12] The latency is the most sensitive and accurate indicator in diagnosing S1 radiculopathy. A difference in latency of 1 ms or more strongly supports the diagnosis of S1 radiculopathy if the history, physical

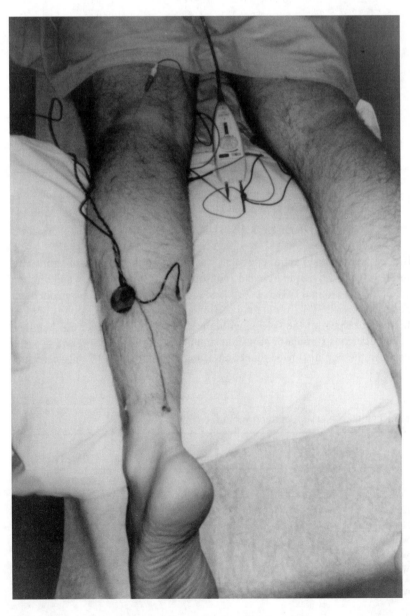

Figure 6.13 Set-up for an H-reflex. The recording electrode is applied over the medial aspect of the soleus and the reference electrode over the Achilles tendon. Needle stimulating electrode is inserted over the tibial nerve in the popliteal fossa.

examination, and EMG are compatible. Side-to-side amplitude differences, on the other hand, are meaningless, because one can alter the amplitude by several maneuvers. In a study by McHugh et al.,[22] the H-reflex amplitude varied with different states of leg muscle activity. Maximal H-reflex amplitudes were obtained with the leg at rest and with mild activation of the agonist. The H-reflex was observed to decline with progressively greater voluntary activation of the antagonist and with isometric maximal co-contraction of the ankle plantar flexors and dorsiflexors.

The formula for predicting the mean expected H-reflex latency of the tibial nerve is the following: $0.46 \times$ [length in cm from medial malleolus to point of stimulation (popliteal area)] + $0.1 \times$ [age in years] + 9.14 (a constant) = predicted mean latency. Greater than 1.0 ms difference is diagnostically significant (3 SD = 1.2 ms side-to-side). If both tibial nerve H-reflex latencies are greater than the predicted mean latency, determine the tibial nerve conduction velocity. The patient could have a peripheral neuropathy. Sural nerve latency is also a sensitive indicator of certain neuropathies. If the history and physical examination and needle EMG are highly suggestive of radiculopathy, always do H-reflex latency on both limbs. More than 1 ms difference side-to-side is diagnostically significant.

The H-reflex latency is useful in the following circumstances:

1. In the first 7–10 days of a suspected S1 radiculopathy, as the H latency may confirm.
2. If needle EMG findings are limited to the paraspinal muscles (posterior primary rami), prolonged or absent H latency is diagnostic of S1 radiculopathy.
3. If needle EMG findings are minimal or inconclusive, prolonged or absent H latency will support S1 radiculopathy.
4. If needle EMG findings do not distinguish between L5 and S1 radiculopathy, H-reflex latency determination will be helpful. Its normality suggests L5, and its absence or prolongation suggests S1 (95% of all lumbosacral radiculopathies are either L5 or S1).
5. In recurrent pain after previous lumbar laminectomy with questionable needle EMG findings, prolonged or absent H latency (unilateral) suggests S1 radiculopathy, if different from preoperative examination.

Pease et al.[23] were the first to test the H-reflex via direct stimulation of the S1 spinal nerve at the foramen (Figure 6.14). This location provides more complete information of the H-reflex pathway by dividing it into its peripheral and spinal conduction portions. In their study, they calculated slowing of the nerve conduction velocity by dividing the latency of the S1 spinal nerve response by the ipsilateral H-reflex latency to get the S1 ratio. This ratio in the control group produced a mean value of 0.48, whereas those patients with S1 radiculopathies had a mean S1 ratio of 0.44. In a related study, Pease et al.[24] established a normal value for the central (spinal) portion of the H-reflex latency. S1 spinal nerve stimulation was performed using standard H-reflex recording technique, as described by Braddom and Johnson.[12] The peak latencies for the two sequential compound CMAPs recorded over the soleus representing the M and H responses were measured. The difference between these two latencies was determined and represents the central (spinal) portion of the H-reflex (Figure 6.15). The normal value for the interpotential latency difference of the H-reflex in the S1 spinal nerve in healthy subjects was 7±0.3 ms. All patients tested who had S1 radiculopathies had central loop latencies greater than 8 ms (Figure 6.16). The normal value of the central loop of the H-reflex determined in this study may allow for earlier and more accurate diagnosis of an acute S1 radiculopathy.

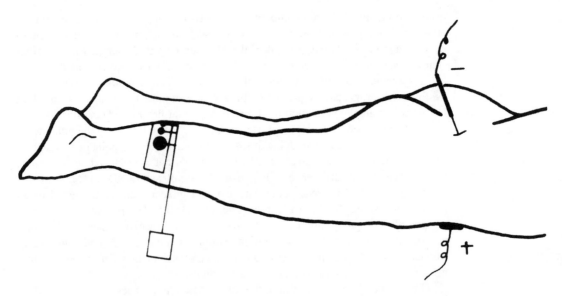

Figure 6.14 S1 spinal nerve stimulation. Recording electrode is over the medial gastrocnemius. Monopolar needle electrode is inserted 1–2 cm medial to the posterior superior iliac spine. The anode is placed on the anterior trunk opposite the needle.

Case 4

A 45-year-old man (from Case 1) who injured his back 2 years ago while moving furniture, and developed an L5 radiculopathy, for which he eventually underwent a diskectomy, presented with a 4-week history of aching pain in his right buttock and calf, which was similar to the pain he had 2 years ago. The patient was referred from the Bureau of Workers' Compensation for EDX studies because the patient's original injury 2 years ago occurred while working, and it was an allowed claim for L5 radiculopathy. The Bureau of Workers' Compensation wanted to know if the patient's recurrent symptoms were related to the original claim or if they were related to a new problem. The patient had his surgery approximately 1½ years ago

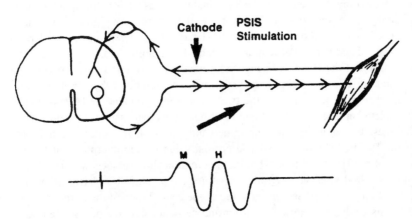

Figure 6.15 S1 spinal nerve stimulation to produce efferent (M) response and afferent activity to evoke H (top). Both responses seen on same recording sweep after careful adjustment of stimulus intensity. (PSIS = posterior superior iliac spine.) (Reprinted with permission from WS Pease, R Kozakiewicz, and EW Johnson. Central loop of the H-reflex: normal value and use in S1 radiculopathy. Am J Phys Med Rehabil 1997;76:183.)

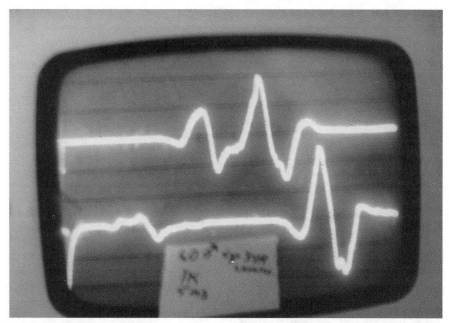

Figure 6.16 Top trace: recording of M and H response in a normal subject with the central loop latency of approximately 7 ms. Bottom trace: recording of delayed H-reflex with central loop latency greater than 8 ms in patient with S1 radiculopathy. (Each square = 5 ms, 1 mV.)

and was doing well until 1 month before presentation. He had been working full time for the past year for a moving company where he did a lot of heavy lifting. He could not recall any preceding event that led to this current episode of pain. On physical examination, he demonstrated sensory deficits to light touch and pinprick over the dorsal aspect of the right foot. Lateral hamstring reflex on the right was diminished. Left lateral hamstring reflex was 2+. Knee jerk and ankle jerk reflexes were 2+ bilaterally. Sitting and supine SLRs were positive bilaterally at 45 degrees. No motor deficits were noted except for right ankle dorsiflexors, which were a 4/5.

EMG of selected muscles in the right lower limb and corresponding paraspinals revealed membrane irritability in an L5 distribution with more irritability in the distal muscles. The size of the fibrillation potentials ranged from 300–600 μV. Motor unit potentials of L5 innervated muscles were of increased amplitude and duration with decreased recruitment. EMG of the left lumbosacral paraspinals were normal. Table 6.6 shows the results of needle EMG in Case 4. Sensory and motor NCSs were within normal limits, and H-reflex was normal bilaterally. Table 6.7 shows the results of NCSs in Case 4.

NCSs were unremarkable. EMG revealed membrane irritability in an L5 distribution with large fibrillation potentials, which was suggestive of an acute process. MUAPs were of increased amplitude and duration as a result of reinnervation, probably related to the old nerve injury of 2 years ago. EDX findings suggested an acute right L5 radiculopathy superimposed on a chronic process. Normal size of EDL response suggested neurapraxic weakness and gave a good prognosis for recovery of nerve function.

Table 6.6 Results of Needle Electromyography in Case 4

Muscle (Right Lower Limb)	Root(s)	Insertional Activity	Spontaneous Activity	Number of MUAPs/Amplitude and Duration
Adductor longus	L2, L3, L4	Normal	None	nl/nl
Vastus medialis	L2, L3, L4	Normal	None	nl/nl
Tensor fascia lata	L4, L5	Few positive waves	1+Fibs	decr/incr
Anterior tibial	L4, L5	Few positive waves	2+Fibs	decr/incr
Peroneus longus	L5, S1	Few positive waves	2+Fibs	decr/incr
Extensor hallucis longus	L5, S1	Few positive waves	2+Fibs	decr/incr
Flexor digitorum longus	L5, S1	Few positive waves	1+Fibs	decr/incr
Lateral gastrocnemius	S1, S2	Normal	None	nl/nl
Abductor hallucis	S1, S2	Normal	None	nl/nl
Biceps femoris	L5, S1, S2	Few positive waves	1+Fibs	decr/incr
Gluteus medius	L4, L5, S1	Normal	Polyphasics	nl/nl
Gluteus maximus	L5, S1, S2	Normal	Polyphasics	nl/nl
Right Lumbosacral Spinals	**Posterior Primary Rami**			
L1–L4	L1–L4	Normal	None	—
L5	L5	Many positive waves	3+Fibs	—
S1	S1	Normal	None	—
Left Lumbosacral Paraspinals	**Posterior Primary Rami**			
L1–S1	L1–S1	Normal	None	—

decr/incr = decreased number of MUAPs with increased amplitude and duration; MUAPs = motor unit action potentials; nl/nl: normal.

RECURRENT RADICULOPATHIES

Evaluation of a patient with a recurrent radiculopathy can often be a difficult task. Analysis of the MUAPs plays a big role in determining the chronicity of a lesion. In chronic lesions, if reinnervation has occurred, there is an increased proportion of polyphasic motor units. Up to 10–12% of MUAPs can be polyphasics in a normal muscle; therefore, to be considered abnormal, they must be present in excess numbers.[25] Reinnervation may be seen as early as 5–6 weeks after onset of an injury. There may also be an increase in amplitude and duration of the MUAPs with reinnervation. If these changes are seen, they are often limited to and more prevalent in the distal limb muscles.[25] The size of fibrillation potentials seen has been shown to be related to the duration of the lesion. Kraft[26] measured the size of fibrillation potentials in patients with radiculopathies. The mean amplitude of the fibrillation potentials during the first 2 months of an injury was 612 µV. By the fifth or sixth month the amplitude decreased to 320 µV, and by 1 year the amplitude was no larger than 100 µV. One may also see complex repetitive discharges in patients with chronic radiculopathies. By carefully analyzing the motor units during needle examination, one should be able to accurately tell the duration of a lesion. If large fibrillation potentials are seen with MUAPs of normal amplitude and duration, the patient probably has a recent-onset radiculopathy. If small fibrillation potentials are seen with MUAPs of increased amplitude and duration, the

Table 6.7 Results of Nerve Conduction Studies in Case 4

Nerve	Peak Latency (ms)	SNAP (μV)	Distal Latency (ms)	CMAP (mV)
Right sural	3.4	15	—	—
Left peroneal (EDL)	—	—	—	6
Right peroneal (EDL)	—	—	—	6.2
Left H-reflex	—	—	29.0	—
Right H-reflex	—	—	29.2	—

CMAP = compound motor action potential amplitude; EDL = extensor digitorum longus; SNAP = sensory nerve action potential amplitude.

lesion will appear to be chronic with evidence of reinnervation. If large fibrillation potentials are seen with MUAPs of increased amplitude and duration, the patient will appear to have either an acute radiculopathy that is superimposed on a chronic lesion or a chronic radiculopathy with ongoing denervation and reinnervation.

Case 5

A 68-year-old man presented with complaint of pain in his low back and posterior thighs for approximately 1 year. Pain was of insidious onset and had been becoming progressively worse. He was only tolerating standing 10 minutes until he developed low back and bilateral buttocks pain and tingling in both feet. These symptoms were improved by sitting. Patient previously could walk 1 mile a day, but had to reduce this to 1 block because of the pain in his buttocks. He denied bowel or bladder symptoms. On physical examination, symptoms were reproducible with extension of the lumbosacral spine, and he noted some relief with flexion. He had diminished sensation to light touch over the dorsal and plantar aspect of both feet. MSRs were diminished bilaterally throughout the lower limbs. SLR was equivocal bilaterally.

Needle EMG of selected muscles in the bilateral lower limbs and paraspinals revealed membrane irritability in L4–S1 distribution with greater irritability noted in the distal muscles. MUAPs displayed increased amplitude and duration with decreased recruitment, also in a L4–S1 distribution. Table 6.8 shows the results of needle EMG in Case 5. Sensory NCSs of the sural nerve were normal bilaterally. Motor NCSs of the peroneal and tibial nerve revealed decreased CMAP amplitudes bilaterally with normal nerve conduction velocities bilaterally. H-reflex was unobtainable bilaterally. Table 6.9 shows the results of NCSs in Case 5.

Needle EMG revealed diffuse membrane irritability in L4–S1 distribution with increased amplitude of the MUAPs and decreased recruitment. NCSs revealed normal sensory responses and decreased CMAP amplitudes of the peroneal and tibial nerve. Findings were consistent with spinal stenosis involving L4–L5 and L5–S1.

LUMBOSACRAL SPINAL STENOSIS

Patients with lumbosacral stenosis most commonly present with buttock and bilateral lower limb pain, which is worse with standing and walking and is relieved by

Table 6.8 Results of Needle Electromyography in Case 5

Muscle (Right Lower Limb)	Root(s)	Insertional Activity	Spontaneous Activity	Number of MUAPs/ Amplitude and Duration
Adductor longus	L2, L3, L4	Normal	None	decr/incr
Vastus medialis	L2, L3, L4	Normal	None	decr/incr
Tensor fascia lata	L4, L5	Normal	Polyphasics	decr/incr
Anterior tibial	L4, L5	Few positive waves	2+Fibs	decr/incr
Peroneus longus	L5, S1	Few positive waves	2+Fibs	decr/incr
Extensor hallucis longus	L5, S1	Few positive waves	2+Fibs	decr/incr
Lateral gastrocnemius	S1, S2	Many positive waves	3+Fibs	decr/incr
Abductor hallucis	S1, S2	Many positive waves	3+Fibs	decr/incr
Biceps femoris	L5, S1, S2	Few positive waves	1+Fibs	decr/incr
Gluteus medius	L4, L5, S1	Normal	Polyphasics	decr/incr
Gluteus maximus	L5, S1, S2	Normal	Polyphasics	decr/incr
(Left Lower Limb)				
Adductor longus	L2, L3, L4	Normal	None	normal
Vastus medialis	L2, L3, L4	Normal	None	normal
Tensor fascia lata	L4, L5	Normal	None	normal
Anterior tibial	L4, L5	Few positive waves	1+Fibs	decr/incr
Peroneus longus	L5, S1	Few positive waves	1+Fibs	decr/incr
Extensor hallucis longus	L5, S1	Few positive waves	1+Fibs	decr/incr
Flexor digitorum longus	L5, S1	Few positive waves	2+Fibs	decr/incr
Lateral gastrocnemius	S1, S2	Few positive waves	2+Fibs	decr/incr
Abductor hallucis	S1, S2	Few positive waves	2+Fibs	decr/incr
Biceps femoris	L5, S1, S2	Normal	Polyphasics	decr/incr
Gluteus medius	L4, L5, S1	Normal	None	normal
Gluteus maximus	L5, S1, S2	Few positive waves	1+Fibs	decr/incr
Right and Left Lumbosacral Paraspinals	**Posterior Primary Rami**			
L1–L3	L1–L3	Normal	None	—
L4–S1	L4–S1	Few positive waves	Polyphasics 2+Fibs	—

decr/incr = decreased number of MUAPs with increased amplitude and duration; MUAP = motor unit action potential; nl/nl = normal; PSWs = positive sharp waves.

sitting or resting. Complaints of numbness or weakness in the legs are common. Walking is limited because of the preceding symptoms. The symptoms are typically made worse with trunk extension and improve with trunk flexion.

Lumbosacral spinal stenosis can cause a wide variety of EMG findings, ranging from normal to bilateral and severe changes. Bilateral multiple lumbosacral radiculopathies are found in approximately 50% of the patients with lumbosacral stenosis.[25] In approximately 20% of the patients, only a single root lesion is found, and in another 20% only limited abnormalities are seen that do not indicate a definite diagnosis. In the remaining patients, no EDX abnormalities are seen.[23]

Table 6.9 Results of Nerve Conduction Studies in Case 5

Nerve	Peak Latency (ms)	SNAP (μV)	Distal Latency (ms)	CMAP (mV)
Left sural	4.0	8	—	—
Right sural	3.9	5	—	—
Left peroneal (EDL)	—	—	—	1.5
Right peroneal (EDL)	—	—	—	1.3
Left tibial (medial gastrocnemius)	—	—	—	2.5
Right tibial (medial gastrocnemius)	—	—	—	2.0
Left H-reflex	—	—	no response	—
Right H-reflex	—	—	no response	—

CMAP = compound motor action potential amplitude; EDL = extensor digitorum longus; SNAP = sensory nerve action potential amplitude.

Dermatomal somatosensory evoked potentials (DSEPs) have been used to evaluate patients with lumbosacral spinal stenosis and may help at arriving at the diagnosis, although their use is still debated among electromyographers. In a study by Snowden et al.,[27] 58 patients with lumbosacral spinal stenosis based on imaging (computed tomography or magnetic resonance imaging) were evaluated with DSEPs (Figure 6.17). The DSEP studies had a 78% sensitivity and 93% predictive value of the anatomic studies positive for lumbosacral spinal stenosis when using multilevel root disease for criteria of the stenosis. When using single root disease as criteria for stenosis, the DSEP studies had a 93% sensitivity and a 94% predictive value. Further studies are needed before the use of DSEPs in patients with lumbosacral spinal stenosis is known.

Case 6

A 65-year-old white man presented with a history of severe right thigh pain, which began approximately 8 weeks ago. He complained of weakness in his right lower limb and had noticed significant atrophy of the thigh. The patient had a history of diabetes mellitus, which began 10 years ago, and was under poor control secondary to noncompliance. On physical examination, the patient had significant atrophy of the right thigh. He had decreased sensation to light touch in a glove and stocking distribution. Muscle strength testing revealed a 3/5 right knee extension and a 5/5 left knee extension. Hip adductors were a 4/5 on the right and a 5/5 on the left. Right ankle dorsiflexion was a 4/5, and left ankle dorsiflexion was a 5/5. Plantar flexion was 4/5 bilaterally. MSRs were normal in upper limbs bilaterally. Right knee jerk was absent and was diminished on the left. Ankle jerk reflex was diminished bilaterally. SLR was negative bilaterally at 90 degrees.

Needle EMG of the right lumbosacral paraspinals revealed diffuse membrane irritability, with the greatest involvement at L3 and L4. EMG of the left lumbosacral paraspinals was normal. Diffuse irritability was seen in muscles supplied by

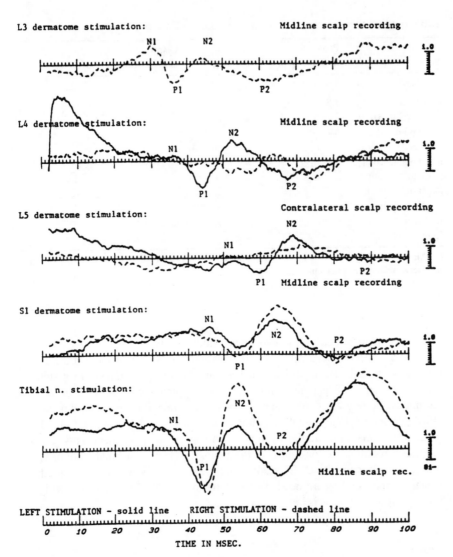

Figure 6.17 An abnormal dermatomal somatosensory evoked potential study of a 77-year-old woman with an 8-year history of bilateral buttock and lower extremity pain referred for spinal stenosis work-up. Scalp responses for lumbar levels L3 through S1 and tibial nerves shown with left stimulation by solid lines and right stimulation by dashed lines. Each waveform is a grand average of two or three trials. Peaks are labeled N1 (onset of P1), P1, N2, and P2. The time axis at the bottom is in ms, and the amplitude calibration on the right is in mV. (Reprinted with permission from ML Snowden, JK Haselkorn, GH Kraft, et al. Dermatomal somatosensory evoked potentials in the diagnosis of lumbosacral spinal stenosis: comparison with imaging studies. Muscle Nerve 1992;15:1038.)

L2, L3, and L4 on the right with no abnormalities seen in the same muscles on the left. There was mild irritability noted in the foot intrinsics bilaterally.

Table 6.10 shows the results of needle EMG in Case 6. Sensory NCSs of the sural were unobtainable bilaterally. Sensory studies of the median, ulnar, and radial nerve of the left upper limb revealed slowed peak latencies and conduction veloci-

Table 6.10 Results of Needle Electromyography in Case 6

Muscle (Right Lower Limb)	Root(s)	Peripheral Nerve	Membrane Irritability	Number of MUAPs/ Amplitude and Duration
Iliopsoas	L2, L3	Few positive waves	1+Fibs	decr/nl
Adductor longus	L2, L3, L4	Few positive waves	2+Fibs	few/mix
Vastus medialis	L2, L3, L4	Many positive waves	3+Fibs	few/mix
Tensor fascia lata	L4, L5	Few positive waves	1+ Fibs	decr/mix
Anterior tibial	L4, L5	Few positive waves	1+Fibs	decr/mix
Peroneus longus	L5, S1	Normal	None	nl/nl
Extensor hallucis longus	L5, S1	Normal	None	nl/nl
Flexor digitorum longus	L5, S1	Normal	None	nl/nl
Lateral gastrocnemius	S1, S2	Normal	None	nl/nl
Abductor hallucis	S1, S2	Few positive waves	None	decr/occ large
First dorsal interossei	S1, S2	Few positive waves	None	decr/occ large
Gluteus maximus	L5, S1, S2	Normal	None	nl/nl
Right Lumbosacral Paraspinals	**Posterior Primary Rami**			
T12–L1	T12–L1	Normal	None	—
L2	L2	Few positive waves	2+Fibs	—
L3–L4	L3–L4	Many positive waves	4+Fibs	—
L5	L5	Few positive waves	None	—
S1	S1	Normal	None	—
Left Lumbosacral Paraspinals	**Posterior Primary Rami**			
L1–S1	L1–S1	normal	none	—

decr/mix = decreased number of MUAPs with normal amplitude and duration and some with increased amplitude and duration; decr/nl = decreased number of MUAPs with normal amplitude and duration; decr/occ large = decreased number of MUAPs, of which some are of occasionally large amplitude and duration; few/mix = few MUAPs with normal amplitude and duration and some with increased amplitude and duration; nl/nl = normal; MUAPs = motor unit action potentials; PSWs = positive sharp waves.

ties, as well as decreased sensory nerve action potential amplitudes. Tibial and peroneal motor studies bilaterally also reveal slowed onset latencies and conduction velocities and decreased CMAP amplitudes. Median and ulnar motor studies of the right upper limb also displayed decreased CMAP amplitudes and slowed conduction velocities. L4 spinal stimulation recording over the vastus medialis showed a 75% decrease in amplitude on the right compared to the left. H-reflex was slowed bilaterally. Table 6.11 shows the results for NCSs in Case 6.

EMG revealed diffuse membrane irritability in an L2–L4 distribution on the right, as well as mild irritability in the foot intrinsics bilaterally. NCSs revealed mildly slowed conduction velocities and decreased amplitudes. EDX testing was consistent with a multilevel lumbar radiculopathy on the right involving L2, L3, and L4. There was also evidence of a mild peripheral neuropathy with both axonal and myelin damage. No other testing could have distinguished the multilevel radic-

Table 6.11 Results of Nerve Conduction Studies in Case 6

Nerve	Peak Latency (ms)	SNAP (µV)	Distal Latency (ms)	CMAP (mV)	NCV (m/s)
Left sural	No response	—	—	—	—
Right sural	No response	—	—	—	—
Left peroneal (EDB)	—	—	6.8	2.0	32
Right peroneal (EDB)	—	—	7.0	2.2	—
Left tibial (abductor hallucis)	—	—	7.1	2.5	31
Right tibial (abductor hallucis)	—	—	6.9	2.3	—
Left femoral	—	—	—	4.0	—
Right femoral	—	—	—	1.0	—
Left H-reflex	—	—	34.5	—	—
Right H-reflex	—	—	34.1	—	—

CMAP = compound motor action potential amplitude; EDB = extensor digitorum brevis; NCV = nerve conduction velocity; SNAP = sensory nerve action potential amplitude.

ulopathy in this patient. This is generally a self-limited condition, and should be treated symptomatically.

SUMMARY

Electrodiagnosis is an important tool in the diagnosis, prognosis, and management of lumbosacral radiculopathy. A skilled electromyographer is aware of early polyphasic motor units, can measure the recruitment interval, measures the H-reflex latency, and compares the CMAP of the involved nerve root to the contralateral leg. This allows the electromyographer to gain valuable information on a patient even before the traditional 3-week period after onset of symptoms. For example, in a patient who presents with 1-week history of foot drop, EDX testing can be performed to help determine if this is true weakness versus conduction block, which can affect the treatment plan. In cases in which the history and physical are equivocal, it will help in the diagnosis. Recognizing early polyphasics can lead to the diagnosis of an acute radiculopathy, which can be beneficial in cases of litigation involving a recent injury.

Electrodiagnosis is useful in evaluating a patient with suspected lumbosacral radiculopathy in the following situations:

1. When radiculopathy is suspected (after 7–10 days) to confirm the diagnosis, establish prognosis, and plan appropriate management.
2. When neurologic deficit is present on physical examination to determine degree of axonal death (after 7–10 days), which will affect how aggressive to be in the treatment plan (i.e., oral steroids versus epidural steroids).
3. Imaging studies show herniated nucleus pulposus, but neurologic deficit is unclear by physical examination. EDX testing will give you information of specific nerve root involvement and will help you know if the herniated nucleus pulposus is causing neurophysiologic dysfunction, and to what degree.
4. Imaging studies show multiple-level disk herniations.
5. Always before surgery to localize the affected nerve root and to establish the existing neurophysiologic deficit.

6. Recurrent radiculopathy or back injury after surgery to establish presence and degree of new compromise.
7. Most medicolegal cases to establish diagnosis and severity.

REFERENCES

1. Haldeman S, Shouka M, Robboy S. Computed tomography, electrodiagnostic, and clinical findings in chronic workers' compensation patients with back and leg pain. Spine 1988;13:345–350.
2. Johnson EW, Melvin JL. Value of electromyography in lumbar radiculopathy. Arch Phys Med Rehabil 1981;62:321–323.
3. Saal JA, Firtch W, Saal JS, et al. The value of somatosensory evoked potential testing for upper lumbar radiculopathy. A correlation of electrophysiologic and anatomic data. Spine 1992;17[Suppl6]:S133–137.
4. Tullberg T, Svansborg E, Isacsson J, et al. A Preoperative and postoperative study of the accuracy and value of electrodiagnosis in patients with lumbosacral disc herniation. Spine 1993;18:837–842.
5. Eisen A. Electrodiagnosis of Radiculopathies. In MJ Aminoff (ed), Neurologic Clinics: Symposium on Electrodiagnosis. Philadelphia: Saunders, 1985;3:495–510.
6. Haymaker W, Woodhall B. Peripheral Nerve Injuries. Philadelphia: Saunders, 1953.
7. Harrell G, Mead S. The problem of spasm in skeletal muscle. JAMA 1950;640–644.
8. Stein J, Baker E, Pine Z. Medial paraspinal muscle electromyography: techniques of examination. Arch Phys Med Rehabil 1993;74:497–500.
9. MacIntosh JE, Valencia S, Bogduk N, Monro RR. The morphology of the human lumbar multifidus. Clin Biom 1986;1:196–204.
10. Micheli LJ, Wood R. Back pain in young athletes: significant differences from adults in causes and patterns. Arch Pediatr Adolesc Med 1995;149:15–18.
11. Colachis SC, Pease WS, Johnson EW. Polyphasic motor unit action potentials in early radiculopathy: their presence and ephaptic transmission as an early hypothesis. Electromyogr Clin Neurophysiol 1992;32:27–33.
12. Braddom RI, Johnson EW. Standardization of H reflex and diagnostic use in S1 radiculopathy. Arch Phys Med Rehabil 1974;55:161–166.
13. Pease WS, Johnson EW, Charles M. Recruitment interval in L-5 radiculopathy: a preliminary report. Arch Phys Med Rehabil 1984;65:654.
14. Clairmont AC, Johnson EW. Evaluation of the Patient with Possible Radiculopathy. In Johnson EW, Pease WS (eds). Practical Electromyography (3rd ed). Baltimore: Williams & Wilkins, 1997;115–130.
15. Johnson EW, Fletcher FR. Lumbosacral radiculopathy. Review of 100 consecutive cases. Arch Phys Med Rehabil 1981;62:321–323.
16. Johnson EW. The positive wave (editorial). Am J Phys Med Rehabil 1997;76:261.
17. Chang CW, Lien IN. Spinal nerve stimulation in the diagnosis of lumbosacral radiculopathy. Am J Phys Med Rehabil 1990;69:318–322.
18. Colachis SC, Klejka JP, Shamir DY, et al. Amplitude of M responses. Side to side comparability. Am J Phys Med Rehabil 1993;72:19–22.
19. Felsenthal G. An overview of the clinical application of electromyography and nerve conduction techniques. Md State Med J 1982;31:60–62.
20. Aiello I, Rosati G, Serra G, et al. The diagnostic value of H-index in S1 root compression. J Neurol Neurosurg Psychiatry 1981;44:171.
21. Baylan SP, Yu J, Grant AE. H-reflex latency in relation to ankle jerk, electromyographic, myelographic, and surgical findings in back pain patients. Electromyogr Clin Neurophysiol 1981;21:201.
22. McHugh DJ, Reeser JC, Johnson EW. H reflex amplitude: effect of leg muscle activity. Am J Phys Med Rehabil 1997;76:185–187.
23. Pease WS, Lagattuta FP, Johnson EW. Spinal nerve stimulation in S1 radiculopathy. Am J Phys Med Rehabil 1990;69:77–80.

24. Pease WS, Kozakiewicz R, Johnson EW. Central loop of the H reflex: normal value and use in S1 radiculopathy. Am J Phys Med Rehabil 1997;76:182–184.
25. Wilbourn AJ, Aminoff MJ. AAEE minimonograph #32: the electrophysiologic examination in patients with radiculopathies. Muscle Nerve 1988;11:1099–1114.
26. Kraft GH. Fibrillation potential amplitude and muscle atrophy following peripheral nerve injury. Muscle Nerve 1990;13:814–821.
27. Snowden ML, Haselkorn JK, Kraft GH, et al. Dermatomal somatosensory evoked potentials in the diagnosis of lumbosacral spinal stenosis: Comparison with imaging studies. Muscle Nerve 1992;15:1036–1044.

PART III
Management and Treatment

Chapter 7

Medication Management of Low Back Pain: A Symptomatic Approach

David J. Tauben

Optimal medication management of back pain relies on attention to its symptomatic presentation. When complaints are associated with well-defined pathologic injury, or even when precise diagnosis may not be established, effective treatment can proceed. Such treatment requires familiarity with current models of pain pathophysiology—how particular symptoms are generated, and how they can be modified pharmacologically.

As in any medical or surgical specialty, symptoms of abnormal function determine treatment approach. To do this correctly, the physician and other providers must first understand how the normal and abnormal pain system works, then, if possible, define the cause of pain in a particular individual, and, finally, design specific drug strategies that favorably modify abnormal pain states. Current progress in pain research allows for treatment interventions that manage challenging clinical symptoms far more effectively than older traditional approaches. This chapter describes clinically useful characteristics of pain, defines common pain types, presents classic and current anatomy and pathophysiology, and outlines theoretical and research models of pain to provide the context of effective pharmacologic management of low back pain symptoms. With this background, optimal drug therapy follows, with the detailing of specific drugs by category, benefit and risk, mechanism of effect, and dose, and then with special review of opioid treatment issues. Quality management of acute and chronic back pain conditions depends on careful elicitation of symptoms, and proceeds rationally and effectively for primary care and subspecialty inpatient and outpatient settings when these symptoms are then heeded.

Because low back pain is the second most common presenting physical complaint in the primary care office,[1] followed only by upper respiratory symptoms, one may expect medication management of low back pain to be well defined and widely agreed on. However, this is not the case. A core curriculum in pain management has been published,[2] and a research-based quality assessment guideline for back pain management has been proposed,[3] although most established practitioners have, of course, individual treatment algorithms based on traditional clinical strategies, historic biases, personal training idiosyncrasies, and anecdotal clinical and life experiences. Although the art of medicine often can deliver effective and safe outcomes after this less-than-fully-scientific approach, continuing quality care requires that physicians, physician extenders, clinical support staff, insurance and regulatory systems, and patients themselves follow medication management practice guidelines based on the most currently accepted scientific principles.

DEFINITION OF PAIN

Pain has been defined best by the International Association for the Study of Pain as *an unpleasant sensory and emotional experience associated with actual or potential tissue damage or described in terms of such damage.*[4] The whole person context of the painful experience is presupposed by this formulation, recognizing at once both the pain sensation and the pain perception. Pain, then, is a biological event within an organism capable, by way of eons of evolutionary pressure, of responding to the injurious experience in an optimally adaptive fashion. Pain is a gift[5] that protects an organism from harm: injurious outcomes from this beneficent loss are seen in leprosy, and insensate peripheral and central neuropathies such as diabetes, spinal cord and nerve entrapment injuries, multiple sclerosis, and syphilis. Normal pain response helps the individual by minimizing exposure to harm. Pathologic pain occurs when the continuing presence of the pain experience no longer confers benefit.

ACUTE PAIN

Acute pain, or pain that occurs soon after an injury and lasts only during the affected tissue recovery time, typically is biologically useful, warns of impending tissue injury, and generally follows a well-defined, and usually predictable, pathoanatomic course.[6] Resolution is expected, and treatment responses are reliable. Although there are normal social and cultural contexts that modify an individual's response to injury, these do not ordinarily interfere with recovery. Regardless, acute pain still consists of a large measure of anxiety, often more than the nociceptive components of the actual injury. Medication management of acute pain requires a comprehensive grasp of how pain affects an individual at a receptor, a whole body, and even whole psychosocial system level.

CHRONIC PAIN

Chronic pain, or pain that persists for either an interval beyond which tissue healing is expected to occur or beyond an arbitrary term of 3–6 months, or continues after reasonable treatments have been unsuccessful,[7] is not biologically useful, and has poorly defined pathophysiologic mechanisms. There are evolving clinical methods that can predict the highest risk individuals who go on to a career of chronic pain.[8–10] Chronic pain management, particularly with opioids, challenges medical providers, patients, third party and disability payers, and regulatory agencies[11] so that often its complex solutions seem not only elusive, but adversarial.[12] At times, multidisciplinary consultation and, infrequently, pain clinic treatment is necessary. Although much published literature on this subject exists,[13–15] medication management in chronic pain remains an area of pathophysiologic uncertainty, and, therefore, clinical disagreement and confusion. Newer models of chronic pain pathophysiology can support and guide the clinician through these treatment challenges.

PAIN MEASUREMENT

Clinicians treating pain largely base their assessments on patients' reports of subjective symptoms. Particularly in chronic pain states, signs seen in acute pain are absent, and vegetative symptoms often predominate.[16] The visual analogue scale provides a relatively consistent measure of an individual patient's pattern of self-report, varying according to that given individual's response to treatment interventions.[17] A convenient and reproducible measuring instrument, the pocket-sized visual analogue scale, should be used frequently, before and after treatment interventions so that pain becomes the fourth vital sign.[18] Many well-known psychological tests can measure pain disorders with strongly associated psychological conditions, to score depression, and to rate disability.[10] No test, psychological or otherwise, can predict medication response, just as no diagnostic imaging study can predict a patient's pain.[19–22] So, the best strategy for management requires eliciting careful symptom history, and treatment is necessarily symptom guided.

PAIN TYPES

Pain symptoms can be categorized as either nociceptive, neuropathic, sympathetic, visceral, central, or psychofunctional. These definitions are essential to formulating a model for the clinical choice of medication (Table 7.1). Distinguishing peripheral sensory receptor activity at a site of tissue injury (nociceptive pain) from stimulation that is more purely neurologically derived (neuropathic pain) is a crucial component of evaluation. Within the category of neuropathic pain, somatosensory can be distinguished from sympathetic. Central pain invokes more complex central nervous system dysfunction, often spontaneous and autonomous, and generally involving many areas of the brain and spinal cord. Comorbid or even primary psychiatric disorders evoke psychofunctional conditions. Although diagnostic tests and clinical examination findings crucially assist these categorizations, symptoms still guide diagnosis and management.

Table 7.1 Types of Pain

Types	Characteristic Symptoms
Nociceptive	Aching
Neuropathic	Burning, shooting, hyperalgic
Sympathetic	Burning, with abnormal swelling, color, temperature, sweating
Visceral	Aching, squeezing, pressure, cramping
Central	Deep ache, burning, hyperalgic
Psychogenic	Wide variety of descriptions

PAIN PATHOPHYSIOLOGY

Classic pathophysiology is soundly based on the anatomic demonstration of peripheral sensory receptors, which typically respond to more than one stimulus modality, either mechanical, thermal, or chemical. Physical stimuli activate specific sensory fiber components of distinct size, myelination, and specialization, such as unmyelinated C-fibers or small myelinated A-delta fibers. Tissue injury triggers an inflammatory response, which then increases the magnitude of the reported pain response evoked by a given stimulus, producing hyperalgesia.[23] The response properties of primary afferent nociceptors are set by individual and cumulative previous stimuli, lowering the threshold for activation or becoming spontaneously active, producing continuous pain that outlasts the initial stimulus.[24] Amidst tissue inflammation, primary afferents also acquire noradrenergic sensitivity, which may lead to coupling between sympathetic and afferent neurons.[25] Entering the spinal cord, the afferent nerves collateralize via somatosensory pathways within the tracts of the dorsal horn, and then distribute via well-defined ascending afferent and descending efferent pathways (Figure 7.1).

Wall and Melzak's classic gate theory[26] celebrated its thirtieth anniversary with uncanny success at predicting complex higher-level modulatory central nervous system function that has been later demonstrated by neurophysiologists.[27] Interesting analogies in diverse fields such as paleontology, cognitive science, and even quantum mathematics, identify complex adaptive systems that also apply to neural plasticity models in pain networks.[28–30] The brain, as the biological organ that medical science attempts to treat, is a physical structure with complex histologic design that can be anatomically, neurochemically, and electrically described. Incomplete current understanding of its complex physiology should lessen restrictions on clinical treatment approaches when symptoms guide chosen therapies.

Chronic pain, particularly when active tissue injury is long resolved, presupposes failure of the central nervous system to successfully respond to some kinds of injuries in some individuals. The human brain, having evolved as an organ intrinsically required to adapt to novel problems, may (if not must) become diseased at times to produce a state of pathologic maladaption, or chronic pain illness. That phantom limb or failed surgical spine pain can occur requires a central nervous system built from an evolutionarily derived biological hardware capable of a situationally plastic functional outcome. Developments in pain research are laying the foundations for this more dynamic model. Research is setting the scientific basis for many newer models of pain pathophysiology, including neurogenic inflammation reverse events at the pain receptor level,[31] wide dynamic range dorsal horn interneuron windup events,[32] spinal cord intermodal and ephaptic crosstalk,[27] and thalamic and other wide-area central brain disturbances.[33] All of these mechanisms participate in the symptom clinicians attempt to modify when they prescribe a pain medicine. The popular lay literature has seen well-selected vignettes of chronic impairments, painful or otherwise, in easily understood and well-written pieces.[34–37]

Pain medications, through elicited patient history, report back to the clinician and aid their diagnosis and management. The altered response to pharmacologic tampering with specific components of the system can and should guide future clinical decision making. By listening to new and changed symptoms,[38] improved medication management follows. Even when diagnosis is elusive, systematic medication trials done with attentive symptom-based analysis of response can provide an outline for successful drug treatment. Additional and concurrent nonpharmaco-

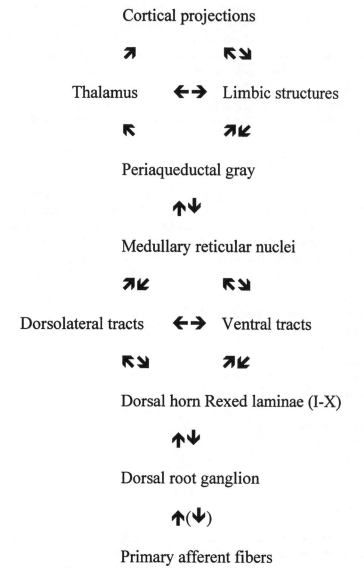

Cortical projections

Thalamus   ←→   Limbic structures

Periaqueductal gray

Medullary reticular nuclei

Dorsolateral tracts   ←→   Ventral tracts

Dorsal horn Rexed laminae (I-X)

Dorsal root ganglion

Primary afferent fibers

Figure 7.1 Ascending and descending pain modulatory network.

logic management further affects symptom presentation. Physical medicine strategies and psychologic interventions modify both assessment and response, and also must be carefully considered and observed throughout the full course of pain medicine treatment.

GOALS OF PAIN CONTROL

The goal of pain control is to relieve an individual's discomfort. This goal is the guiding principle of pharmacologic management of pain. When successful, improvement in functional status follows. Pain medicine thus enhances functional restoration programs for both acute and chronic pain problems. Adequate analgesia in acute care settings allows more rapid recovery by permitting more easily tolerated passive and active movement. Longer-term therapies, when effective, reduce chronic pain–induced complications, such as: global deconditioning; depression, including suicide; family, marital, and vocational dysfunction; and sleep deprivation and fatigue. Correct choice, dose, route, frequency, and time or symptom contingent dosing of pain medication dictates good practice. All of these decisions are better made within the context of a systematic review of the pharmacopoeia of pain medicines.

PAIN TREATMENT PHARMACOLOGY

Clinicians do best by categorizing pain drugs by pharmacologic class. This helps structure any treatment based on presenting symptom complex and by presumed pathophysiologic mechanism, or pain generator. Accurate categorization also avoids the commonly made error of duplication within drug type, and, hence, avoids needless toxicity. It also optimizes synergy of treatment as the layers of a painful complaint are revealed. The following is a list of categories of drugs:

- Acetaminophen
- Nonsteroidal anti-inflammatory drugs (NSAIDs)
- Corticosteroids
- Antidepressants
- Benzodiazepines
- Muscle relaxers
- Central agents
- Topicals
- Oral anesthetics
- Sympatholytics
- Opioids

Acetaminophen

Acetaminophen is the cheapest, safest, and most readily available effective analgesic. Its site and mechanism of action remains undetermined, with central nervous system inhibition of prostaglandin synthesis, but only minimal peripheral prostaglandin effect. Many patients may already be using this agent before presenting to the clinician, especially in chronic pain states. As a result, it is crucial to elicit all nonprescription agents that an individual may be taking, because toxicity to both liver and kidney is risked at dosages in excess of 4 g daily, particularly when alcohol is coadministered.[39]

Acetaminophen is also part of many combination opioid products, generally permitting them to remain a Drug Enforcement Administration schedule III or IV, rather than the more prescriptively cumbersome schedule II agent. Beware of toxicity of the acetaminophen component when repeated doses of these are required, such as acetaminophen with codeine (Tylenol #3), acetaminophen with hydrocodone (Vicoden, Lortab, or Norco), and acetaminophen with oxycodone (Percocet or Tylox). For instance, a fixed combination product with 500 mg acetaminophen taken two doses six times daily (vis. 2 tab q4h), accumulates a 6-g total daily acetaminophen dose, a potentially toxic routine exposure, particularly if the patient is self-supplementing 8 to 12 500-mg over-the-counter (OTC) extra-strength pain relievers (6 g already), and possibly consuming admitted recreational quantities of routine alcohol. By ascertaining all ingested prescribed and OTC agents, and calculating the total acetaminophen content, safe prescription of this important agent can be assured. Adding the OTC 500 mg product to a pure opioid regimen (i.e., morphine slow release) enhances the opioid analgesia and is an effective adjunct, as is historically done with liquid pain cocktails. Many clinicians periodically measure liver function and creatinine, and evaluate a urinalysis for protein or active sediment for any patient routinely on 4 g per day acetaminophen regimens, particularly if any other risk factors are present. If there are any abnormalities, a 24-hour creatinine clearance can be measured. Some patients, due to pre-existing analgesic nephropathy or idiosyncratic intolerance, present greater risk of complication from acetaminophen than from opioids. These patients should be identified and managed off acetaminophen, or they risk renal injury.

Nonsteroidal Anti-Inflammatories

Aspirin remains a gold-standard analgesic compound, although largely replaced by the ever-increasing armamentarium of nonselective NSAIDs and the newer cyclooxygenase selective (COX-2) drugs. The most widely purchased and prescribed category of analgesic, with more than 70 million prescriptions and more than 30 billion OTC tablets sold annually in the United States,[40] NSAIDs offer a variable degree of pain relief independent of their anti-inflammatory properties,[41] often somewhat idiosyncratically. Although there is no single predictor of patient response, the symptomatic presentation of predominantly nociceptive pain, certainly with any inflammatory characteristics such as swelling, warmth, erythema, with or without laboratory markers, such as elevated sedimentation rate or C-reactive protein, justifies a trial with one or, if needed, several sequential subcategories of NSAIDs. Table 7.2 presents most currently used agents, divided by pharmacologic category, listing typical and maximum dosage. Despite a hope by many clinicians that drugs in the same chemical class should share a similar benefit and side effect profile, this is not a consistent clinical practice finding. Therefore, familiarity with a number of agents from several classes is required for optimal care without presupposition of outcome until empirical trial.

Anti-inflammatories interfere with prostaglandin synthesis and cyclooxygenase (COX) activity (Figure 7.2). COX-1 regulates physiologic prostaglandin levels for normal cellular processes; COX-2 activity is induced by mediators of inflammation. Although all available NSAIDs share the property of COX inhibition, and bind to both COX-1 and COX-2, there is significant variation of selectivity.[42] New highly selective COX-2 inhibitors, celecoxib and rofecoxib, offer anti-inflammatory effect without disrupting the homeostatic local organ and tissue actions of prostaglandins and thromboxane, although still interfering with the induction of the inflammatory cascade. This may lessen their renal and gastrointestinal toxicity. Inhibition of lipoxygenase, leukotriene synthesis, lysosomal enzyme release, neutrophil aggregation, and suppression of rheumatoid factor production and other cell mediated activities contribute to additional effects. Which physiologic mechanism predominates for pain relief is not yet established because there is no direct correlation between anti-inflammatory potency and analgesic effect. Nabumetone may produce more potent anti-inflammatory effects than analgesia, for instance. Intracellular G-

Table 7.2 Nonsteroidal Anti-Inflammatory Drugs

Drugs	Interval	Maximum Daily Dose
Salicylates		
Aspirin	325 q4h	6,000 mg
Diflunisal (Dolobid)	250–500 q12h	1,500 mg
Salsalate (Disalcid)	500–1,000 q8–12h	3,000 mg
Magnesium salicylate (Doan's)	325–500 q4–6h	4,800 mg
Choline salicylate (Arthropan)	870/5 ml q4–6h	5,220 mg
Combinations (Trilisate)	500–1,000 q6–8h	3,000 mg
Pyrazolines		
Phenylbutazone	Rarely recommended due to toxicities	
Propionic Acids		
Fenoprofen (Nalfon)	200–600 q4–6h	3,200 mg
Flurbiprofen (Ansaid)	50–100 q6–12h	300 mg
Ibuprofen	200–800 q4–6h	3,200 mg
Ketoprofen (Orudis, Oruvail)	12.5–75 q6h	300 mg
Naproxen (Naprosyn, Anaprox)	220–550 q4–24h	1,500 mg
Oxaprozin (Daypro)	600–1,200 q24h	1,800 mg
Indoles		
Etodolac (Lodine, Lodine XL)	200–500 q6–12h	1,200 mg
Indomethacin	25–75 q8h	200 mg
Ketorolac (Toradol)	10 p.o. after 15–30 i.v. q6 × 5 days only	
Sulindac (Clinoril)	150–200 q12h	400 mg
Tolmetin (Tolectin)	200–600 q8h	2,000 mg
Fenamates		
Meclofenamate (Meclomen)	50–100 q4–8h	400 mg
Mefenamic Acid (Ponstel)	250 q6h	1,000 mg
Oxicams		
Piroxicam (Feldene)	10–20 q24h	20 mg
Phenylacetic Acids		
Diclofenac (Voltaren, Cataflam)	25–100 q6–24h	200 mg
Naphythylalkanones		
Nabumetone (Relafen)	500–750 1–2 q24h	2,000 mg
COX-2 Selective		
Celecoxib (Celebrex)	100–200 q12h	400 mg
Rofecoxib (Vioxx)	12.5–25 q12h	25 mg long term

protein signal disruption[43] and direct pain receptor inhibition, in part by inhibiting retrograde neurogenic inflammation, also participate in their analgesic effect.[44] Analgesia comparable to opioids has been demonstrated with parenterally administered ketorolac,[45] and oral ibuprofen has been shown to provide comparative analgesia to ketorolac in emergency room patients with acute musculoskeletal pain.[46] Prescribers should be aware, however, that like all NSAIDs, ketorolac can cause serious renal injury, particularly when volume depleted, and gastrointestinal injury even with only parenteral exposure.

Cell membrane phospholipase ➔ Arachadonic acid ➔Leukotrienes

⬇

Cyclooxygenase ⬅ Prostaglandin synthetase (COX)

↙   COX-1 (regulatory) variably inhibited by different nonsteroidal anti-inflammatory drugs

↙   COX-2 (inflammatory) induction inhibited by steroids and nonsteroidal anti-inflammatory drugs

Prostaglandin G2

⬇

Peroxidase   ➔ Prostaglandin H2 ➔ Prostaglandin synthesis

⬇⬇⬇

Prostacyclin ➔   Blood vessel

Thromboxane A2➔ Platelets

Prostaglandin E2➔ D2➔ Stomach, kidney

Prostaglandin F2➔ I2➔ Stomach, kidney

Figure 7.2 Prostaglandin production.

Side effects of NSAIDs are usually broadly shared among the full group, although with higher risk for some drugs. Ibuprofen, naproxen, and ketoprofen have been reported to have less gastrointestinal risk[47]; yet, even here there are wide variations of intolerance and adverse outcome. Dyspepsia, nausea, heartburn, bloating, or cramping are common, occurring in up to 25% of NSAID users.[48] Symptomatic ulcers, visible bleeding, or perforation ranges from 1% to 4%, depending on duration of therapy,[49] with epidemiologic evidence of 7.3 serious gastrointestinal side effects per 1,000 patients per year.[50] The estimated 16,500 annual U.S. number of NSAID-related deaths compares similarly with the 1997 mortality from acquired immunodeficiency syndrome, making it the fifteenth most common cause of death in the United States.[51] New COX-2 agents show significant reductions in endoscopic ulcer incidence—6–8% versus 17–35% in a variety of COX-1 agents[52,53]; however, because there has been serious clinically significant bleeding reported with coxibs, vigilance regarding gastrointestinal side effects should be maintained.

Treatment of NSAID-related dyspepsia and gastrointestinal ulcers should be both vigilant and, at times, preemptive. Use of histamine H_2-receptor antagonists may simply mask symptoms rather than protect against serious mucosal injury.[51] Proton-pump inhibitors may offer more effective prevention and treatment of NSAID-associated gastroduodenal ulcers.[54,55] Mucosal protection with sucralfate has no proven benefit. Misoprostol, a replacement prostaglandin, at doses of 200 μg four times daily reduces NSAID-associated ulcers by 40% compared to placebo,[56] but with its high incidence of nonulcer abdominal symptoms (e.g., bloating, diarrhea) and contraindication in any woman who might become pregnant has a somewhat limited clinical role. Arthrotec combines the NSAID, diclofenac, with misoprostol in a single formulation.

All category NSAID-induced renal injury can be significant and severe, particularly in volume-depleted postoperative circumstances and in the elderly or otherwise chronically ill medical patient. Ketorolac has such a significant risk that long-term administration beyond more than a week is not recommended. Many physicians routinely monitor renal function, including periodic measurement of creatinine clearance when abnormalities are suspected by history or screening studies.

Hepatic transaminases rise in a small number of cases, and clinical judgment is required to determine when significant enough to discontinue their use. When clinical benefits were previously demonstrated, rechallenge with the same or an alternative subcategory NSAID can be considered after an interval sufficient for either creatinine or liver function to recover, usually within 2–4 weeks. COX-2 drugs should be prescribed similarly. Severe idiosyncratic toxicities prompted bromfenac (Duracet), a COX-1 agent, to be recalled by the manufacturer after four deaths and eight liver transplants within 11 months on the market. Phenylbutazone is so poorly tolerated, with adverse effects on the gut, bone marrow, and kidney, so as to be rarely indicated, even for anti-inflammatory purposes; it is best avoided as an analgesic. Table 7.3 shows NSAID monitoring recommendations.

Anticoagulant side effects are based on the irreversible inhibition of platelet aggregation by acetylation of cyclooxygenase, preventing thromboxane A2 production. Acetyl-based agents, like aspirin, prolong bleeding time for the 7–10 day life of the platelet. Other nonacetylated NSAIDs disrupt platelet function less intensively and for shorter duration. Clinical trials have shown no COX-2 agent antiplatelet effect. They probably can be cautiously used in patients with coagulation defects or who are on rigorously monitored anticoagulant therapy. Older COX-1 agents are best avoided in patients with any form of coagulopathy. Celecoxib interacts less with warfarin dosing than rofecoxib, and both COX-2 drugs interact less than do all COX-1 drugs.

Drug interactions with NSAIDs include diminished antihypertensive effect of angiotensin-converting enzyme inhibitors, and reduced natriuretic response to furosemide and thiazides. Celecoxib plasma concentration is increased with concomitant fluconazole, and lithium levels rise with either coxib administered.

Corticosteroids

Corticosteroids are useful in acute traumatic or inflammatory settings, especially when a short course can aid in diagnosis by defining response, allowing a rapid taper, or later prompting a selective injection strategy. This is a useful approach to acute lumbar disk and facet symptoms, particularly when radicular pain or motor symptoms, or both, are present. Many rheumatologic disorders in which spine pain symptoms predominate respond favorably to a challenge with 40–60 mg oral prednisone. A commonly prescribed prepackaged methylprednisolone product (Medrol Dosepack, or generics) contains only 24 mg at peak, then tapers, perhaps an insufficient dose for some conditions that could respond to higher doses. A clear-cut

Table 7.3 Nonsteroidal Anti-Inflammatory Drug Monitoring Recommendations

Age (yr)	Use Pattern	Test	Frequency
20–60	Intermittent	Creatinine, U/A	Annual
	Regular low dose	Creatinine, AST, U/A	Twice yearly
	Regular high dose	Creatinine, AST, U/A	3× yearly
		Creatinine clearance	Every 2–3 years
60+	Intermittent	Creatinine, U/A	Annual
	Regular low dose	Creatinine, AST, U/A	3× yearly
	Regular high dose	CBC, creatinine, AST, U/A	Quarterly
		Creatinine clearance	Every 1–2 years

AST = aspartate amino transferase; CBC = complete blood cell count; U/A = urinalysis.

response can prompt a rheumatologic workup or referral. Caution must be exercised regarding both short- and long-term side effects. Short-term side effects include agitation, edema, gastrointestinal upset, sleep disorder, and glucose intolerance with marked hyperglycemia in some diabetics. Avascular necrosis is a catastrophic side effect, which can rarely occur, even with short-term use at high doses, probably in excess of 60–80 mg; therefore, some clinicians may pursue more complete informed consent regarding this side effect. Long-term more common side effects include promotion of accelerated osteoporosis, cataracts, weight gain, and myopathies. Corticosteroids also must be withdrawn slowly after daily use longer than several weeks. For patients on longer term treatments, increased dosage must be considered for other comorbid medically acute physiologic stress states. These compelling adverse outcomes with serious complications must be considered relative contraindications for anything but short-term corticosteroid use for primarily pain symptoms.

Antidepressants

Antidepressant agents are exceptionally effective medications in the management of both acute and chronic low back pain, in both nondepressed and depressed individuals. Up to 80% of patients without mental health disorders documented by an array of clinical tests report up to 50% reduction in pain when treated with a tricyclic antidepressant drug.[57,58] Depressed patients respond even better, due to improvement in both states. The predominant mechanism of analgesia from antidepressant drugs derives from their down-regulatory effect on descending inhibitory pain pathways above and within the spinal cord dorsal horn noradrenergic and serotonergic interneuron network.[59]

Many antidepressants provide sedation, helping and often immediately restoring normal sleep. Fatigue and dysphoria from sleep deprivation are more rapidly resolved than the usual 2–3 week delay encountered for measurable analgesic response, the typical response time also observed for their antidepressant effect. Many antidepressants can be activating, enhancing functional restoration efforts independent of mood effect. Selection of an antidepressant drug should carefully target medication to an historically elicited symptom. That is, an individual with disturbed sleep does well on a more sedating agent (e.g., amitriptyline, doxepin, or nefazodone), whereas those for whom sleep is less of a problem do better on a more stimulating agent (e.g., nortriptyline, desipramine, or venlafaxine.)

Table 7.4 lists antidepressant drugs by pharmacologic category and offers typical dosing ranges. Generally, one-half the usual antidepressant dosing is necessary to achieve analgesic effect. Patient size, age, and gender do not reliably predict therapeutic dosing, so periodic drug level monitoring remains an important guide to optimal tricyclic dose selection. Although some individuals respond idiosyncratically, mixed serotonin and noradrenergic agents seem to offer the best chance of clinical improvement.[57] Familiarity with the monoaminergic profile of antidepressant drugs is thus clinically relevant and important, as is anticipating their side effects. Predictable problems include anticholinergic (dry mouth, dry eye, visual accommodation difficulties, urinary retention, constipation, tachycardia), sedative or stimulant, and orthostatic side effects (Table 7.5). Weight gain is common with most tertiary and secondary amines (tricyclics) and tetracyclics. Sexual dysfunction in both men and women occurs in approximately 10% of selective serotonin reuptake inhibitor users. An electrocardiogram is indicated when higher dose ranges are required, and probably for all elderly patients and patients with underlying cardiac disease. Venlafaxine can raise blood pressure, so this should be monitored, particularly in patients predisposed by history of prior elevation. Nefazodone and venlafaxine both have modest incidences of nausea. Bupropion and nefazodone have the lowest incidences of sexual dysfunction. Of note is the tricyclic pharmacology of cyclobenzaprine (Flexeril), probably accounting for its historical use in low back pain management. Its antidepressant potency has not been studied, and it should not be coadministered with other tricyclics for fear of cumulative tricyclic toxicity, including arrhythmias. Tramadol, with both opioid and antidepressant monoaminergic receptor effects, is discussed later, in the section on opioids.

Benzodiazepines and Sedatives

Benzodiazepines are best limited to acute low back pain treatment and are largely contraindicated in chronic pain. A brief course (i.e., less than 2 or 3 weeks of sedative and antianxiety benefits) can be justified for acute sprain strain injuries and disk herniations. Longer treatment significantly complicates management by confounding depressant and habituating side effects. True skeletal muscle relaxation, not consistently demonstrated in clinical trials, is better accomplished by analgetically treating the pain that prompts the muscle pain symptom. Sleep aid can be more safely accomplished with tricyclic antidepressants, without potentially producing physiologic dependency and central nervous system depression. Zolpidem (Ambien) and zaleplon (Sonata) are nonbenzodiazepine hypnotics, probably modulating gamma-aminobutyric acid (GABA)-benzodiazepine receptors, useful for transient insomnia and probably does not lead to rebound insomnia even after chronic use. Zaleplon can be given to patients who awaken and cannot resume sleep, even as late as 3 AM without daytime sedation.

Certainly, in the setting of chronic pain, benzodiazepines and sedatives present significant pharmacologic impediments to ultimate recovery.[60] Tolerance; rebound sleep disturbance; exacerbated depression; confusion, particularly in the elderly; complicated withdrawal syndromes; and, in some cases, true addictive disorders restrict this category of treatment to a limited number of individuals who have established comorbid and psychiatrically confirmed diagnoses of panic or anxiety

Table 7.4 Antidepressant Drugs

	Typical Analgesic Dosage/Day (mg)
Tertiary amines	
Amitriptyline (Elavil)	10–150 qhs
Cyclobenzaprine (Flexeril)	10 t.i.d. or 10–20 qhs
Doxepin (Sinequan)	10–150 qhs
Imipramine (Tofranil)	10–150 qhs
Secondary amines	
Amoxapine (Asendin)	25–150 qhs
Desipramine (Norpramin)	10–50 b.i.d. or qhs
Nortriptyline (Aventyl, Pamelor)	10–100 qhs
Protriptyline (Vivactil)	5–10 up to q.i.d.
Tetracyclic compounds	
Maprotiline (Ludiomil)	25–75 usually qhs
Mirtazapine (Remeron)	15–60 qhs
Serotonin specific reuptake inhibitors	
Citalopram (Celexa)	10–60 qAM
Fluvoxamine (Luvox)	50–100 qhs
Fluoxetine (Prozac)	10–40 qAM
Paroxetine (Paxil)	10–40 qAM
Sertraline (Zoloft)	25–200 qAM
Cyclohexanol	
Venlafaxine (Effexor)	25–150 b.i.d. or qAM
Phenylpiperazine	
Trazodone (Desyrel)	25–300 qhs
Nefazodone (Serzone)	50–300 b.i.d. or qhs
Monocyclic	
Bupropion (Wellbutrin)	37.5–150.0 b.i.d.
Monoamine oxidase inhibitors	Rarely indicated
Isocarboxazid (Marplan)	
Phenelzine (Nardil)	
Tranylcypromine (Parnate)	
Mixed opioid effect	
Tramadol (Ultram)	50–100 q.i.d.

disorders, or both. Chronic insomnia may be treated more safely with zolpidem or zaleplon for longer courses than with other hypnotic drugs, particularly when other treatments fail to resolve this, at times, refractory problem. Guidelines have been provided that explicitly require a specific psychiatric diagnosis and treatment plan to support the use of benzodiazepine agents beyond a several-week course.[61] Many

Table 7.5 Relative Side Effects of Selected Antidepressants

Drug	Side Effects			Amine Uptake Profile	
	Sedation	Orthostasis	Anticholinergic	Noradrenaline	Serotonin
Amitriptyline	4+	2+	4+	2+	4+
Doxepin	3+	2+	2+	1+	2+
Imipramine	2+	3+	2+	2+	4+
Nortriptyline	2+	1+	2+	2+	3+
Desipramine	1+	1+	1+	4+	2+
Venlafaxine	0	0	0	3+	3+
Trazodone	2+	2+	1+	0	3+
Nefazodone	2+	1+	0/1+	0/1+	5+
Fluoxetine	0/1+	0/1+	0/1+	0/1+	5+
Paroxetine	0/1+	0	0	0/1+	5+
Sertraline	0/1+	0	0	0/1+	5+
Mirtazapine	3+	2+	2+	2+	4+
Bupropion	0	1+	2+	0/1+	0/1+

clinicians treating chronic pain, especially those in multidisciplinary pain centers, early in treatment withdraw patients off these drugs in a systematic fashion, by substituting a moderately long-acting agent, either as a scheduled fixed dose, or by prescribing the equivalent dosing in a blinded liquid pain cocktail, and then tapering by 10% decrements approximately weekly, or more rapidly if abstinence symptoms are to be anticipated and managed concurrently. Table 7.6 lists benzodiazepine agents by category, and Table 7.7 lists equipotency equivalencies, relevant for conversions and tapers, to avoid serious abstinence syndromes, the signs and symptoms of which are listed in Table 7.8.

Muscle Relaxers

Muscle relaxers are a mixed group of predominantly sedative drugs that have pharmacologic potential to modulate muscle stretch receptor response.[62] Whether the sedative, and, hence, mild anxiety relief, is the active clinical event, or any direct muscle stretch receptor effect provides benefit, remains largely undetermined. Because they span several groups, they differ in side effect potential. It is important also to recognize that muscle relaxers of the fenemate class (i.e., carisoprodol) share many of the benzodiazepine cautions, including major withdrawal and psychological dependencies[63]; they are best avoided except short term for acute low back sprains and strains. Again, the inclusion of the tricyclic agent cyclobenzaprine (Flexeril) in this category reinforces the clinical observation that tricyclic antidepressants as a group have substantial analgesic and antianxiety benefits, thereby producing secondary muscle relaxant effects. Coadministration of cyclobenzaprine with other tricyclics should be avoided, and caution should be exercised when prescribed to the elderly or those with comorbid cardiac conditions. Exceeding the recommended 24-hour dose limit of 30 mg of cyclobenzaprine also risks significant tricyclic toxicity. Muscle relaxer side effects include sedation, depression, anticholinergic and auto-

Table 7.6 Benzodiazepines

	Usual Dosage (mg)
Short acting	
Alprazolam (Xanax)	0.25–1.0 t.i.d.
Estazolam (ProSom)	1–2 qhs
Lorazepam (Ativan)	0.5–1.0 t.i.d.
Oxazepam (Serax)	10–30 qhs
Quazepam (Doral)	7.5–15.0 qhs
Triazolam (Halcion)	0.125–0.5 qhs
Long acting	
Chlordiazepoxide (Librium)	5–25 q.i.d.
Clorazepate (Tranxene)	3.75–7.5 b.i.d.
Clonazepam (Klonopin)	0.5–1.0 b.i.d.
Diazepam (Valium)	2.5–5.0 b.i.d.
Prazepam (Centrax)	5–10 qhs
Temazepam (Restoril)	15–30 qhs

nomic side effects, and potential for withdrawal and dependency in the fenemate group. Table 7.9 lists muscle relaxers by category and standard dose ranges.

Anticonvulsants and Central Agents

Anticonvulsants and other central agents probably reduce pain by the same mechanisms that underlie their anticonvulsant actions, suppression of paroxysmal discharges, neuronal hyperexcitability, or spread of abnormal discharges,[64] and by blocking voltage-dependent sodium channels. Their benefits are seen chiefly in neuropathic pain conditions, such as radicular pain after impingement injuries. Table 7.10 lists these agents. Rarely recommended immediately after injury, they are useful in chronic management of especially lancinating, but also burning, stinging, hyperalgic, and allodynic symptoms. Antihistamines offer sedation and may augment analgesia from other drug categories, and, importantly, reduce nausea related to opioids. Antipsychotic drugs are now rarely prescribed for pain, in part because of their serious long-term dyskinesia toxicities and because of superior efficacy of other central category agents.

Table 7.7 Sedative Hypnotic Equivalent Dosage

Butalbital (in Fiorinal, Fioricet)	100 mg
Carisoprodol (Soma)	350 mg
Chlordiazepoxide (Librium)	25 mg
Diazepam (Valium)	10 mg
Meprobamate (Equanil)	400 mg
Phenobarbital	30 mg
Whiskey	3–4 oz

Table 7.8 Sedative Hypnotic Abstinence Symptoms

Hypertension, often severe
Orthostatic hypotension, often severe
Fever
Tachycardia
Tremor
Organic delirium with confabulation and hallucinosis
Seizures

Anticonvulsants have a long history of effective use in the management of neuropathic pain, such as diphenylhydantoin for peripheral neuropathies and carbamazepine for tic doloreaux. There is little literature that addresses their role in radiculopathic pain, and they are not frequently used for this indication, although they can be considered. Carbamazepine has unique hepatic and bone marrow toxicity, and these risks require regular monitoring, although the rare aplastic anemia presents typically without warning, and routine but stable reduction in hematologic parameters is generally the rule. At times, carbamazepine causes clinically important disturbances of lipid metabolism, and, when occurring, cholesterol should be monitored.

Gabapentin, structurally related to GABA, but without known GABA receptor interactions, is gaining wide use as an antiseizure drug of choice in the management of neuropathic pain. It can be quite effective in a wide dose range, and enjoys low toxicity, absent blood monitoring requirements and minimal drug-to-drug interactions. Idiosyncratic sensitivity to its sedation side effects can be problematic, because analgesic benefits generally are not seen in doses below 1,800 mg divided per 24 hours, with rare patients requiring and tolerating doses up to 6,000 mg.

Table 7.9 Muscle Relaxants

	Typical Dosage
Sedative hypnotics	
Barbiturates/butalbital combinations (Fiorinal, Fioricet)	50 mg/tab q.d.–q.i.d.
Benzodiazepines (i.e., Valium)	2–10 mg t.i.d.
Tricyclics	
Cyclobenzaprine (Flexeril)	10 mg t.i.d. or 10–30 qhs
Carbamates	
Carisoprodol (Soma)	350 mg t.i.d.
Meprobamate (Equanil, Miltown, Robaxisal)	200 mg t.i.d.
Other centrally acting	
Baclofen (Lioresal)	10–20 mg q.i.d.
Chlorzoxazone (Parafon)	250–500 mg t.i.d.
Metaxalone (Skelaxin)	400 mg t.i.d.-q.i.d.
Methocarbamol (Robaxin)	750–1,000 mg q.i.d.
Orphenadrine (Norflex, Norgesic, Banflex)	100 mg b.i.d.
Tizanidine (Zanaflex)	1–4 mg t.i.d.
Peripherally acting	
Dantrolene (Dantrium)	25–50 mg up to q.i.d.

Table 7.10 Centrally Acting Drugs

	Typical Dosage
Anticonvulsants	
Carbamazepine (Tegretol)	50–200 mg up to t.i.d.
Gabapentin (Neurontin)	100–2,000 mg up to t.i.d.
Phenytoin (Dilantin)	100 mg t.i.d. or 300 mg qhs
Valproic Acid (Depakene, Depakote)	125–500 mg t.i.d.
Antipsychotics	
Phenothiazines (Fluphenazine, et al.)	Used rarely
Butyrophenones (Droperidol)	For nausea, 0.625–1.25 mg i.v.
Antihistaminics	
Diphenhydramine (Benadryl)	25–50 mg up to q.i.d.
Phenothiazines (Phenergan)	25–50 mg up to q.i.d.
Piperazines (hydroxyzine: Vistaril)	25–50 mg up to q.i.d.

Topical Analgesics

Topical analgesics are of only limited benefit in the management of low back pain, and can be prescribed when local tissue sensitivity predominates or triggers a myofacial response. Capsaicin induces a burning counter-stimulant when applied, possibly through interference with Substance P pain pathways.[65] Topical salicylates (Aspercreme or Panalgesic) interact with local tissue prostaglandin mechanisms. Topical lidocaine products, such as EMLA cream or Lidoderm, are useful only in neuropathic pain localized to limited areas, and are rarely effective for relief of low back pain symptoms.

Mexiletine

The oral local anesthetic mexiletine, an antiarrhythmic derivative of lidocaine, has been found effective at managing a number of neuropathic pain conditions, and could be considered an adjuvant in the management of refractory radicular pain. Some experts recommend a monitored intravenous lidocaine infusion before instituting an oral treatment trial.[66] Proceeding directly to a clinical trial is more convenient, but may take several weeks to define a negative response. Significant proarrhythmic complications can occur with any class 1A antiarrhythmic, an issue for anyone with ischemic heart disease or predisposed to arrhythmias due to intrinsic conduction system disease. In such cases, it is either best to avoid use of this only occasionally effective agent, or to pursue inpatient monitoring while the drug is being introduced. Patients who may be candidates for such an approach are best studied by intravenous lidocaine protocol before adding this agent.

Sympathetic Agents

Rarely, low back pain presents with neuropathic symptoms that include sympathetically mediated pain in the involved extremity. Burning pain, abnormal sudomotor responses, altered temperature response, and edema are characteristic presentations of abnormal sympathetic nervous system participation in the pain symptomatology. Sympathetically mediated symptoms, when present, can justify trials with sympathetically active agents such as phenoxybenzamine, clonidine, prazosin, and, at times, by calcium channel blockers such as nifedipine.[64] Gabapentin may also be tried in these circumstances, although often treatment is refractory to any single category of drug, and best outcome is achieved with a number of drug- and activity-based therapies.

Opioids

Opioids are potent analgesics, generally lessening pain in most back pain disorders, yet remain controversial for all but acute low back injuries. Different opioid drugs interact with different chords of opioid receptor subtype to produce their unique analgesic and side effect profiles, which can idiosyncratically lead to a wide range of individual clinical responses. Mu receptor analgesia is the predominant desired pharmacologic response. However, individual patient benefits can be seen with other receptor emphasis, although adverse side effects seem to be the rule with kappa specific profiles. Table 7.11 lists opioid receptor subtypes and typical side effects. Table 7.12 lists opioids by receptor effects. Sigma receptors are no longer considered to be of opioid class. *N*-methyl-D-aspartate (NMDA) receptors interact with opioid receptors, and although NMDA receptors are nonopioid, they are bound by the opioids dextromethorphan and pentazocine.[67] Table 7.13 groups opioids by dose, route, and dosage interval. Table 7.14 lists opioids by equianalgesic dosing. Shared category toxicities can be expected: sedation; acute respiratory suppression; nausea; constipation; anticholinergic responses (dry mouth, urinary retention, orthostatic hypotension); and withdrawal on abstinence after prolonged period of administration (usually 4–6 weeks of regularly maintained blood levels). Occasionally, pruritus occurs, and, because it is usually a direct cutaneous mast cell effect rather than a generalized allergic problem, it can be managed with antihistamines.

Although waning effect, or tolerance, to dose and side effect is seen acutely, long-term management should not require indefinite dose escalations to achieve satisfactory pain relief. In fact, unlimited prescribed dose increases are often predictors of poor responsiveness, and, hence, adverse outcome with longer term use. The anticipated dose increases seen in management of cancer and acquired immunodeficiency syndrome–related pain reflects progressive and malignant tissue injury, because those patients with stable disease remain at level plateaus until objective disease progression is otherwise clinically evident. Peak analgesic dose ranges for a representative group of opioids is seen in Table 7.15, which gives the upper-end ranges typically encountered in the management of even long-term nonmalignant pain. Significant variance beyond these doses is encountered infrequently, at times prompting second diagnostic and, occasionally, addiction consultations to assure they are clinically appropriate.

Despite apparent benefit from opioids in many clinical presentations of acute low back pain, with and without radiculopathy, controversy remains. For instance, the Agency for Health Care Policy and Research low back pain guideline, with its dependence on prospective studies to validate recommended use, specifically advises against the use of opioids in acute back pain management.[3] In fact, most pain experts, and certainly most clinicians, prescribe opioids safely and effectively for this common complaint. Many clinical presentations do, however, best without

Table 7.11 Opioid Receptor Effects

Mu	Kappa	Delta
Analgesia	Analgesia	No analgesia
Apnea	Apnea	Apnea
Indifference	Sedation	Nausea
Miosis	Miosis	Pruritus
Nausea	Diuresis	Tolerance
Constipation	No tolerance	
Urinary retention		
Pruritus		
Tolerance		

opioids, particularly myofascial pain without underlying injury and fibromyalgia (see the section Myofascial Pain Management).

Inpatient Opioid Use

Patients with acute low back pain do not typically require hospitalization for uncontrolled pain, but more commonly for other related or unrelated medical or surgical conditions. Opioid use in hospitalized patients is managed differently than in the outpatient setting. Intravenous continuous and intermittent delivery systems, a tightly controlled setting, and high intensity of service require familiarity with a parenteral formulary, skill at selecting dosing schedule and route, and ability to convert any effective regime into an outpatient strategy. Use of intramuscular injections offers no advantage over intravenous administration, because punitive injections play no role in controlling intake. Patient-controlled analgesia pumps can deliver smaller dose increments more frequently on demand, and can be set to provide basal infusion for opioid-tolerant individuals or for nighttime intervals to promote undisturbed sleep. Transition from parenteral to oral agents can be done with relative ease in this controlled environment, using long half-life slow release products in those for whom more prolonged prescribing is necessary. Short-acting oral opioids are used when discontinuation of the drug is expected shortly after discharge, or for bolus peak dosing of incident pain superimposed on basal sustained release formulations.

Table 7.12 Opioid Receptor Interactions

Drug	Mu	Kappa	Delta
Morphine	3+	1+	2+
Fentanyl	4+	1+	1+
Meperidine	2+	—	2+
Hydromorphone	3+	—	2+
Methadone	3+	—	2+
Pentazocine	—	3+	?

1+ = minimal; 2+ = mild; 3+ = moderate; 4+ = marked; — = no effect, ? = undetermined.

Table 7.13 Opioids

	Typical Dosage/Typical Interval
Agonists	
Short acting low/moderate potency	
Codeine	30–60 mg q3–4h
Propoxyphene (Darvon)	65-200 mg q4–6h
Hydrocodone (Vicodin, Norco, Lortab)	5–10 mg q4–6h
Tramadol (Ultram)	50–100 mg q6h
Short acting high potency	
Hydromorphone (Dilaudid)	p.o.: 1–4 mg q4h
	i.v.: 0.25–2.0 mg q3h
Meperidine (Demerol)	p.o.: 50–300 mg q2–3h
	i.v.: 50–150 mg q2–3h
Morphine	p.o.: 10–60 mg q4h
	i.v.: 5–15 mg q3–6h
Oxycodone (Percodan, Percocet, Tylox)	p.o.: 5–15 mg q3–4h
Long-acting high potency	
Levorphanol (Levo-Dromoran)	p.o.: 2–4 mg q6h
Methadone	p.o.: 5–20 mg q6h
Sustained release morphine (i.e., MS Contin)	p.o.: 15–60 mg q8–12h
Sustained release oxycodone (Oxycontin)	p.o.: 10-40 mg q8–12h
Transdermal fentanyl (Duragesic)	Topically: 25–150 mcq q72h
Agonist–antagonist	
Short acting (**All rarely recommended**)	
Pentazocine (Talwin)	p.o.: 50 mg q6h
Butorphanol (Stadol)	Nasal/i.m./i.v. 1 mg q4h
Nalbuphine (Nubain)	i.m./i.v. 5–10 mg q3h
Buprenorphine (Buprenex)	i.m./i.v. 0.3–0.6 mg q4–6h

Outpatient Opioid Use

Most acute low back pain, of course, is managed in the outpatient setting. In the outpatient setting, opioid use requires patient compliance and medical record documentation that facilitates and supports such care. It also demands prescriber expertise. Familiarity with several opioid agents of differing duration of action is necessary, due to both idiosyncratic patient intolerance, as well as anticipated short-term side effects.

Hydrocodone has an analgesic duration of 4–6 hours, and a relatively low incidence of nausea. Codeine's duration of effect is a bit shorter, and it may cause more nausea. Hydromorphone may have the least associated nausea of all oral and parenteral products, but is a Drug Enforcement Administration schedule II agent, requiring more regulatory precautions for its prescription. Immediate-release oxycodone offers a higher potency 4–6 hour opioid effect, with or without admixed acetaminophen (all formulations schedule II). Delayed release oral formulations of oxycodone and morphine facilitate smoother dosing in long-term and higher-dose circumstances. Pharmacokinetically, long-acting levorphanol offers analgesia of 6 or more hours, and methadone has an analgesic effect of up to 8 hours, shorter lived than its 24–48 hour antiwithdrawal and sedative effects. Long-acting agents can

Table 7.14 Opioid Equianalgesic Dosage (Compared to Morphine)

Morphine	i.v. = 1
	p.o = 3–6
Codeine	p.o. = 30
Hydrocodone	p.o. = 5
Hydromorphone	i.v. = 0.1–0.2
	p.o. = 0.2–0.4
Oxycodone	p.o. = 3
Levorphanol	p.o. = 0.2
Methadone	p.o. = 0.8–1.0
Propoxyphene	p.o. = 3.2–6.5
Meperidine	i.v. = 7.5–10.0
	p.o. = 20–30
Fentanyl	Topical = 1.5–1.8

take up to 24–96 hours, usually four times their half-lives, to reach equilibrium state when their full analgesic effect can then be determined. This delay can reduce benefits, because adverse side effects also persist for longer duration than with short-acting or delivery system–delayed products. Topical fentanyl patches may be associated with less nausea, and are typically reserved for long-term steady-state opioid management strategies, because several days are required to build skin depot availability and because less costly and more flexible alternative oral products are available. Managing chronic low back pain with long-term opioid dosing is better done by converting short duration agents into time-contingent long-acting alternatives as needed. This management smooths the analgesic effect, much like a parenteral patient controlled analgesia system, and lessens between dose withdrawal symptoms that can confuse symptom presentation.

Tramadol has low affinity binding with mu receptors, hence, it is an opioid. Tramadol also inhibits both serotonin and noradrenergic reuptake, synergistically providing an antidepressant-like analgesia. This unique pharmacodynamic, although lessening abuse potential, does not fully avert both psychological and physiologic dependency.[68] It has no anti-inflammatory effects. It offers some monoaminergic advantage in combination with other opioid mu receptor agents. At full dose, there is a low but potential risk of seizures when mixed with other antidepressant agents. Its predominant side effects are dizziness, nausea, constipation, headache, and somnolence. Although more expensive than an equianalgesic prescription of codeine plus nortriptyline, its unique role is for patients with chronic low back pain who risk abuse with long term opioids or who cannot tolerate other less costly alternatives.

Table 7.15 Typical Maximum Daily Opioid Doses in Chronic Nonmalignant Pain

Sustained release morphine	90–240 mg
Sustained release oxycodone	120–240 mg
Methadone	60–120 mg
Topical fentanyl	50–100 µg

Tolerance

Tolerance, an expected biological event, describes the subcellular modifications requiring an increased dose to achieve a physiologic effect previously seen at lower doses. Tolerance routinely occurs with benzodiazepines and opioids when continuous treatment duration exceeds several weeks. It is not seen with antidepressants, anticonvulsants, and NSAIDs. Muscle relaxants of the fenemate class (e.g., carisoprodol) exhibit some degree of clinical tolerance. Tolerance to the opioid side effects of sedation and respiratory depression develops much more rapidly than to its analgesic effects, as quickly as several days, permitting rapid dose escalations that may be required for therapeutic efficacy. Tolerance to opioid-related constipation typically never develops, requiring concomitant stimulant (not just bulk type fiber) laxative use. Autonomic side effects to opioids wane at varying rates, somewhat idiosyncratically and often incompletely. Development of tolerance is not indicative of addiction, it is an expected biological event.

Abstinence syndromes, the adverse physiologic feeling experienced on abrupt discontinuation off opioids and benzodiazepines after their continuous use for longer than 4–6 weeks, is also not indicative of addiction. Opioid abstinence is never life threatening, although certainly uncomfortable, due to muscle pain and large motor myoclonus (literally, kicking the habit) and heightened back pain symptoms (Table 7.16). Benzodiazepine withdrawal, on the other hand, has the potential to be serious, with abstinence causing seizures, hallucinations, and major autonomic derangement, including severe hypertension, and even death from status epilepticus, arrhythmias, and vasomotor instability (see Table 7.8). Withdrawal off antidepressants may also be seen, usually as mild dysphoria and sleep disturbance, although generally not a significant clinical problem, less so when tapered over 7–10 days. Serious abstinence syndrome, including delirium tremens, can occur with discontinuation off fenemate sedatives.

Tapering schedules that reduce benzodiazepines and sedatives by 10% every 5–7 days are generally safe, although less hurried withdrawal is better tolerated in the more dynamic outpatient setting. Reductions of up to 25% every 3–5 days can be accomplished with opioids, again with less rapid schedules better tolerated. Often, clonidine, a centrally acting α_2-adrenergic agonist, prescribed as its topical long-acting formulation with or without its short-acting oral tablet (i.e., *Catapress TTS-1 or -2*, with prn clonidine 0.1 q4–8h, watching for orthostatic hypotension, tachycardia, and anticipating dry mouth) is effective because of its locus ceruleus action, because many autonomic components of opioid withdrawal may arise from this central brain structure.[69] Liquid pain cocktails, which substitute short-acting opioids with long-acting methadone and replace tablet form benzodiazepines with more flexibly dosed liquid diazepam, may be useful to blind the dose reductions and smooth the pharmacokinetically by fractional decrements not possible with available oral preparations. Incomplete cross-tolerance may be seen with both opioid and benzodiazepine conversions and should be anticipated to some degree. Tablet form methadone has a long history of effectiveness because of its pharmacologically prolonged half-life, as has the benzodiazepine chlordiazepoxide, because of its biologically active prolonged metabolites. Slow-release oral delivery products can also be titrated down more easily because these formulations effectively deliver short-acting morphine (MS Contin) or oxycodone (Oxycontin) at controlled slow rates.

Most low back pain patients are withdrawn, or detoxified, in the usual outpatient setting by the physician pharmacologically treating the low back pain problem. Multidisciplinary consultation can be sought when a psychiatric diagnosis or addic-

Table 7.16 Opioid Abstinence Symptoms

"Kicking the habit," myoclonic jerking
Abdominal cramps
Diarrhea
Sweats
Lacrimation
Sneezing
Yawning
Piloerection
Sleep disturbance
Dysphoric mood
Heightened back pain symptoms

tion, or both, is a comorbid condition. Prescription of opioids for the sole purpose of managing a substance abuse problem requires federal Drug Enforcement Agency licensing as a special drug treatment program, and should never be attempted except in that context. Prescription of opioids, even primarily on a detoxification schedule, if done in the context of low back pain management, is legal and medically appropriate low back pain care. Some patients with prolonged opioid or benzodiazepine use, or both, who are not experiencing addictive illness require inpatient hospital settings to withdraw off these agents, in which benzodiazepines represent the more challenging agent to eliminate. This treatment approach is most effectively done in a dedicated multidisciplinary pain unit, instead of drug and alcohol abuse programs, because substance abuse settings are designed to diagnose and manage addiction disorders, not patients iatrogenically dependent on physiologically habituating agents in the course of their low back pain management.

Addiction

Addiction is drug abuse, an occasional accompaniment to both acute and chronic low back pain problems. Symptoms and signs of addiction must be heeded, and are listed in Table 7.17.

Risk of addiction is reinforced by euphoria or by neglect of other life difficulties while medicated with an opioid. Past history of alcoholism or other addictions is an important risk factor, although not an absolute contraindication for acute or chronic opioid use. Family history of addiction may also increase a patient's own personal risk. Ongoing cigarette use may also predict addictive risk.[70] A well-defined treatment duration, agreed on in advance and based on anticipated routine clinical outcome experience, is particularly helpful when treating active addicts, or for those in recent recovery. Incidence of addiction in the general population is estimated to be between 5% to 16% of the general population,[71] so prevalence among pain patients can be assumed to be at least this high. However, prescription of opioids for appropriate conditions, at appropriate dose, for an appropriate duration does not produce addictive outcomes in the vast majority of cases. The incidence of iatrogenic addiction in hospitalized patients receiving opioids in older studies has been a remarkably rare 4 of 11,882[72]; whereas a study of 2,002 consecutive admits to Johns Hopkins Medical Center detected a 19–25% incidence of alcoholism on neurology, general surgery, and medical services.[73]

Pseudoaddiction

Pseudoaddiction, excessive concern about acquisition, including manipulation and other deceits, can be seen when a patient has benefited from, but is insufficiently treated with, opioids. These patients can behave like addicts until they are properly diagnosed and treated with adequate analgesics. Often, previously disturbing patterns of use dramatically resolve with stable and reliable opioid management strategies.

Opioids for Chronic Pain

Opioids as a long-term palliative treatment of chronic low back pain remains controversial. There are a number of excellent reviews of the subject offering a diverse range of opinion regarding chronic opioids in the management of nonmalignant chronic pain.[74–76] Several state regulatory agencies have actively participated in the published production of appropriate guidelines for treating with chronic opioids, theoretically reducing prescriber risk of sanctions, but not always their fears of sanction.[77,78] Standard quality care strategies practiced in the management of other chronic medical conditions also using agents capable of serious adverse events should be followed. Proper treatment requires completely obtained and recorded history and appropriately directed examination; careful and ongoing documentation of efficacy; regular review of adverse effect; diagnosis and management of comorbid depression; and attention to functional outcome measures. Reasonable efforts to find alternative nonopioid treatments should have been unsuccessful due to documented poor efficacy, intolerance, or unacceptable risk. Time-contingent long-acting dosing, occasionally with as needed short acting agents for incident pain flares, is recommended. Alterations in clinical course or changes in "clinical tempo" merit systematic reevaluation, because new conditions may supervene. Consultants' recommendations should be duly noted in the medical record, and significant variance from their advice, solicited or otherwise, should be supported by differing clinical evidence and documented in the patient's medical record. Regular visits for follow-

Table 7.17 Addiction: Symptoms and Signs

Symptoms
    Intense desire for the drug of choice
    Overwhelming concern about a drug's availability
    Inability to control intake
    Compulsive use despite adverse physical, psychosocial consequences
    Drug euphoria
    Drug used to treat other symptoms, i.e., depression, sleep disorders, other medical conditions
      for which opioids were not advised
Signs
    Use during periods of reduced symptoms
    Acquisition of a drug from nonmedical sources or by manipulation
    Unsanctioned dose escalation
    Drug hoarding
    Unapproved concurrent use of unsanctioned drugs (i.e., alcohol, marijuana, and other illicits)

up evaluation and refills should occur, and only one provider should write for any and all analgesics. Evidence of abuse, misuse, or addictive behavior prompts immediate discontinuation after taper ideally with addiction medicine consultation or referral to a substance abuse treatment program.

DRUG SELECTION STRATEGY

The typical clinical presentations of low back pain, with and without radiculopathy, can be pharmacologically managed with a variety of agents once adequately diagnosed and primary symptoms are assessed. There can be no understating the importance of a detailed systematic review of a particular patient's unique presenting complaints. Questions regarding intensity and character of pain, presence or absence of neuropathic symptoms, associated sleep and mood disorders, and past responsiveness to previously offered prescriptive remedies are essential to proper management. Understanding particular pain mechanisms involved in the given clinical situation guides prescriptive choice. For example, acute or subacute diskogenic or facet pain syndromes more often respond to NSAIDs than do myofascial, neuropathic, or central pain processes. Back pain of fibromyalgia does not respond to the same drug treatment regimes as the back pain of traumatic, repetitive, or degenerative injury. Pain complaints when associated with psychologic conditions, such as depression or even somatization, respond to different drug strategies and interventions than do less complicated presentations.

Drug Management of Low Back Pain

A symptom-guided approach to uncomplicated low back sprain or strain, often involving acute nociceptive injury to disk, facet, and ligamentous structures, merits a trial with an NSAID agent. If gastrointestinal intolerance is a problem, then concurrent treatment with either a prescriptive strength H_2-blocking antiulcer agent, such as cimetidine, or a proton pump inhibitor, such as omeprazole, is worth trying. Alternatively, misoprostol, either alone or as the combination NSAID product with diclofenac, Arthrotec, can be attempted. Acetaminophen can be coadministered with an NSAID or used alone, although renal risk may be increased in combination. Alcohol use must be discouraged and ongoing use considered a potential barrier to recovery and treatment. Expected sleep disturbances should be managed when short term, either with benzodiazepines, zolpidem or zaleplon or sedating antidepressants. Longer term sleep problems are best treated with sedating antidepressants, particularly if depression is present. Benzodiazepines and other potential dependency producing sedatives are to be avoided unless prescribed for less than 7–14 days. Opioids are helpful despite the lack of academically controlled clinical outcome studies justifying their use. Practical clinical experience supports opioid prescription for low back pain. Short-acting, as needed dosing is effective for short-term use. Long-acting scheduled dose opioids are recommended when opioid responsive benefits are seen during a more prolonged course and functional improvement is maintained. Stimulant laxative agents (e.g., Senokot, Dulcolax, Lactulose) are recommended whenever opioids are prescribed, bulking agents (e.g., Metamucil) are usually not sufficient.

Radiculopathic Pain Management

Low back pain with significant radiculopathic symptoms can also be effectively treated with NSAIDs. Corticosteroids can be considered when acute neurologic symptoms or signs, or both, are present, administered either orally or via selective injection. Opioids should be targeted to diminish the back pain component. Neuropathic shooting, burning, lancinating pain is treated with tricyclics, frequently useful even in acute settings, recognizing that maximum antidepressant analgesia is established only over several weeks. The sedation side effects can be immediately exploited to assist sleep. Gabapentin or other anticonvulsants may also be coadministered. Rarely, mexiletine may be useful.

Myofascial Pain Management

Myofascial low back pain and fibromyalgia-related low back pain symptoms typically do not respond to NSAIDs, and characteristically have complicating fatigue components often exacerbated by opioids. Although most patients describe subjective relief, opoids are not ordinarily recommended for anything but acute short-term use due to frequently worsened functional outcomes. Table 7.18 lists the American College of Rheumatology criteria for the diagnosis of fibromyalgia. Response to antidepressant drugs of mixed receptor types and to other centrally acting agents, such as anticonvulsants and antispasticity agents, describes a complex pain system disturbance for these conditions. Abnormal central pain mechanisms modulated by sensitized and chemically coupled peripheral systems may account for the nociceptive symptoms of fibromyalgia.[79] Nondermatomal and often spreading pain symptoms tend to respond idiosyncratically, but with enough frequency to consider serotonergic, noradrenergic, GABA-ergic, and sodium channel modulation. More stimulating noradrenergic tricyclics such as desipramine, serotonin specific drugs such as fluoxetine, or dopaminergic agents such as bupropion are particularly beneficial for alleviating accompanying fatigue and depression complaints. Neurontin can lessen dysesthetic and allopathic symptoms. Baclofen can help relieve spasticity complaints when present, and can occasionally reduce myalgias, and enhance restorative sleep. The anticonvulsants carbamazepine, valproic acid, and diphenylhydantoin typically are too sedating to be helpful.

DIFFERENTIAL DIAGNOSIS OF MEDICAL LOW BACK PAIN

Clinicians should attend to the more complete differential diagnoses that low back symptoms may accompany. Careful history and examination aim to exclude myriad medical causes of low back pain, some listed in Table 7.19. Absence of trauma or overuse history; fever; prior diagnosis of malignancy; significant risk for, or actual presence of, vascular disease; preceding corticosteroid use merit further consideration, workup, or consultation. When focusing on pain symptomatically, it is essential that an assured diagnosis has been established and alternative serious causes ruled out. Suppressing symptoms aggressively requires confidence that clinical complaints are best relieved, not pursued. Lack of response to expected management or sudden change of a previously stable regimen may indicate a need for additional diagnostic evaluation or consultation.

Table 7.18 Fibromyalgia Diagnostic Criteria

History of widespread pain:
  Defined by bilateral, above and below the waist, and axial skeletal pain
    Pain in 11 of 18 tender point sites on digital palpation (bilateral):
      Suboccipital
      Low cervical anterior intertransverse C5-7 space
      Trapezius upper border midpoint
      Medial supraspinatus origin
      Second rib upper costochondral surface
      2 cm distal to lateral epicondyle
      Upper outer gluteal, anterior fold
      Posterior greater trochanteric prominence
      Medial knee proximal joint line fat pad

Source: Wolfe F, Smythe HA, Yunus MB, et al. The American College of Rheumatology 1990 Criteria for the Classification of Fibromyalgia. Arthritis Rheum 1990;33:160–172.

Mood Disorders

Mood disorders are important clinical conditions associated with low back pain. Whether the pain problem precedes, follows, exacerbates, or is concurrent with depressive symptoms, it must be treated diligently, with or without antidepressant drugs. Inadequately addressing and ineffectively managing depression often significantly impairs treatment outcome. This point cannot be understated.

Symptoms of depression are managed with well chosen antidepressant drugs, selecting activating or neutral agents, such as desipramine or nortriptyline when fatigue is prominent, and sedating agents, such as doxepin or amitriptyline, when sleep is a problem or anxiety is an active symptom. Selective serotonin reuptake inhibitor–category drugs may be less effective for pain control than mixed-receptor category agents. Familiarity with antidepressant drugs as analgesics allows parallel use as agents that can lift mood, reduce or eliminate vegetative and somatic complaints, and lessen the anxiety that so often accompanies both acute and chronic low back pain.

In the setting of acute or chronic low back pain, major depressive episodes are characterized by either depressed mood, the loss of interest or pleasure in nearly all activities, irritability, or any combination of these symptoms. Additional symptoms required for diagnosis are listed in Table 7.20. Dysthymia, a mood disorder often encountered in the setting of chronic low back pain, is characterized by at least 2 years of depressed mood for more days than not, accompanied by depressive symptoms not severe enough to qualify for a major depressive episode.[80] Either mood disorder can be treated with any of the antidepressants useful for pain, although the doses generally should be in the fully therapeutic range, rather than the lower doses required for analgesia alone.

Anxiety disorders include panic conditions, post-traumatic stress disorder, acute stress disorder, generalized anxiety disorder, and anxiety related to medical conditions or side effects of treatment.[81] Patients with both acute, and certainly chronic, low back pain often have some features of anxiety; when severe, treatment is generally indicated. Symptoms of a panic attack are listed in Table 7.21. Symptoms of a generalized anxiety disorder are listed in Table 7.22. Use of antidepressants with sedating characteristics are recommended first-line approaches when managing anxiety symptoms associated with

Table 7.19 Causes of Medical Low Back Pain

Infectious	Diskitis
	Epidural abscess
	Acute or postherpetic
Vascular	Abdominal aortic aneurysm
	Ischemic disease: cardiac, mesenteric, aortoiliac
Gynecologic	Endometriosis
	Pelvic inflammatory disease
	Ectopic pregnancy
Genitourinary	Nephrolithiasis
	Prostatitis
Gastrointestinal	Pancreatitis
	Duodenal ulcer
Rheumatologic	Fibromyalgia
	Spondyloarthropathies
	Polymyalgia rheumatica
	Diffuse idiopathic skeletal hyperostosis
Metabolic	Diabetic neuropathy
	Osteomalacic or osteoporotic fracture
	Paget's disease
Hematologic	Sickle cell, myeloma
Malignant	Metastatic breast, prostate, colon, lung, etc.

low back pain conditions. Even the nonsedating drugs, such as the selective serotonin reuptake inhibitors, can be effective. Only when no other treatment proves effective, and only when an assured diagnosis of a mood disorder preferably supported by a psychiatric or psychological consultation should a benzodiazepine be prescribed.

Pain Disorders

Pain disorders are a new diagnostic entity in the context of psychiatric diagnosis, and have earned a specific listing in the *Diagnostic and Statistical Manual of Mental Disorders, Fourth Edition*, including those with and without complicating psychological factors, and with and without both psychological factors and medical conditions.[82] Criteria for diagnosis of a pain disorder are listed in Table 7.23. Categorizing chronic pain symptoms according to anatomic region; organ system; temporal and pattern characteristics; intensity; and etiology permits the crucial differentiation from somatization disorder. Somatization occurs when multiple somatic complaints occur over several years and cannot be accounted for by any known pathophysiologic disturbance. Chronic pain is treated quite differently than somatization, which is best managed psychiatrically.

Substance-induced mood disorder is a prominent and persistent disturbance in mood, judged to be due to the direct physiologic effect of a medication, prescribed or otherwise. It prevails on any prescriber to be confident that his or her prescription for pain control is not the cause of this iatrogenic complication. When in doubt, psychiatric or addiction medicine consultation is required.

Table 7.20 Symptoms of Depression

Sadness
Emptiness
Diminished interest or pleasure in activities (anhedonia)
Weight loss or gain
Appetite loss or gain
Insomnia or hypersomnia
Psychomotor agitation or retardation
Fatigue or loss of energy
Feelings of worthlessness, excessive or inappropriate guilt
Diminished ability to think or concentrate, or indecisiveness
Recurrent thoughts of death
Suicidal ideation with/without plan with/without attempt

Headache Symptoms

Headache, whenever accompanying low back pain complaints, requires concurrent symptomatic management. It may be due to comorbid cervical spine disease—cervicogenic headache. Headache may be a somatic symptom of depression. When due to analgesic potentiation or rebound that occurs with acetaminophen, sedative, or opioid use, these drugs should be eliminated. Anti-inflammatories are effective for many headaches, and probably do not cause rebound. Antidepressants are effective prophylaxis for many headache types, and gabapentin and valproic acid are useful for muscle tension as well as migraine headaches.

DISABILITY MANAGEMENT

Disability from low back pain can be worsened by excessive sedation from not only opioids, but any of the potentially sedating agents used in its management. Functional capacity deterioration, progressive weight gain, and persistent depression all signal poor treatment response. Impairment and disability can be assessed by care-

Table 7.21 Symptoms of Panic

Palpitations, pounding heart, or accelerated heart rate
Sweating
Trembling or shaking
Sensations of shortness of breath or smothering
Feeling of choking
Nausea or abdominal distress
Feeling dizzy, unsteady, lightheaded, or faint
Feelings of unreality or depersonalization
Fear of losing control or going crazy
Fear of dying
Paresthesias
Chills or hot flushes

Table 7.22 Symptoms of Generalized Anxiety Disorder

Excessive anxiety and worry, occurring more days than not
Difficulty controlling the worry
Restlessness, feeling keyed up or on edge
Easy fatigue
Difficulty concentrating or mind going blank
Irritability
Muscle tension
Sleep disturbance

ful symptom review done frequently while under pain drug treatment. Assurance that these are not adverse outcomes from prescribed therapy is crucial, and if so, alternative drugs and strategies must be considered. Multidisciplinary intervention is often required when disability is disproportionate to impairment.

ADDICTION MANAGEMENT

Addiction management depends on accurate and timely addiction diagnosis. Urine toxicology can confirm presence of prescribed and absence of illicit or unsanctioned drugs, useful when patient candor is uncertain. Ordering a drug screen requires informed patient consent, at times challenging the doctor-patient relationship. When addiction is diagnosed, prompt referral to specialty addiction treatment is crucial and treatment should not be attempted by the clinician treating the low back pain condition, without such specialty support.

GERIATRIC PAIN MANAGEMENT

Geriatric pain medicine practice recognizes and integrates multisystem degenerative medical conditions, anticipating increased vulnerability to drug toxicity and side effects, with complicated comorbidities and concomitant treatments. Back pain is also consistently more challenging to treat in the elderly, because of more complex diagnosis and more prolonged course of recovery. The International Association for the Study of Pain has published a comprehensive monograph on this subject.[83]

Special caution must be exercised when prescribing NSAIDs to this population, because of increased renal, gastric, and hepatic toxicity, as well as interference with many commonly prescribed cardiovascular agents, such as reduced angiotensin-

Table 7.23 Diagnostic Criteria for Pain Disorder

Pain in one or more anatomic sites prompting clinical attention
Pain causes significant distress or impairment
Psychological factors are judged to have important role in onset, severity, exacerbation, or maintenance of the pain
Symptom or deficit is not intentionally produced or feigned
Pain not better accounted for by mood disorder

converting enzyme inhibitor effect, reduced digoxin clearance, and lessened diuretic activity. Increased frequency and intensity of monitoring for toxicity are advised (see Table 7.3).

Drug metabolism and clearance are routinely delayed, so choosing half the dose at twice the interval is a good general rule. Avoiding drugs, particularly opioids with pharmacokinetically long half-life or sedating agents with long acting metabolites in preference for short-acting drugs without active metabolites is safer. For example, morphine is preferable to methadone, and lorazepam is preferable to chlordiazepoxide or even diazepam. When long-acting effects are desired, preparations that are manufactured for slow delivery can be more reliably cleared because the active drug is itself short acting once released (e.g., morphine or oxycodone). Topical fentanyl can accumulate in skin depot and produce prolonged sedation, and impaired skin perfusion can make absorption less reliable.

Drugs used for younger age groups can be supplemented with specific treatments for comorbid osteoporosis, particularly in elderly women, such as Miacalcin nasal spray or alendronate. Subcutaneous calcitonin injection can provide analgesia for the first few weeks after acute osteoporotic compression fractures in addition to facilitating bone recovery. Malignancy should be considered in many cases, and a relatively recent comprehensive medical examination should be part of any low back pain workup in the elderly.

SUMMARY

Comprehensive symptomatic analysis—cause of pain as assessed by type of pain complaint—permits successful management when drugs are chosen for specifically targeted ability to control particular character of symptoms. Accurate diagnosis must be presumed, with continuous reappraisal of efficacy, side effects, function, and mood. Optimal drug selection minimizes same-category agents and maximizes symptomatic benefits. Skilled clinical drug management of low back pain follows thoughtful understanding of the origin of a patient's complaints—a symptom-guided approach.

REFERENCES

1. Deyo RA, Rainville J, Kent DL. What can the history and physical examination tell us about low back pain? JAMA 1992;268:760–765.
2. Fields HL (ed). Core Curriculum for Professional Education in Pain (2nd ed). Task Force on Professional Education, International Association for the Study of Pain. Seattle: IASP Press, 1995.
3. Bigos S, Bowyer O, Braen G, et al. Acute Low Back Pain in Adults. Clinical Practice Guideline No. 14. AHCPR Publication No. 95-0642. Rockville, Maryland: Agency for Health Care Policy and Research, Public Health Service, U.S. Department of Health and Human Services, 1994.
4. Merskey H. Pain terms: a list with definitions and notes on usage. Recommended by the IASP Subcommittee on Taxonomy. Pain 1979;6:249–252.
5. Brand PW, Yancey P. The Gift of Pain. Grand Rapids, Michigan: Zondervan Publishing House, 1993.
6. Wilson PR, Lamer TJ. Pain Mechanisms: Anatomy and Physiology. In PP Raj (ed), Practical Management of Pain (2nd ed). St. Louis: Mosby Year Book, 1992;66.
7. Wilson PR, Lamer TJ. Pain Mechanisms: Anatomy and Physiology. In PP Raj (ed), Practical Management of Pain (2nd ed). St. Louis: Mosby Year Book, 1992;75.

8. VonKorff M, Ormel J, Keefe FJ, Dworkin SF. Grading the severity of chronic pain. Pain. 1992;50:133–149.
9. Shelton JL. Psychological Considerations. In AJ Cole, SA Herring (eds), The Low Back Pain Handbook. Philadelphia: Hanley and Belfus, 1997:245–252.
10. Shelton JL, Robinson JP. Psychological aspects of chronic back pain. Phys Med Rehabil Clin North Am 1991:2;1:127–144.
11. Joranson DE. Federal and state regulation of opioids. J Pain Symptom Manage 1990;5:s12–s23.
12. Clark HW, Sees KL. Opioids, chronic pain, and the law. J Pain Symptom Manage 1993;8:297–305.
13. Abram SE (ed). The Pain Clinic Manual. Philadelphia: JB Lippincott, 1990.
14. Cohen MJ, Campbell JN (eds). Pain Treatment Centers at a Crossroads. Seattle: IASP Press, 1996.
15. Loeser JD, Egan KJ. Managing the Chronic Pain Patient: Theory and Practice at the University of Washington Multidisciplinary Pain Center. New York: Raven Press, 1989.
16. Sternbach RA. Acute Versus Chronic Pain. In PD Wall, R Melzack (eds), Textbook of Pain, Edinborough: Churchill Livingstone, 1984;173–177.
17. Turk DC, Melzack R (eds). Handbook of Pain Assessment. New York: Guilford Press, 1992.
18. Quality improvement guidelines for the treatment of pain. American Pain Society Quality of Care Committee. JAMA 1995;274:1874–1880.
19. Weisel SW, Tsourmas N, Feffer HL, et al. A study of computer-assisted tomography: I. The incidence of positive CAT scans in an asymptomatic group of patients. Spine. 1984;9:549–556.
20. Powell MC, Szypryt P, Wilson M, Symonds EM. Prevalence of lumbar disc degeneration observed by magnetic resonance in symptomless women. Lancet 1986;2:1366–1367.
21. Jensen MC, Brant-Zawadzki M, Obuchowski N, et al. Magnetic resonance imaging of the lumbar spine in people without back pain. N Engl J Med 1994;331:69–73.
22. Boden SD, Davis DO, Dina TS, et al. Abnormal magnetic-resonance scans of the lumbar spine in asymptomatic subjects: a prospective investigation. J Bone Joint Surg Am 1990;72A:403–408.
23. Bennett GJ. Update on the neurophysiology of pain transmission and modulation: focus on the NMDA-receptor. J Pain Symptom Manage 2000;19[Suppl]:S2–S6.
24. Raja SN, Meyer RA, Campbell JN. Hyperalgesia and Sensitization of Primary Afferent Fibers. In HL Fields (ed), Pain Syndromes in Neurology. Boston: Butterworth–Heinemann, 1990:19–45.
25. Baron R. The influence of sympathetic nerve activity and catecholamines on primary afferent neurons. IASP Newsletter. May/June 1998:3–8.
26. Wall PD. Comments after 30 years of the gate control theory. Pain Forum 1996;5:12–22.
27. Devor M, Rappaport ZH. Pain and the Pathophysiology of Damaged Nerve. In HL Fields (ed), Pain Syndromes in Neurology. Boston: Butterworth–Heinemann, 1990:47–83.
28. Edelman, GM. Neural Darwinism, The Theory of Neuronal Group Selection. New York: BasicBooks, 1987.
29. Gell-Mann M. The Quark and the Jaguar, Adventures in the Simple and the Complex. New York: WH Freeman, 1997:235–305.
30. Gould SJ. Wonderful Life, The Burgess Shale and the Nature of History. New York: WW Norton, 1989.
31. Heller PH, Green PG, et al. Peripheral Neural Contributions to Inflammation. In HL Fields, JC Liebeskind (eds), Progress in Pain Research and Management (vol 1). Seattle: IASP Press, 1994:31–60.
32. Price DR, Mao J, Mayer DJ. Central Neural Mechanisms of Normal and Abnormal Pain States. In HL Fields, JC Liebeskind (eds), Progress in Pain Research and Management (Vol 1). Seattle: IASP Press, 1994:61–84.
33. Craig AD. A new version of the thalamic disinhibition hypothesis of central pain. Pain Forum 1988;7:1–14.
34. Sacks O. The Man Who Mistook His Wife for a Hat and Other Clinical Tales. Duckworth, London, 1985.
35. Sacks O. An Anthropologist on Mars. New York, Vintage Books, 1996.
36. Gawande A. The pain perplex. The New Yorker September 21, 1998:86–94.

37. Damasio, A. The Feeling of What Happens: Body and Emotion in the Making of Consciousness. Chapter 2: Emotion and Feeling. New York: Harcourt Brace, 1999:35–81.
38. Kramer PD. Listening to Prozac. New York: Penguin Books, 1993.
39. Perneger TV, Whelton PK, Klag MJ. Risk of kidney failure associated with the use of acetaminophen, aspirin, and nonsteroidal antiinflammatory drugs. N Engl J Med. 1994;331:1675–1679.
40. Lichtenstein D, Syngal S, Wolfe M. Nonsteroidal antiinflammatory drugs and the gastrointestinal tract: the double-edged sword. Arthritis Rheum 1995;38:5–18.
41. McCormack K, Brune K. Dissociation between the antinociceptive and anti-inflammatory effects of the nonsteroidal anti-inflammatory drugs. Drugs 1991;41:533–547.
42. Scheiman JM. Gastrointestinal Effects of NSAIDs; Therapeutic Implications of COX-2 Selective Agents. Managing Arthritis, Postgraduate Medicine Special Report. New York: McGraw-Hill, 1998:17–22.
43. Weissman G. The action of NSAIDs. Hosp Pract 1991;26:60–76.
44. Heller PH, Green PG, et al. Peripheral Neural Contributions to Inflammation. In HL Fields, JC Liebeskind (eds), Progress in Pain Research and Management (vol 1). Seattle: IASP Press, 1994:31–60.
45. Drug Facts and Comparisons 2000, 54th Edition. In Olin BR, Blasing S, Beltrun JT, et al. Ketorolac Tromethamine. St Louis, Missouri, 845.
46. Turturro MA, Paris PM, Seaberg DC. Intramuscular ketorolac versus oral ibuprofen in acute musculoskeletal pain. Ann Emerg Med 1995;26:117–120.
47. Abramowicz M (ed). Drugs for pain. The Medical Letter 1993;35:2.
48. Bjorkman DJ. Nonsteroidal anti-inflammatory drug-induced gastrointestinal injury. Am J Med 1996;101[Suppl1A]:25S–32S.
49. Drug Facts and Comparisons 2000, 54th Edition. In Olin BR, Blasing S, Beltrun JT, et al. Nonsteroidal Anti-Inflammatory Agents. St Louis, Missouri, 838–848.
50. Singh G, Triadafilopoulus G. Epidemiology of NSAID-induced GI complications. J Rheumatol 1999;26[Suppl26]:18–24.
51. Wolfe M, Lichtenstein D, Singh G. Gastrointestinal toxicity of nonsteroidal antiinflammatory drugs. N Engl J Med 1999;340:1888–1899.
52. Celebrex FDA package insert, G.D. Searle & Co./Pfizer, Skokie, IL, 12/31/98.
53. Vioxx FDA package insert, Merck & Co. Inc, West Point, PA, 5/99.
54. Hawkey C, Karrasch J, Szczepanski L. Omeprazole compared with misoprostol for ulcers associated with nonsteroidal antiinflammatory drugs. N Engl J Med 1998;338:727–734.
55. Lanza F. A guideline for the treatment and prevention of NSAID-induced ulcers. Am J Gastroenterol 1998;93:2037–2046.
56. Silverstein F, Graham D, Senior J, et al. Misoprostol reduces serious gastrointestinal complications in patients with rheumatoid arthritis receiving non-steroidal anti-inflammatory drugs: a randomized, double-blind, placebo-controlled trial. Ann Intern Med 1995;123:241–249.
57. Onghena P, Van Houdenhove B. Antidepressant-induced analgesia in chronic non-malignant pain: a meta-analysis of 39 placebo-controlled studies. Pain 1992;49:205–219.
58. Max MB. Antidepressants as Analgesics. In HL Fields, JC Liebeskind (eds), Progress in Pain Research and Management (Vol 1). Seattle: IASP Press, 1994:229–246.
59. Hammond DL. Pharmacology of Central Pain-Modulating Networks (Biogenic Amines and Nonopioid Analgesics). In HL Fields, R Dubner, F Cervero (eds), Advances in Pain Research and Therapy (vol 9). New York: Raven Press, 1985:499–513.
60. Haddox JD. Neuropsychiatric Drug Use in Pain Management. In PP Raj (ed), Practical Management of Pain. St. Louis: Mosby Year Book, 1992:652.
61. Guidelines for Outpatient Prescription of Controlled Substances, Schedules II-IV for Workers on Time-Loss, Washington State Medical Association and the Washington State Department of Labor and Industries, 1992.
62. Drug Facts and Comparisons 2000, 54th Edition. In Olin BR, Blasing S, Beltrun JT, et al. Skeletal Muscle Relaxants. St Louis, Missouri, 838–848.
63. Littrell RA, Hayes LR, Stillner V. Carisoprodol (Soma): a new and cautious perspective on an old agent. South Med J 1993;86:753–756.
64. Portenoy RK. Management of Neuropathic Pain. In CR Chapman, KM Foley (eds), Current and Emerging Issues in Cancer Pain: Research and Practice. New York: Raven Press, 1993:351–369.

65. Guzzo CA, Lazarus GS, Werth VP. Dermatologic Pharmacology. In JG Hardman, LE Limbird, PB Molinoff, et al. (eds), The Pharmacological Basis of Therapeutics (9th ed). New York: McGraw Hill, 1996;1612.

66. Gaylor BS, Miller KV, Rowbotham MC. Response to intravenous lidocaine infusion differs based on clinical diagnosis and site of nervous system injury. Neurology 1993;43:1233–1235.

67. Price DD, Mayer DJ, Mao J, Caruso FS. NMDA-receptor antagonists and opioid receptor interactions as related to analgesia and tolerance. J Pain Symptom Manage 2000;19[Suppl]:S7–S11.

68. Norton LL, Ferrill MJ. Tramadol: Establishing a place in therapy. Am J Pain Manage 1996;6:42–50.

69. Gold MS, Redmond DE Jr, Kleber HD. Clonidine blocks acute opiate-withdrawal symptoms. Lancet 1978;2:599–602.

70. Burling TA, Ziff DC. Tobacco smoking: a comparison between alcohol and drug abuse patients. Addict Behav 1988;13:185–190.

71. Savage SR. Addiction in the treatment of pain: significance, recognition, and management. J Pain Symptom Manage 1993;8:265–278.

72. Porter J, Jick H. Addiction rare in patients treated with narcotics. N Engl J Med 1980;302:133.

73. Moore RD, Bone LR, Geller G, et al. Prevalence, detection, and treatment of alcoholism in hospitalized patients. JAMA 1989;261:403–407.

74. Portenoy RK. Opioid Therapy for Chronic Nonmalignant Pain: Current Status. In HL Fields, CL Liebeskind (eds), Progress in Pain Research and Management (Vol 1). Seattle: IASP Press, 1994:229–246.

75. Turk DC. Clinicians' attitudes about prolonged use of opioids and the issue of patient heterogeneity. J Pain Symptom Manage 1996;11:218–230.

76. Portenoy RK. Current pharmacotherapy of chronic pain. J Pain Symptom Manage 2000;19 [Suppl]:S16–S20.

77. Joranson DE. State medical board guidelines for treatment of intractable pain. APS Bulletin 1995;5:1–5.

78. Policies for Management of Pain. Olympia, WA: Washington State Department of Health, Quality Improvement Administration, 1112 SE Quince St., Olympia, WA, 1996.

79. Yunus MB. Towards a model of pathophysiology of fibromyalgia: aberrant central pain mechanisms with peripheral modulation. J Rheumatol 1996;19:846–850.

80. American Psychiatric Association Mood Disorders. In Diagnostic and Statistical Manual of Mental Disorders (4th ed). American Psychiatric Association, 1994:317–391.

81. American Psychiatric Association Anxiety Disorders. In Diagnostic and Statistical Manual of Mental Disorders (4th ed). American Psychiatric Association, 1994:393–444.

82. American Psychiatric Association Somatoform Disorders. In Diagnostic and Statistical Manual of Mental Disorders, (4th ed). American Psychiatric Association, 1994:445–469.

83. Ferrell BR, Ferrell BA (eds). Pain in the Elderly. Seattle: IASP Press. 1996.

Chapter 8
Physical Therapy Treatment for Low Back Pain

Mark R. Bookhout and Marla M. Bookhout

Prescriptions for physical therapy treatment for low back pain have traditionally consisted of hot packs or ice, ultrasound, diathermy, massage, and generalized exercise programs, such as William's flexion exercises. Since the 1970s, however, therapists have become skilled in assessing the spine and pelvis for mechanical dysfunction, basing treatment on the premise that improvement of mobility and function can provide relief from pain. The purpose of this chapter is to discuss the present state of the art of physical therapy treatment for patients with low back pain, exploring the various theories and rationales for treatment. In the long run, the shared treatment goal of all physical therapists, regardless of their training, is for the patient to achieve self-management capability.

As discussed in Chapter 4, physical therapy treatment should not be initiated for low back pain without a comprehensive neurologic and biomechanical evaluation of the patient. The treatment plan is based on the clinical behavior of the patient's signs and symptoms in the context of the findings from the biomechanical examination, because the true mechanism of production of low back pain is often unclear.[1,2] Because low back pain is usually a multifactorial problem, a specific diagnostic label is of limited assistance when choosing physical therapy treatment,[3,4] but can help to delineate contraindications for conditions such as fractures, osteoporosis, neoplasm, infection, rheumatoid arthritis, or progressive neurologic signs. A clinical treatment strategy based on knowledge of which tissues can be a source of pain, and how each tissue may respond to mechanical stresses produced with sustained postures or test movements, is fundamental to determining the treatment approach to be used.

Wyke[5] describes pain as an unpleasant emotional state that is aroused by unusual patterns of activity in specific (nociceptive) afferent systems. This morphologically distinct system of nociceptive nerve endings is sensitive to mechanical and chemical tissue dysfunction. Normally, the nociceptive receptor system remains largely quiescent, but it is activated when its unmyelinated nerve fibers are depolarized by the application of mechanical forces such as pressure, distraction, distension, abrasion, contusion, laceration, or tearing of the containing tissue. Nociceptors also become active when exposed to sufficient concentrations of irritating chemical substances, such as lactic acid, potassium ions, polypeptide kinins, 5-hydroxytryptamine, prostaglandins, and histamine, that are released from traumatized, inflamed, necrosing, or metabolically abnormal tissues.[5] Although Wyke denied the existence of nociceptors in the intervertebral disk, research supports the innervation of the outer one-third to one-half of the annulus fibrosus, making the disk a possible source of low back pain.[6,7] Other tissues containing nociceptive fibers include skin and subcutaneous tissue, fat, joint capsules and ligaments, periosteum, fascia, tendons, dura mater, and the walls of blood vessels.

Wyke[5] believes that inflammatory disorders are seldom the cause of low back pain, except as a complication of some acute febrile illness, suggesting that the majority of low back pain is a sequelae of injury, be it chemical irritation or mechanical deformation. Treatment selection is, therefore, based on the clinical presentation of the patient's symptoms, the response to active and passive test movements, and the tissues that are perceived to be the source of the patient's pain (i.e., joints, intervertebral disk, muscle, and soft tissue).

RATIONALE FOR TREATMENT

Joints

The effects of immobilization on articulating joints have been extensively studied.[8–10] A spinal joint that has been strained may, like a peripheral joint, develop an acute synovitis with reactive muscle guarding and spasm in an attempt to immobilize the joint to allow healing to occur. If this same joint does not become remobilized either through movement or exercise, it may become hypomobile, and, therefore, be at risk should certain quick, unexpected movements occur that stretch the joint beyond its new and limited physiologic barriers. Theoretically, a hypomobile joint may also place excessive stress or strain on neighboring joints and may, if long standing, promote hypermobility in a neighboring joint similar to the transitional hypermobility that sometimes occurs at a level adjacent to a lumbar or cervical spinal fusion. Disagreement among practitioners may exist as to which spinal segment (hypermobile versus hypomobile) is responsible for the patient's symptoms, but most would generally favor the restoration of normal motion to the hypomobile joint by some type of mobilization. The use of selectively applied forces (joint mobilization and manipulation) has, therefore, emerged as a physical therapy treatment modality to address hypomobile spinal joints, based on the belief that many patients experience low back pain as a consequence of dysfunctional spinal joint mobility. Hypermobile joints are treated by addressing any neighboring hypomobility and then using some type of external support or stabilization exercise program, or both, to prevent additional stresses and strains on the hypermobile joint.

Janda[11] noted that altered joint function (movement restriction) affects the quality of muscle function across the involved joint, influencing muscles either in an inhibitory or facilitatory way. Jull and Janda[12] state that the proprioceptive input required for good motor control may be diminished when there is pain or stiffness in a lumbar motion segment; therefore, the practitioner must make every attempt to achieve free and painless mobility of the lumbar motion segments to promote successful motor rehabilitation.

Disks

The most common symptomatic injury to the intervertebral disk appears to be a torsional injury resulting from excessive axial rotation of a lumbar segment.[13] Structurally and mechanically, the annulus fibrosus resembles a ligament, susceptible to mechanical injury, and capable of being a source of pain if torn or over-stretched.[14] Many patients relate the onset of their low back pain to a lifting incident in which they were bent forward and rotated to one side. It is in this position that the annulus fibrosus is at the greatest risk for torsional injury.[14,15] In cadaveric experiments with artificially induced injuries to the posterolateral annulus, Panjabi and coworkers[16] found that flexion and lateral bending away from the side of injury produced the greatest tensile stresses to the injured area; they speculated that these movements should be blocked or avoided to prevent further tensile loading at the injury site. Part of the physical therapy evaluation is thus directed toward determining whether tensile forces produced by flexion, side bending, rotation, or a combination thereof aggravate the patient's symptoms. The treatment program is then designed to avoid these movements, especially during the healing phase immediately after injury, and to encourage movements that decrease tensile loading (i.e., extension and lateral bending toward the side of injury).

Soft Tissue

Controversy exists as to the role of muscle and other soft tissues in the production of back pain. Imbalances between opposing muscle groups could conceivably result in abnormal stresses to the joints and the intervertebral disks of the lumbar spine. Soft tissue responses, such as spasm, overactivity, or inhibition, occur in the surrounding musculature when there is acute or chronic dysfunction in a spinal segment.[5,12,17] If these soft tissue responses persist, they will alter the patterns of movement locally, eventually changing the way the entire body moves and functions. In 1994, Hides et al.[18] found evidence of lumbar multifidus muscle wasting ipsilateral to the side of symptoms in patients with acute or subacute low back pain. They measured the cross-sectional area of the multifidus from L2–L5 and found asymmetry confined to one vertebral level. In a subsequent study in 1996, Hides et al.[19] found that without a specific exercise program designed to target the multifidus muscle, subjects in a control group continued to exhibit marked asymmetry in a cross-sectional area of the multifidus, even after their low back symptoms subsided. These authors proposed that this inhibition of multifidus function could lead to recurrence of low back pain.

Janda[12,20] observed that the muscular response to dysfunction in the locomotor system is not random, but rather, occurs in predictable patterns of muscle overactivity or tightness versus inhibition or weakness (Table 8.1). In support of Janda's observations, research has demonstrated the role of the transversus abdominis in lumbar spinal stability.[21] In patients with low back pain, there is a delay in firing (inhibition) of the transversus abdominis, indicating a change in motor control in this population.[22] Once abnormal motor patterns have been established, treatment must be carefully chosen and properly sequenced to reverse this process.

Table 8.1 Typical Reactions of Various Muscles to Dysfunction

Muscles Prone to Tightness	Muscles Prone to Weakness
Gastrocnemius/soleus	Peroneals
Posterior tibialis	Anterior tibialis
Short hip adductors	Vastus medialis and lateralis
Hamstrings	Gluteus maximus, medius, minimus
Rectus femoris	Rectus abdominis
Iliopsoas	Serratus anterior
Tensor fasciae latae	Rhomboids
Piriformis	Lower trapezius
Erector spinae	Short cervical flexors
Quadratus lumborum	Extensors of the upper limb
Pectoralis major	
Upper trapezius	
Levator scapulae	
Sternocleidomastoid	
Scalenes	
Flexors of the upper limb	

Source: Reprinted with permission from GA Jull, V Janda. Muscles and Motor Control in Low Back Pain: Assessment and Management. In LT Twomey, JR Taylor (eds), Physical Therapy of the Low Back. New York: Churchill Livingstone, 1987;253–278.

TREATMENT APPROACHES

Joint Mobilization and Manipulation

The selection of joint mobilization and manipulation technique can vary depending on the desired result, be it mechanical or neurophysiologic.[23] Mechanical approaches to mobilization are aimed at improving accessory movements in a joint—that is, those movements that normally occur between joint surfaces when a joint is moved, but the person is unable to perform actively.[24,25] Maitland[24] advocates the use of graded oscillations of movement, whereas others, such as Kaltenborn,[26] Stoddard,[27] and Paris,[25] use specific direct pressures applied to the spinal segment, either as a slow, sustained stretch, or a low-amplitude, high-velocity thrust. Bourdillon et al.,[28] Greenman,[29] and Mitchell et al.[30] are proponents of muscle energy technique, an osteopathic technique that uses precise positioning with contraction and relaxation of the muscles affecting the segment to achieve an increase in range and a normalization of movement (Figure 8.1). Theoretically, skilled practitioners in any of these schools of thought should be able to achieve successful mobilization of a particular joint if an appropriate evaluation has been performed to determine which joint is dysfunctional.

Exercise can also be used as a form of self-mobilization, presuming that the therapist is skilled in observation and is able to teach the patient the correct individualized movements to address a given dysfunction. McKenzie,[31] probably one of the best known proponents of self-mobilization exercises, bases the direction of mobilization on the patient's response to repeated test movements.

In addition to the mechanical effects of spinal mobilization, neurophysiologic effects have also been proposed. Wyke[32] reported the existence of four types of

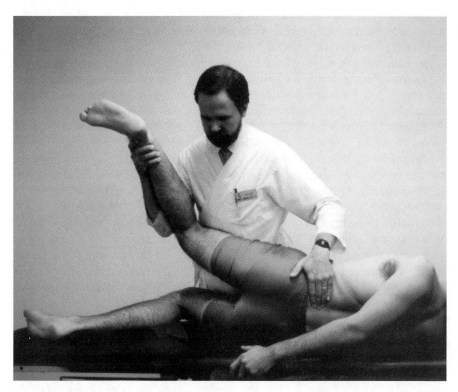

Figure 8.1 Position of therapist and patient for correction of flexed, right side bent, right rotated L5 on S1 with muscle energy techniques. Patient is asked to contract and relax appropriate musculature to achieve an increase in motion at the specific segment.

synovial joint receptors. Types I, II, and III are classified as mechanoreceptors, which relay positional and kinesthetic information from the joint to the central nervous system. The type IV receptors are the free unmyelinated nociceptive nerve endings previously described. Mechanoreceptor discharge from stimulation of type I, II, and III receptors has an inhibitory effect on the presynaptic cells that are responsible for the transmission of nociceptor activity, thus modulating the nociceptor afferent input. The perception of pain can therefore be modulated by increasing the activity in the type I, II, and III mechanoreceptors by the use of various joint mobilization techniques, particularly those that are oscillatory in nature, by the use of certain exercises, or by the use of such modalities as transcutaneous electrical nerve stimulation and electrogalvanic stimulation, or a combination of these techniques.

Treatment for Soft Tissue Dysfunction

Various types of treatments that address soft tissue dysfunction include exercise, massage and soft tissue mobilization, myofascial release, craniosacral therapy,[33] and indirect techniques, such as counterstrain[34] and functional techniques.[35]

Exercise programs should be individualized and directed toward addressing the muscular imbalances noted during the evaluation. There are three stages to an exercise program: (1) restoration of muscles that are overactive or tight to their normal length; (2) strengthening of muscles that have been inhibited and are weak; and (3) establishing optimal motor patterns to secure the best possible protection of the spine.[12] Jull and Janda[12] found that it is important to lengthen the tight muscles first, because the shortened muscle often inhibits its antagonist, not allowing strengthening to occur. When attempting to strengthen a weak muscle, the therapist must watch for poor movement patterns created by substitution. An example is the overuse of the hip flexors rather than the abdominals to do a sit-up exercise. Each patient's exercise program must be individually designed so that the correct muscles are activated during any given movement. In addition to lengthening and strengthening muscles, treatment must be aimed at giving the patient good coordination and control of muscular activity. This is achieved by first promoting conscious control during exercise movements with the use of appropriate facilitation techniques, and then working toward proper movement on a subcortical or automatic basis. Jull and Janda[12] suggest the use of rhythmic stabilization techniques and stimulation of the basic righting reactions to bring in more normal automatic postural adjustments. They advocate using balance boards and minitrampolines during this process.

TREATMENT EXAMPLES FOR VARIOUS CLINICAL PRESENTATIONS

Rather than rely on diagnostic labels, we discuss patients with clinical symptoms and signs that are seen in an everyday practice and propose approaches to treatment that are based on these signs and symptoms. Patients with pain of mechanical origin typically present with restrictions in mobility of the spinal column. The patient may also have dysfunction in the joints of the pelvis, including the pubic symphysis, the sacroiliac joints, and the hips. The treatment plan includes mobilizing the hypomobile spinal segments or pelvic joints, or both, in conjunction with addressing any soft tissue dysfunction and re-educating functional movement patterns.

Low Back or Leg Pain, or Both, Accompanied by a Lateral Shift

The patient may present with a loss of normal lumbar lordosis and a lateral shift either toward or away from the side of pain. As discussed in Chapter 4, the first approach is to attempt correction of the patient's lateral shift and note pain response (Figure 8.2). Centralization of the pain is the desired goal. If centralization of pain can be achieved by shift correction followed by lumbar spinal extension, the patient's prognosis for full recovery is good.[36,37] At times, it is necessary to fit the patient with an elastic lumbosacral corset with a molded plastic insert to help hold the patient in the corrected position for a few days. If attempts at correcting the patient's shift in a standing position are unsuccessful, shift correction must then be attempted in the prone position. This may be done initially with the patient prone over several pillows and the therapist working slowly to restore lumbar spinal extension by removing the pillows one at a time. Occasionally, the use of lumbar traction is helpful to facilitate shift correction. Saunders[38] advocates pelvic traction in the prone position with one-half to three-fourths body weight statically for 5–7

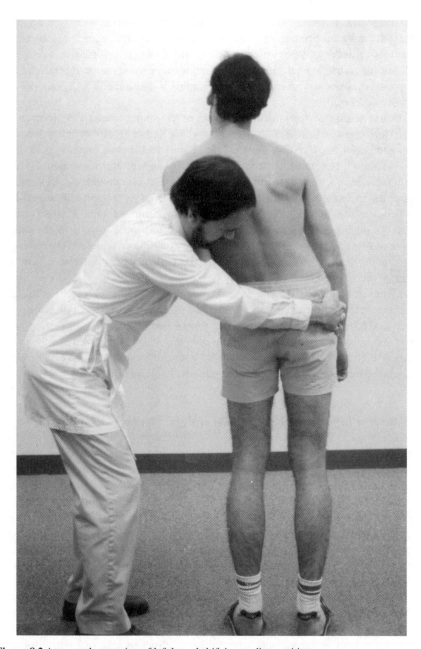

Figure 8.2 Attempted correction of left lateral shift in standing position.

minutes; however, in the acute stage, a patient may not tolerate this amount of pull. The patient's response to traction should be closely monitored; some increase in back pain is acceptable, but increase in leg pain is not. Traction should be followed immediately by attempted shift correction and prone press-ups. The goal of treatment in these cases generally is to enable the patient to correct his or her lateral shift and restore the normal lumbar lordosis so as to promote healing in a physiologically correct position.

If the patient has no obvious lateral shift, but complains of increased unilateral pain with backward bending in a standing or prone position, a less obvious restriction in side gliding may be present. One should always check passive side gliding mobility for restriction before initiating backward bending, as peripheralization of symptoms may occur with extension movements if the side gliding component has not been addressed.[31]

The use of shift correction and extension or flexion movements to promote centralization of pain has been advocated by McKenzie.[31] He believes that disk derangements are responsible for the lateral shift and loss of lumbar spine extension, and he further states that centralization of pain with test movements is absolutely reliable in indicating which movements should be chosen for treatment to reduce the mechanical deformation. Kopp et al.'s study[37] supports the use of lumbar extension in the treatment of patients with herniated lumbar intervertebral disks, but other possible causes for this clinical syndrome, such as facet dysfunction or spasm involving the iliopsoas muscles, could be considered. Therefore, the protocol for treatment should be based on the patient's behavior rather than on a pathologic concept.[39]

After shift correction is achieved and some type of lumbar extension is initiated, the patient can be further educated in the use of a lumbar support pillow or roll in sitting and lying, and can be instructed in proper body mechanics for getting in and out of a chair or bed. Once centralization of symptoms has occurred and the patient appears to be stable, a more individualized exercise program can be established to address the return of normal movement patterns in all directions.

Low Back or Leg Pain, or Both, with Neurologic Findings

Patients with neurologic findings (e.g., motor weakness, objective sensory deficits, and depressed or diminished reflexes) may respond favorably to conservative treatment if the neurologic signs are not progressing.[40] Treatment is directed toward centralizing the patient's symptoms while carefully monitoring neurologic findings. Caution is advised when monitoring only the patient's pain level, as progressive nerve root compression results in numbness and decreased pain perception, which can be interpreted erroneously as a favorable outcome. The use of lumbar spinal traction is sometimes helpful in the treatment of patients with neurologic findings.[41] Saunders[38] advocates traction of short duration for herniated disks, with treatment times of 10 minutes for intermittent traction and less than 8 minutes for sustained traction, working up to a pull of one-half to three-fourths of the patient's body weight. When neurologic symptoms are caused by a herniated disk, the patient often presents with a lateral shift and loss of lumbar lordosis. The use of traction may allow these patients to more easily correct their shift and restore lumbar spinal extension.

Positional distraction[25] (Figure 8.3) or Cottrell 90/90 traction[42] may be helpful for the patient whose neurologic signs are caused by central or lateral stenosis. These patients typically achieve centralization of symptoms with flexion movements, rather than extension, coupled with side bending away and rotation toward the side of pain.

High-velocity thrust manipulation of the spine in the presence of neurologic findings is not advocated, but contract and relax or muscle energy techniques can often be beneficial to treat any associated joint dysfunction.

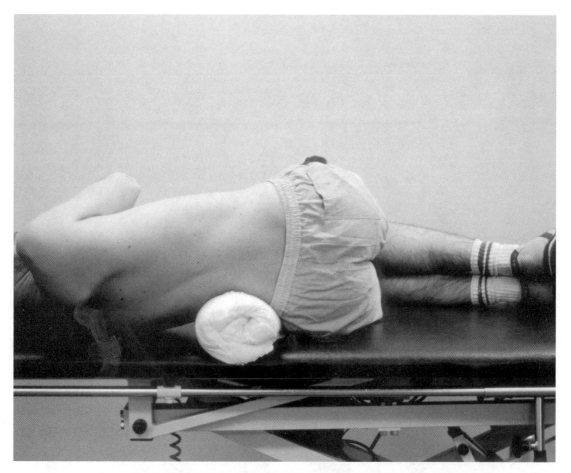

Figure 8.3 Positional distraction with patient's lumbar spine flexed, left side bent, and right rotated to open foramen on right side of spine.

Low Back Pain with Signs and Symptoms of Adherent Nerve Root

A patient with low back pain with signs and symptoms of adherent nerve root presents with pain in the low back, buttocks, and lower extremity, which is accentuated with forward bending or straight leg raising. As the patient bends forward in standing, the knee bends on the affected side and the trunk deviates toward that side (Figure 8.4).[43] Deviation does not occur with forward flexion in sitting, and repeated knees-to-chest motion does not accentuate the patient's pain, because, in these positions, tension has been taken off the nerve root. The slump sit test[24] (Figure 8.5) is positive, as are Kernig's and Lasegue's signs. Treatment for these patients consists of a slow, progressive on and off stretch to promote gliding or sliding of the adherent nerve root in the supine position, using hamstring stretching with the gradual addition of ankle dorsiflexion and adduction with internal rotation of the hip. Eventually, the more aggressive slump sitting stretch can be added, including straight leg raising and ankle dorsiflexion.[24,44]

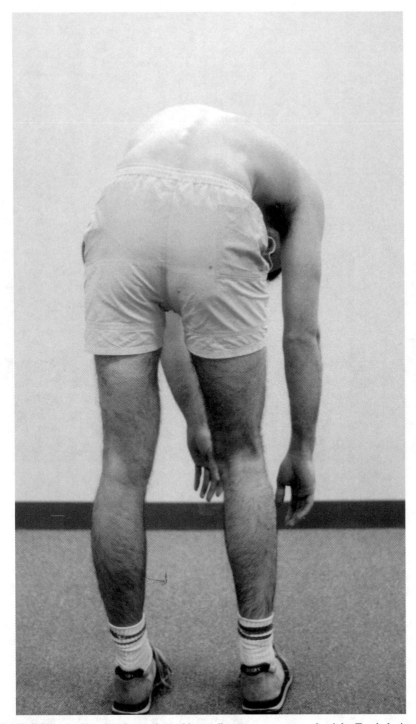

Figure 8.4 Forward bending in a patient with an adherent nerve root on the right. Trunk deviates to the right and patient flexes right knee as forward bending is attempted.

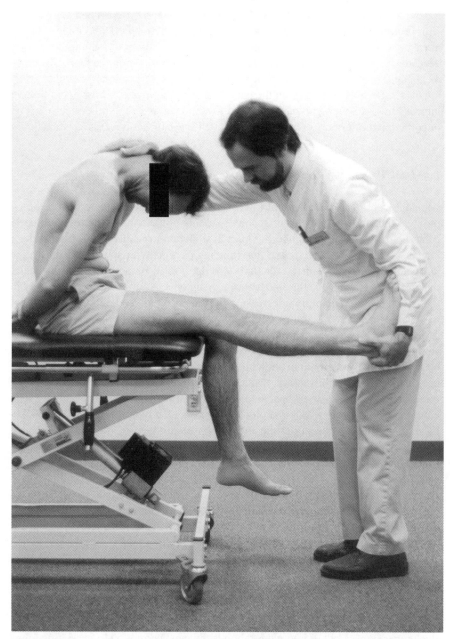

Figure 8.5 Slump sit test. Patient is asked to let the spine slump through its full range of thoracic and lumbar flexion. Cervical flexion is then added and held by the therapist as knee is fully extended and foot is dorsiflexed. If patient's symptoms diminish appreciably with release of cervical flexion, test is considered positive for adverse dural tension.

Postural Dysfunction

McKenzie[31] states that postural pain may arise from any pain-sensitive tissue in the lumbar spine, and occurs from over-stretching of normal tissues. The pain is usually felt as a dull ache, and, according to McKenzie, is never referred. The pain is worse with prolonged sitting, standing, or bending, but is never produced or felt during movement. There is no loss of range of motion, and the onset of symptoms is time-dependent, with only sustained end range positions reproducing the pain. The treatment consists of instructing the patient in modification of posture, particularly during those activities that bring on the pain. The use of a lumbar pillow to control the lumbar lordosis is of significant value. Active and passive postural correction is an important part of treatment for patients with all types of lumbopelvic dysfunction.

Low Back Pain in the Presence of Spondylolisthesis

Although care must be taken not to cause further slippage of a spondylolisthesis, physical therapy has much to offer these patients in the way of improving muscle balance and decreasing neighboring joint dysfunction to reduce stress on the lower lumbar segments. We have found that in many patients with spondylolisthesis, the upper lumbar spinal segments or the sacroiliac joints, or both, are mechanically dysfunctional and may be the source of the symptoms. Normalization of mobility in these joints is often helpful in decreasing the patient's pain and allowing him or her to work toward better stability with appropriate exercises. These patients usually respond well to stretching of the iliopsoas and rectus femoris, accompanied by strengthening of the abdominals and the gluteus maximus and gluteus medius muscles. Traditionally, abdominal strengthening exercises have been prescribed for low back pain patients with spondylolisthesis. O'Sullivan et al.[45] have reported on the effectiveness of a 10-week specific exercise treatment program in patients with chronic low back pain with a radiologic diagnosis of spondylolysis or spondylolisthesis. The specific training group focused on recruitment of the deep abdominal muscles, especially the transversus abdominis, with coactivation of the lumbar multifidus proximal to the pars defect. The specific training exercise group showed a statistically significant reduction in pain intensity and functional disability levels, compared to a control group that had been treated with traditionally prescribed general exercise (i.e., swimming, walking, and trunk curl-ups) and modalities, such as heat and ultrasound. The authors also reported that the specific exercise group was able to maintain their improvement at a 30-month follow-up.[45]

Low Back Pain in the Presence of Lower Kinetic Chain Dysfunction

Studies[46,47] have correlated reduced mobility in the hips with increased loading on the lumbar spine. Loss of internal rotation is the most common hip restriction found in patients with low back pain.[47] Mobilization of the hip joints, especially the posterior hip capsule, and restoration of length in the external rotator muscles is necessary for the patient who demonstrates these findings on evaluation.

The pelvis and lumbar spine may assume a variety of different compensatory positions in response to a leg length discrepancy, placing abnormal stresses on the tissues of the low back.[48] Giles and Taylor[49] found that leg length inequality of 10 mm or more appears to be twice as common in persons experiencing low back pain than in the normal asymptomatic population. Treatment should be aimed at normalizing the alignment of the sacral base[50] by whatever methods are deemed necessary after a thorough evaluation of the lower kinetic chain. This may include lift therapy, mobilization or stabilization of the joints of the lower extremity, exercises to improve muscle balance, and correction of biomechanical dysfunction of the feet with orthotics.

Clinically, we have noted a prevalence of chronic ankle sprains in patients with low back pain. Bullock-Saxton et al.[51] looked at the function of the hip extensors in subjects who had experienced previous unilateral ankle sprain. They noted through the use of surface electromyography a delay in onset of activation of gluteus maximus on both the uninjured and injured sides of the body compared to normal control subjects. In a subsequent study, Bullock-Saxton[52] also noted local sensory deficits associated with severe ankle sprain that could interfere with normal motor control, thus affecting not only the ankle but the whole lower kinetic chain.

SUMMARY

Although a specific diagnostic label may delineate general guidelines, physical therapy treatment for low back pain is ultimately based on the patient's clinical presentation. Reassessment is a constant part of therapeutic intervention, and modification of the treatment plan is carried out in accordance with the patient's subjective and objective responses.

The goals of treatment are to initially relieve stress on injured tissues to allow healing to take place, and then to normalize joint and soft tissue mobility and re-educate faulty movement patterns in the locomotor system. This method of rehabilitation is based on the premise that pain is often caused by faulty mechanics and can be relieved by the restoration of normal neuromotor control.

Patient education plays a large part in the treatment of low back pain and includes an explanation of the findings from the biomechanical examination, the type of therapeutic intervention necessary, and the anticipated prognosis for recovery, with clear instructions to the patient regarding his or her role in the rehabilitation process. Ultimately, the goal is for the patient to achieve independent self-management with a clear understanding of his or her condition and the knowledge to control, and hopefully reduce, future reoccurrences.

REFERENCES

1. Nachemson A. A Critical Look at the Treatment for Low Back Pain. In M Goldstein (ed), The Research Status of Spinal Manipulative Therapy. Bethesda, Maryland: U.S. Department of Health, Education and Welfare, 1975;76–998.
2. Haldeman S. The Clinical Basis for Discussion of Mechanisms of Manipulative Therapy. In IM Korr (ed), The Neurobiological Mechanisms in Manipulative Therapy. New York: Plenum Press, 1978;53–75.
3. Trott PH, Grant R, Maitland GD. Manipulative Therapy for the Low Lumbar Spine: Technique Selection and Application to Some Syndromes. In LT Twomey, JR Taylor (eds), Physical Therapy of the Low Back. New York: Churchill Livingstone, 1987;199–224.
4. Lamb DW. A Review of Manual Therapy for Spinal Pain with Reference to the Lumbar Spine. In GP Grieve (ed), Modern Manual Therapy of the Vertebral Column. Edinburgh: Churchill Livingstone, 1986;605–621.
5. Wyke B. The Neurology of Low Back Pain. In M Jayson (ed), The Lumbar Spine and Back Pain (2nd ed). Turnbridge Wells, Kent: Pitman Medical, 1980;265–331.
6. Bogduk N, Tynan W, Wilson AS. The nerve supply to the human lumbar intervertebral discs. J Anat 1981;132:39–56.

7. Yoshizawa H, O'Brien JP, Smith WT, Trumper M. The neuropathy of intervertebral discs removed for low back pain. J Pathol 1980;132:95–104.
8. Salter RB, Field P. The effects of continuous compression on living articular cartilage. J Bone Joint Surg Am 1960;42A:31–39.
9. Enneking WF, Horowitz M. The intraarticular effects of immobilization on the human knee. J Bone Joint Surg Am 1972;54A:973–985.
10. Evans EB, Eggers GW, Butler JK, Blume LJ. Experimental immobilization and remobilization of rat knee joints. J Bone Joint Surg Am 1960;42A:737–758.
11. Janda V. Muscle Weakness and Inhibition (Pseudoparesis) in Back Pain Syndromes. In GP Grieve (ed), Modern Manual Therapy of the Vertebral Column. New York: Churchill Livingstone, 1986;197–201.
12. Jull CA, Janda V. Muscles and Motor Control in Low Back Pain: Assessment and Management. In LT Twomey, JR Taylor (eds), Physical Therapy of the Low Back. New York: Churchill Livingstone, 1987;253–278.
13. Farfan HF. Mechanical Disorders of the Low Back. Philadelphia: Lea & Febiger, 1973.
14. Bogduk N. Pathology of lumbar disc pain. J Manual Med 1990;5:72–79.
15. Pearcy MS. Inferred strains in the intervertebral discs during physiological movements. J Manual Med 1990;5:68–71.
16. Panjabi MM, Krag MH, Chung TQ. Effects of disc injury on mechanical behavior of the human spine. Spine 1984;9:707–713.
17. Korr IM. The Facilitated Segment. In B Kent (ed), Proceedings of the International Federation of Orthopaedic Manipulative Therapists. Hayward, California: IFOMT, 1977;81–92.
18. Hides JA, Stokes MJ, Saide M, et al. Evidence of lumbar multifidus muscle wasting ipsilateral to symptoms in patients with acute/subacute low back pain. Spine 1994;19:165–172.
19. Hides JA, Richardson CA, Jull GA. Multifidus muscle recovery is not automatic after resolution of acute, first-episode low back pain. Spine 1996;21:2763–2769.
20. Janda V. Muscles, Central Nervous Motor Regulation and Back Problems. In IM Korr (ed), The Neurobiological Mechanisms in Manipulative Therapy. New York: Plenum Press, 1978;27–41.
21. Cresswell AG, Oddsson I, Thorstensson A. The influence of sudden perturbations on trunk muscle activity and intra-abdominal pressure while standing. Exp Brain Res 1994;98:336–341.
22. Hodges PW, Richardson CA. Delayed postural contraction of transversus abdominis in low back pain associated with movement of the lower limb. J Spinal Disord 1998;11:46–56.
23. Nyberg RE. Role of Physical Therapists in Spinal Manipulation. In JV Basmajian (ed), Manipulation, Traction, and Massage (3rd ed). Baltimore: Williams & Wilkins, 1985;22–46.
24. Maitland GD. Vertebral Manipulation (5th ed). London: Butterworth–Heinemann, 1986.
25. Paris SV. The Spine: Course Notebook. Atlanta: Institute Press, 1979.
26. Kaltenborn F. Mobilization of the Extremity Joints: Examination and Basic Treatment Techniques. Oslo: Olaf Norlis Bokhandel, 1976.
27. Stoddard A. Manual of Osteopathic Technique. London: Hutchinson Medical Publishers, 1959;212–213.
28. Bourdillon JF, Day EA, Bookhout MR. Spinal Manipulation (5th ed). Oxford, UK: Butterworth–Heinemann, 1992.
29. Greenman PE. Principles of Manual Medicine (2nd ed). Baltimore: Williams & Wilkins, 1996.
30. Mitchell FL, Moran PS, Pruzzo NA. An Evaluation and Treatment Manual of Osteopathic Muscle Energy Procedures. Valley Park, Missouri: Mitchel, Moran and Pruzzo Associates, 1979.
31. McKenzie RA. The Lumbar Spine: Mechanical Diagnosis and Therapy. Waikanae, New Zealand: Spinal Publications, 1981.
32. Wyke B. Articular neurology: a review. Physiotherapy 1972;58:94–99.
33. Upledger JE, Vredevoogd JD. Craniosacral Therapy. Chicago: Eastland Press, 1983.
34. Jones LH. Strain and Counterstrain. Colorado Springs: American Academy of Osteopathy, 1981.
35. Bowles CH. Functional technique: a modern perspective. J Am Osteopath Assoc 1981; 80:326–331.
36. Donelson R, Silva G, Murphy K. Centralization phenomenon: its usefulness in evaluating and treating referred pain. Spine 1990;15:211–213.

37. Kopp JR, Alexander AH, Turocy RH, et al. The use of lumbar extension in the evaluation and treatment of patients with acute herniated nucleus pulposus. Clin Orthop 1986;202:211–218.
38. Saunders HD. Evaluation, Treatment and Prevention of Musculoskeletal Disorders. Minneapolis: Viking Press, 1985.
39. Oliver MJ, Lynn JW, Lynn JM. An Interpretation of the McKenzie Approach to Low Back Pain. In LT Twomey, JR Taylor (eds), Physical Therapy of the Low Back. New York: Churchill Livingstone, 1987;225–251.
40. Saal JA, Saal JS. Non-operative treatment of herniated lumbar intervertebral disc with radiculopathy: an outcome study. Spine 1989;14:431–437.
41. Onel D, Tuzlaci M, Sari H, Demir K. Computed tomographic investigation of the effect of traction on lumbar disc herniations. Spine 1989;14:82–90.
42. Cottrell GW. 90/90 Traction in the Treatment of Common Back Problems. In Proceedings Western Orthopedic Association, Hawaii. 1980.
43. Rask M. Knee flexion test and sciatica. Clin Orthop 1978;134:221.
44. Butler DS. Mobilization of the Nervous System. Melbourne: Churchill Livingstone, 1991.
45. O'Sullivan PB, Twomey LT, Allison GT. Evaluation of specific stabilizing exercise in the treatment of chronic low back pain with radiologic diagnosis of spondylolysis or spondylolisthesis. Spine 1997;22:2959–2967.
46. Mellin G. Correlations of hip mobility with degree of back pain and lumbar spinal mobility in chronic low back pain patients. Spine 1989;13:668–670.
47. Ellison JB, Rose SJ, Sahrmann SA. Patterns of hip rotation range of motion: a comparison between healthy subjects and patients with low back pain. Phys Ther 1990;70:537–541.
48. Beal MC. A review of the short-leg problem. J Am Osteopath Assoc 1950;50:109–121.
49. Giles LGF, Taylor JR. Low back pain associated with leg length inequality. Spine 1981;6:510–521.
50. Greenman PE. Lift therapy: use and abuse. J Am Osteopath Assoc 1979;79:238–250.
51. Bullock-Saxton JE, Janda V, Bullock MI. The influence of ankle sprain injury on muscle activation during hip extension. Int J Sports Med 1994;15:330–334.
52. Bullock-Saxton JE. Sensory changes associated with severe ankle sprain. Scand J Rehab Med 1995;27:161–167.

Chapter 9
Injection Therapy

Susan J. Dreyer and Paul Dreyfuss

Fluoroscopically guided, contrast-enhanced selective lumbar spinal injections provide diagnostic information about the precise pain generator(s), and may also be of therapeutic value in the patient's pain management. A careful history and physical examination allow the clinician to develop a presumptive diagnosis and specific treatment plan. The clinical impression is often refined by judicious use of diagnostic studies (e.g., radiographs, electromyography, and magnetic resonance scans). Patients who do not improve with time and do not respond to interventions as anticipated, or those with multiple structural abnormalities in whom the primary pain generator remains unclear, are candidates for diagnostic fluoroscopically guided, contrast-enhanced, lumbar spinal injections. Persons with inflammatory pathology unresponsive to more conservative treatment may benefit from a therapeutic spinal injection with a corticosteroid preparation (e.g., an epidural steroid injection [ESI] for radiculopathy).

The accurate diagnosis of low back pain may be complicated by overlapping clinical signs and symptoms and lack of correlation between imaging studies and clinical presentation. Magnetic resonance imaging (MRI) may not reveal an obvious anatomic defect despite symptoms that limit a patient's activities. In other cases, false-positive testing results when pathology identified on imaging does not correlate with the clinical presentation. The incidence of clinically asymptomatic, false-positive MRI abnormalities increases with the age of the patient.[1] When the diagnosis remains unclear, selective spinal injections may provide a more precise diagnosis and may be used to optimize the treatment plan.

Selective spinal injections produce a controlled and focused blockade of a particular anatomic structure based on the principles of regional anesthesia. These techniques require skillful needle placement under fluoroscopic control and use of small quantities of local anesthetics to prevent diffuse anesthetic spread and loss of diagnostic specificity. The addition of corticosteroids to the local anesthetic of selective injections may provide therapeutic benefits beyond the temporary effect of the local anesthetic. Injections are not generally used in therapeutic isolation; they provide diagnostic information and analgesia. With less pain, patients are better able to participate in other aspects of their treatment. All injection procedures require thorough patient assessment to determine appropriateness of the injection.

PATIENT SELECTION

Injection therapy is generally reserved for patients who do not respond to traditional, conservative treatments such as oral medications, physical or manual therapy, rest, and time. Although there are no studies to indicate the optimal time for injections, they are generally reserved for use after several weeks of unsuccessful conservative therapy. However, patients with acute, painful radiculopathy may benefit from an ESI early in the course of treatment. Epidural corticosteroid injections appear to be more effective early, when there is a stronger inflammatory component to the pain.[2,3] They often provide dramatic analgesia and may allow a patient to avoid regular use of narcotics or even hospitalization.

History, physical examination, and, if indicated, diagnostic studies, can help guide the clinician to the source of the patient's pain. Selective spinal injections may support or refute the role of the suspected structure as the pain generator for an individual patient and may provide some therapeutic analgesia.

Patients presenting with primarily axial pain may have an acute central disk herniation, anular tear, painful sacroiliac or zygapophysial joints (z-joints), muscular strain, ligamentous sprain, or referred pathology. Chapters 1–5 discuss differentiating these sources of pain. Painful central disk herniations or anular tears may be treated with epidural corticosteroid injections on occasion, although the clinical response is not believed to be as great as when ESIs are performed for radicular pain. Piriformis syndrome can also present as pain radiating down the posterior leg and may be effectively treated with stretching and local injection into the piriformis muscle. Controlled injections into a z-joint or sacroiliac joint (SIJ) are the diagnostic criterion for these sources of axial pain, and may be beneficial for associated refractory axial and pseudoradicular referred pain.[4] Confirmatory blockade of a structure with a different anesthetic agent of different duration of action may be used in clinical practice to reduce the need for true placebo injection.[4]

The diagnostic or therapeutic benefit of a planned injection should be greater than the potential risk for any given patient. Contraindications to injections include bleeding disorders, systemic or local infections, grave or life-threatening medical problems, and allergy to the proposed injectants.

Generally, individuals who have a bleeding diathesis or who are on anticoagulant therapy are not candidates for injections. On occasion, the potential benefit justifies discontinuing the anticoagulant before the injection. In addition to Coumadin and heparin, patients on the newer low-molecular-weight heparins (e.g., enoxaparin [Lovenox], ardeparin [Normiflo] or other antithrombotic agents, including danaparoid [Orgaran]) are at increased risk of bleeding complications and should generally not receive selective spinal injections. Antiplatelet agents, such as ticlopidine (Ticlid) and clopidogrel (Plavix), are also relatively contraindicated. To minimize the risk of bleeding, some clinicians recommend withholding all aspirin-based products for 7–10 days before an injection and all nonsteroidal anti-inflammatory drugs for 2–3 days. The location and expected difficulty of the injection often dictate whether a practitioner withholds platelet-inhibiting drugs.

Injections are also contraindicated in the presence of local or systemic infections because of the risk of spreading the infection. At times, a local skin infection necessitates an alternate route of injection or delay of the procedure. Spinal injections are elective and should be performed in the safest manner for the individual. For this reason, medically unstable patients should have their illnesses treated appropriately before elective injections.

Patients with diabetes mellitus may experience a decline in blood sugar control after injections of corticosteroids. Likewise, patients with congestive heart failure, renal failure, hypertension, or significant cardiac disease may decompensate clinically after corticosteroid injections due to effects on fluid and electrolyte balance. Appropriate monitoring and adjustments of medication regimens help to minimize these effects. Because patients with mitral valve prolapse are at increased risk for cardiac infections, antibiotic prophylaxis is sometimes given before the procedure, although this is not routine because the procedures are considered sterile. Prophylaxis is generally not given to patients with total joint replacements or pacemakers.

Patients with a known drug hypersensitivity should not receive that medication in a parenteral form. Exceptions may be made if the reaction was mild and the potential benefit is high. In such cases, one should consider premedicating with corticosteroids and histamine blockers. Also, the smallest possible dose and careful monitoring should be used. Appropriate resuscitative equipment, trained personnel, and medications must be readily available.

The routine use of intravenous access and cardiopulmonary monitoring in selective spinal injections remains controversial. The authors routinely place intravenous access and monitor pulse oximetry throughout the procedure. Blood pressures are monitored preinjection and postinjection and during the injection, if clinically warranted. Without fluoroscopic guidance, the need for monitoring increases because the potential for inadvertent vascular or subarachnoid injection increases.

EPIDURAL STEROID INJECTIONS

ESIs are probably the most common of the specialized spinal injections and are actually a family of related injections involving the injection of corticosteroids into the epidural space for diagnostic and therapeutic purposes. ESIs have become an integral part of nonoperative management of lumbar disk herniations[5] and are endorsed by the North American Spine Society and the Agency for Health Care Policy and Research.[6,7] Epidural steroid injections are generally safe to administer, but the potential risks and benefits should be weighed for each patient. For review of the literature regarding the efficacy of ESIs, see the references by Kepes,[8] Benzoin,[9] Haddox,[10] and Koes.[11] The most commonly quoted beneficial response rates are that 60–75% of patients receive at least some relief.[8,12] Meta analysis before Carrette's study[13] have shown a small but statistically significant benefit of corticosteroid epidural injections over placebo injections for radicular pain.[14–16] A randomized control trial shows the greatest benefit of corticosteroid ESIs to occur in the first 6 weeks after treatment; however, this study found no long-term difference in the active versus placebo group at 3 months post injection.[13] Due to this fact, most clinicians use this window of pain reduction in the first 1–2 months after an epidural corticosteroid injection to facilitate an active rehabilitation plan. Epidural steroids are believed to work through their potent anti-inflammatory effects. Acute disk injuries release phospholipase A2, a potent proinflammatory enzyme that results in the production of leukotrienes and prostaglandins via the inflammatory cascade of arachidonic acid. The role of inflammation in the production of radicular pain is now well documented.[17–20] In addition to chemical irritation, a herniated disk may exert pressure on an exiting nerve root. Periradicular swelling from the pressure of the actual herniated disk produces significant discomfort when an inflamed nerve root is placed under tension. Corticosteroids may relieve pain by reducing the edema and subsequent deformity. Another mechanism proposed for the palliative actions of ESIs is the direct blockade of nociceptive nerves. Corticosteroids have been shown to inhibit nociceptive axons directly, much like a local anesthetic.[21,22]

The best response to ESIs is reported in the first 3 months of radicular pain.[2,3,12] Postsurgical patients without recurrent disk herniation tend to respond less favorably. Postsurgical patients often have postoperative scarring of the ligamentum flavum to the dura; therefore, midline injections at the previous surgical site should be avoided because a higher incidence of inadvertent dural puncture exists. Transforaminal or caudal approaches are favored in these postoperative patients, unless the site of new pathology is believed to be remote from the site of the original surgery, such as new L5–S1 disk herniation with the remote history of L1–L2 fusion due to fracture.

The epidural space may be entered from a traditional interlaminar route, a caudal approach, or a more anterior transforaminal avenue. The caudal approach is the oldest approach to the epidural space and has the lowest incidence of inadvertent dural punctures because the dura typically extends only to S2. However, it is difficult to reliably achieve spread of the injectant past the L4–L5 level without excessive volumes. Also, the aperture of the sacral hiatus varies and may be absent in rare individuals. The caudal epidural steroid is often performed when fluoroscopic guidance is unavailable, although fluoroscopy greatly improves the technical success rate of actually entering the epidural space and instilling medication at the desired location.[23,24] Some prefer the caudal approach in postoperative patients with lower disk pathology because it avoids the technical difficulty of going around a fusion mass laterally to achieve a transforaminal injection and the risk of dural puncture in an area of postoperative scar for the interlaminar approach. Caudal epidural steroids may also be indicated when there are significant anatomic abnormalities of the lumbar spine from congenital malformations or trauma. On occasion, proximal flow is not obtained with needle placement through the sacral hiatus, and a catheter technique may be used at this location to place the catheter tip and injected medications more proximal to the site of pathology.

The interlaminar ESI is performed from a midline or paramidline approach. It localizes the medication to the level of the pathology but does not localize the medication anteriorly by the disk and inflamed nerve root. Other investigators have determined that dorsally placed medicine typically concentrates only dorsally and may not spread anteriorly to the target tissue.[25] Fluoroscopic monitoring for this approach improves both its accuracy and safety as inadvertent soft tissue injections, intradural injections, and vascular uptake not otherwise noticed can be avoided. Spinal stenosis with radiculopathy may occasionally worsen after interlaminar injections, presumably due to increased pressure associated with the volume of injectant.

Although no controlled studies exist comparing the efficacy of caudal, interlaminar, and transforaminal ESIs, the authors prefer the transforaminal approach. Transforaminal ESIs require fluoroscopic control, and they allow instillation of the medication closest to the herniated disk and inflamed nerve root interface. Unilateral unilevel radiculopathy, large central disk herniations (due to inherent decreased dorsal epidural space), foraminal disk herniations, foraminal stenosis, or lateral recess stenosis may respond best to a transforaminal ESI.[26,27] It appears that most clinicians have adopted the transforaminal (selective) epidural injection as the procedure of choice for lumbosacral radiculopathy.[26,28]

Fluoroscopy to confirm epidural placement for treatment of radiculopathy is strongly advised, but not universally accepted.[29] Even in experienced hands, without fluoroscopic guidance, studies show 20–30% of interlaminar ESIs may miss the epidural space.[23,30,31] In 9–10% of injections, venous penetration may occur despite a negative aspiration for blood. The injectionist may erroneously perceive epidural location at an inadequate depth of tissue penetration, especially when there are abundant soft tissue planes. An absent or thin ligamentum flavum may result in inappropriately deep injections into the subarachnoid space with serious consequences, including unintended spinal anesthesia and possibly delayed arachnoiditis. The epidural space is highly vascular, and inadvertent vascular injections are not uncommon, despite failure to aspirate blood.[31]

Often the patient selected for an ESI has a degenerative spine with narrowing or scoliosis, or both. Fluoroscopic guidance helps minimize trauma from the needle in such patients. Fluoroscopic visualization and confirmation with a contrast agent are recommended to assure that the medication is properly placed within the epidural space and that flow occurs to the target location.

Inadvertent dural puncture reportedly occurs in 0.1–5.0% of all epidural injections. It can result in a persistent spinal fluid leak that imposes tension on intracranial structures; this is manifested by a headache when the individual assumes an upright posture. In general, postdural puncture headaches respond to rest in the supine position, adequate hydration, and analgesics. Occasionally, they require repair by an autologous epidural blood patch. Significant problems may occur if the injectionist does not recognize the subarachnoid position and injects medications intended for the epidural space into the intrathecal space. Respiratory depression can occur from unintentional spinal anesthesia, and intrathecal injection of medications with preservatives may cause arachnoiditis and pain. Inadvertent intravascular injections can cause local anesthetic toxicity, including seizures, cardiac arrest, and death. Intravascular injection of corticosteroids may cause burning, pain, and even anaphylactic reactions.

Strict adherence to aseptic technique is critical to avoid superficial and deep infections from ESIs. Epidural steroids suppress the adrenal system for 2–3 weeks, which may unmask a systemic infection or allow it to spread. Development of an epidural abscess is heralded by increased back pain, fever, and leukocytosis. An epidural abscess requires rapid investigation, decompressive surgery, and antibiotic treatment to minimize the risk of permanent neurologic sequelae.

As with all spinal injections, coagulopathies or altered bleeding states increase the risk of bleeding complications. This can be especially deleterious in the epidural space in which bleeding, with resultant hematoma, may cause neurologic injury. Unrecognized arteriovenous malformations may also cause bleeding complications after epidural blockade. Relaxation of the patient to avoid venous distention from Valsalva maneuvers and placement of the epidural puncture in the less vascular midline region will reduce the risk of venous puncture. Injection of a contrast agent further confirms extravascular location before instilling the active medications.

Bladder dysfunction, with decreased awareness of distention, may result from prolonged local anesthetic blockade of the sacral roots. Over distension of the bladder may weaken the detrusor muscle, with persistent symptoms after epidural injections. This is presumably more typical with long-lasting anesthetics used operatively or for labor epidurals than for ESIs.

Neurologic complications can result from direct penetrating trauma to the spinal nerves or spinal cord by the epidural needle, neurotoxicity of medications injected, ischemia, or compression from a hematoma or abscess. Patients may also experience a transient increase in back and radicular pain after ESIs in the absence of other complications.

ESIs can be repeated but should not be done as a series of three without regard to response. Most practitioners limit the number of epidurals to three per year. This limit is based on desire to limit total corticosteroid dose, rather than studies of adverse reactions after three injections. Patients who obtain a good response initially and later have a recurrence of radicular pain may benefit from an additional injection at that time. Other patients improve after only one or two injections and should not automatically receive a series of three injections. Patients who experience only transient relief of hours, but no sustained relief, probably represent a population of primarily mechanical, not dural or radicular, inflammatory pain.

Caudal ESIs place a spinal needle in the sacral hiatus. Even in experienced hands, one study reported blind caudal epidural injections are unsuccessful in 40% of patients and do not deliver the medication to the epidural space; therefore, fluoroscopic control is recommended.[12] Without the use of fluoroscopy, even in experienced hands, the rate of inappropriate needle placement (noncaudal canal penetration) is as high as 34% with caudal ESIs.[24] Fluoroscopy allows one to guard against inadvertent intravascular injections and to assess the flow of injectant in relation to the site of pathology. If fluoroscopy reveals the contrast to be spreading only unilaterally, out of the ventral sacral foramina, or to the side opposite the majority of the patient's pain, the needle should be repositioned in the caudal epidural space, or a catheter should be used to advance to the target tissue. Alternatively, a lumbar approach could be considered.

Interlaminar Epidural Steroid Injection Technique

The lumbar epidural space can be approached directly by introducing a needle into the interlaminar space between spinous processes, passing it through the interspinous ligament and ligamentum flavum into the epidural space. The epidural space is at its maximum in the midline of the midlumbar spine, measuring 5–6 mm. It tapers again caudally and measures approximately 2 mm at S1. The epidural space becomes more vascular, as well as narrow, as one moves lateral to the midline. The ligamentum flavum is greatest in the midline also, measuring up to 6 mm, and can offer substantial resistance to the needle. This resistance is one important guide to needle depth during interlaminar ESIs. Alternatively, a paramedian approach directs the epidural needle through the interspinous space just lateral to the interspinous ligament and through the ligamentum flavum (Figure 9.1).

Typical epidural injectants include 6–18 mg of betamethasone (Celestone Solu-span), local anesthetic (1–2 ml of 2% preservative-free lidocaine or 1–5 ml of 1% preservative-free lidocaine or 1–2 ml of 0.5% of preservative-free bupivacaine) for a total of 2–10 ml. Some clinicians also add preservative-free normal saline as a diluent. Most clinicians use a volume of 5–10 ml, because 1 ml typically spreads one segmental level.[32,33] Thus, volume is dictated by the number of segments affected by symptomatic pathology.

Transforaminal Epidural Steroid Injection Technique

Transforaminal, or selective, epidural injections instill the medication along the desired nerve root and into the anterior epidural space adjacent to the disk herniation (Figure 9.2). This procedure requires fluoroscopic visualization of the regional

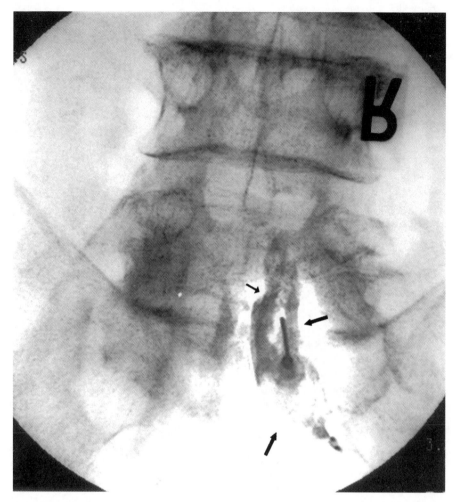

Figure 9.1 Lumbar L5–S1 paramedian epidural steroid injection using a 20-g epidural needle (dark vertical line with circular hub). Epidural placement is confirmed. (arrows = localized epidurogram of nonionic contrast as visualized with fluoroscopy.)

bony anatomy to allow proper direction of the needle under the pedicle and exit zone of the nerve roots. Transforaminal injections may occasionally provide clues regarding the pathology causing the acute radiculopathy, such as a displaced nerve root, or negative dye pattern from a far lateral disk herniation.

SELECTIVE NERVE ROOT INJECTIONS

Selective nerve root injections may be used to help isolate the primary pain generator in a degenerative spine with multiple possible sights of pathology, as a surgical planning tool, or when the imaging studies do not correlate well to clinical symptoms.[26,34] An excellent review on selective nerve root blocks has been performed and should be read by individuals with further interest in this technique.[34] Substantial support exists for using nerve root blocks to prognosticate a positive outcome

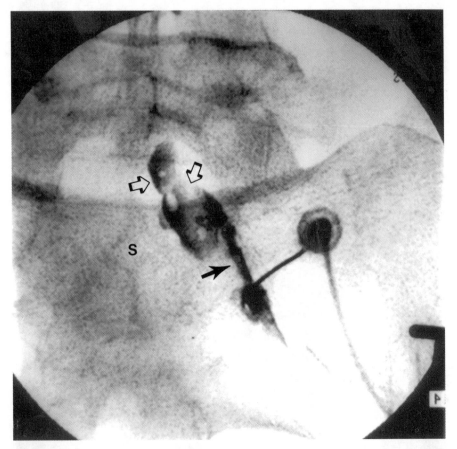

Figure 9.2 Posteroanterior radiograph during an S1 selective epidural injection. (closed black arrow = S1 nerve root; open black arrows = selective epidural flow; S = S1 spinous process.)

after decompressive surgery.[34,35] Selective nerve root injections are performed in a fashion similar to transforaminal epidural injections, except the needle can be kept slightly more lateral, inferior, and anterior, and volume of injectants should be kept to 2 ml or less to avoid spread to adjacent levels (Figure 9.3). Others distinguish selective nerve root block versus selective epidural solely by using a higher concentrated anesthetic to allow for a more focal nerve root blockade. In this fashion, needle placement is the same for both procedures, but volume and spread of the injectant are limited. Fluoroscopic visualization of contrast outlining the nerve root without spread to the adjacent levels via the epidural space is essential.

Zygapophysial (Facet) Joint Injections

Injections into the z-joints, or around their nerve supply, were developed to localize and treat low back pain emanating from these posterior, paired synovial joints. Literature regarding z-joint injections has been reviewed.[36–39] It is well established that the lumbar z-joints can produce low back and referred lower extremity pain with a prevalence from 15% to 40% using controlled injection techniques.[40,41] Presently,

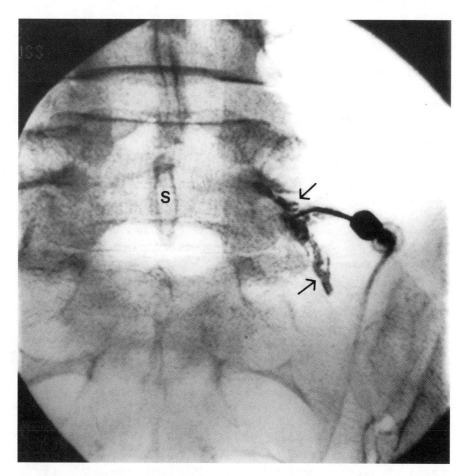

Figure 9.3 Radiograph of an L5 nerve root block using a 22-g spinal needle and imaged posterior to anterior. Contrast outlines the nerve *(arrows)*. No epidural flow to adjacent levels is appreciated. (S = spinous process of L5.)

diagnostic blockade of the joint is the only reliable means of establishing which patients with low back pain experience z-joint pain. Specifically, history and physical examination, bone scan, and computed tomography/MRI have not been able to identify symptomatic facet joints.[36,42,43] Knowledge of the precise pain generator can help guide therapeutic intervention and prevent unnecessary surgery on radiographically abnormal but asymptomatic disk herniations. A current randomized controlled trial has not validated the use of intra-articular corticosteroid z-joint injections in treatment isolation.[44] However, current guidelines recommend one not to use corticosteroid facet injections in treatment isolation, but as a facilitator to a more comprehensive rehabilitation plan.[36]

Lumbar z-joints may be anesthetized in one of two ways: (1) intra-articular joint injections or (2) blockade of the joints' nerve supply, the medial branch division of the dorsal ramus. Blockade of the medial branch division of the dorsal ramus is better known as medial branch blocks. Injections into the lumbar z-joints are analogous to the more common peripheral joint injections. Both require a thorough knowledge of the regional anatomy and injection techniques. Both are used to block pain from the involved joint and, if steroids are injected, to relieve presumed inflammation. However, unlike their peripheral counterparts, lumbar z-joint injections require fluoroscopy to ensure an intra-articular placement. Medial branch blocks can exclude or implicate the lumbar z-joint as the source of low back pain and are a diagnostic test only as therapeutic value of these injections have not been established.[45,46] The nerve supply to the lumbar z-joints is via the medial branches of the dorsal rami at the level of the specific joint and the level above. For example, the L4–L5 z-joint is innervated by the medial branches of the L3 and L4 dorsal rami. The dorsal rami innervate primarily the z-joint and a segmental multifidus muscle. Thus, anesthesia of these nerves blocks the z-joint without interrupting sensation from other important nociceptors, such as the ventral root, dura, disk, or ligaments.

Medial branch, radiofrequency neurotomies, also inaccurately known as *rhizotomies*, denervate the lumbar z-joints. In cases in which the z-joint is the proven pain generator, and more conservative forms of treatment have not brought relief, radiofrequency neurotomies may provide significant relief.[47–50] In radiofrequency neurotomies of the lumbar z-joints, the medial branch nerves innervating the joint are targeted, as they are for medial branch nerve blocks. However, instead of only injecting a local anesthetic, as is done for a temporary block, the nerve is heated by application of radiofrequency current. This results in long-lasting (months to years) denervation and interruption of the afferent pain signals from that z-joint.

The risks of z-joint injections include general risks of bleeding, infection, local tissue damage, allergic reaction, or drug adverse effects, as discussed earlier in the section Patient Selection. Poorly placed injections may cause subarachnoid spread of local anesthetics and subsequent spinal anesthesia.[51,52] In addition, radiofrequency neurotomies carry the risk of dysesthetic pain or root pain and injury from a misplaced lesion. Careful testing before lesioning, combined with excellent technique, minimizes the chance of misplaced denervations.

Precise localization of z-joint injections requires fluoroscopic imaging and confirmation of position with contrast medium (Figure 9.4). There are no reliable, palpable landmarks for lumbar z-joint injections. Only through radiographic visualizations can one ensure the needle has reached the desired location within the joint or at the medial branches of the appropriate dorsal rami. In addition to confirming location, injection of a contrast medium identifies inadvertent venous cannulizations that may occur despite negative aspiration for blood.[53]

All lumbar z-joint injections require informed consent, sterile field preparation, and sterile technique. Light sedation may improve an anxious patient's tolerance, but is not routinely required. If conscious sedation is given, appropriate monitoring of pulse, oxygenation, and blood pressure must be performed. Patients undergoing diagnostic injections should not receive analgesic agents.

Medial Branch Blocks

The specificity for medial branch blocks is comparable to intra-articular joint blockade.[53,54] In theory, medial branch blocks may be more accurate because intra-articular injections may not anesthetize the posterior joint capsular nociceptors. Using contemporary methodology, the target specificity of lumbar medial branch blocks has been established.[53] The ability of lumbar medial branch blocks to anesthetize the z-joints occurs at a rate of 89%, provided inadvertent venous uptake does not occur. Conversely, an 11% false-negative rate may exist with lumbar medial branch blocks.[55,56] In general, medial branch blocks require precision, but

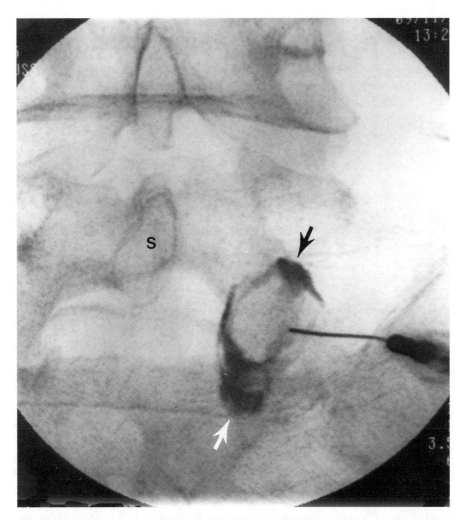

Figure 9.4 Posteroanterior radiograph of an L5–S1 zygapophysial joint arthrogram. The dark contrast is seen to fill the superior joint recess *(black arrow)* and the larger inferior joint recess *(white arrow)* confirming intra-articular placement. The spinal needle is seen as a nearly horizontal black line extending from the right lateral edge of the radiograph to the posterolateral aspect of the L5–S1 joint. (S = spinous process.)

are less technically demanding than their intra-articular counterparts. The target for medial branches of the primary dorsal rami that innervate the lumbar z-joints lies at the mid-aspect of the junction of the subjacent transverse process and the superior articular process. On oblique imaging, the target point is generally in the eye of the Scottie dog. Each lumbar z-joint is innervated by the ipsisegmental medial branch of the dorsal ramus and the level above. Due to the inferior course of the medial branch, the target locations are at the base of the transverse processes of the involved joint. For example, the L4–L5 joint is innervated by the L3 and L4 medial branch nerves crossing the transverse processes of L4 and L5, respectively.

The L5 dorsal ramus block is technically different from the other lumbar levels because this nerve lies on the sacral base and not at the root of the transverse process. The L5 dorsal ramus lies in the junction of the sacral ala and the superior articular process of S1. The medial branch does not divide from the dorsal ramus until the nerve travels below the inferior portion of the L5–S1 joint. Therefore, this level is technically a block of the dorsal ramus and not the medial branch. The dorsal ramus is larger than the L1–L4 medial branches and a light touch should reduce the possibility of traumatizing the nerve and causing referred lower extremity pain. A small branch from the dorsal ramus of S1 may contribute to the innervation of the L5–S1 joint. The medial branch of the S1 dorsal ramus can be blocked just above the S1 neural foramen.[57] However, a provocative physiologic study refutes innervation to the L5–S1 z-joint via an ascending branch of the S1 dorsal ramus.[55,56]

The patient is re-examined for pain relief after blockade of the selected nerves. A pain diary kept for the next 12–72 hours can facilitate accurate recall. The most objective results are recorded using standardized pain assessment tools by an independent observer querying the patient at discharge.

Radiofrequency Neurotomies

Medial branch radiofrequency neurotomies may provide pain relief for recalcitrant lumbar facet pain. A radiofrequency current is delivered via an insulated needle placed over the medial branch nerve in an attempt to coagulate the medial branch nerve and interrupt transmission of the painful afferent nerve signals from the facet joint to the brain such that one is no longer aware of underlying joint pathology. Medial branch blocks are an important diagnostic tool, and a positive response is used as the selection criterion for radiofrequency neurotomy.[47,49,58] A successful outcome has been reported in 45–86% of patients undergoing medial branch neurotomy after single or dual medial branch blocks as the main selection criterion at 1-year follow-up or longer.[47,49,59] Higher success rates are seen in those selected with dual versus single medial branch blocks.[47,50,59] Although methodologic flaws exist, there is one double-blind, randomized control trial that shows lumbar radiofrequency neurotomy to be beneficial.[48] Pain that is reproducibly relieved by medial branch blocks should emanate from the blocked joints. However, joint injection procedures are associated with approximately a 35% placebo response.[60] Caution should be exercised and care should be taken to avoid overinterpretation of a favorable response to a single block because there is a 38% false-positive rate associated with single z-joint blocks.[60] Substantial pain relief after two sets of medial branch blocks with different duration anesthetics more reliably implicates the z-joint as the source of low back pain. This methodology does not compromise sensitivity, although it improves the specificity of these procedures without the use of a placebo.[4] Medial branch blocks are performed with local anesthesia; therefore, their effect is temporary. For unknown reasons, patients who respond favorably to medial branch blocks occasionally achieve long-lasting relief of their chronic low back pain.

The target location for medial branch radiofrequency neurotomies is identical to that for medial branch blocks. Placement of the radiofrequency probe tangential to the nerve optimizes the overlap of the elliptical burn and the nerve (Figure 9.5). The nerve is stimulated before application of the current, which may reproduce usual discomfort, but, more important, confirms lack of spinal nerve root stimulation.

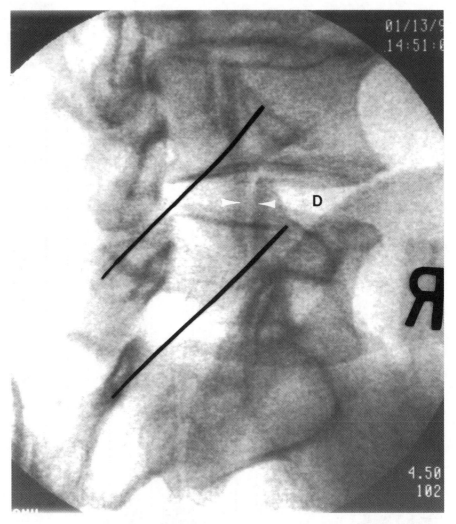

Figure 9.5 Oblique radiograph of the lumbar spine during a radiofrequency neurotomy. The 20-g radiofrequency needles are placed parallel to the L3 and L4 medial branch nerves to denervate the L4–L5 joint. The area of denervation is elliptical and parallels the needle. (D = L4–L5 disk; short white arrows = L4–L5 zygapophysial joint.)

Sacroiliac Joint Injections

The SIJ can cause pain in the low back, buttocks, and lower extremities.[61] The prevalence of SIJ pain is approximately 15%, as determined by controlled analgesic procedures; thus, this diagnosis cannot be denied.[62,63] When the majority of pain is below the L5 segmental level and the patient has sacral sulcus tenderness or points to the posterior superior iliac spine as the source of his or her pain, or both, there is a 60% chance the SIJ is the underlying pain source.[64] Although there are no pathognomonic historical, physical examination, or radiographic signs of SIJ pain,[62,64–67] many patients with sacroiliac pathology localize their pain with one finger over their posterior superior iliac spine.[68] Injection of the SIJ should be considered in cases of chronic low back and buttock pain not attributable to other causes. Specifically, tumor, infection, and a painful herniated disk should be excluded before considering SIJ injections. Pain that is not relieved by local blockade suggests a different etiology.

Controlled studies exist only in those patients with documented inflammatory spondyloarthropathies in which benefit of the corticosteroids has been demonstrated.[69] In those patients with traumatic idiopathic SIJ pain, no randomized controlled trial exists on the benefit of isolated intra-articular corticosteroid injections (Figure 9.6). These injections are analogous to corticosteroid injections in peripheral joints for control of chronic inflammation and pain. Pain from inflammatory sources (e.g., inflammatory arthropathies or osteoarthritis) that is not relieved by conservative measures may respond favorably to intra-articular SIJ injections of corticosteroids.

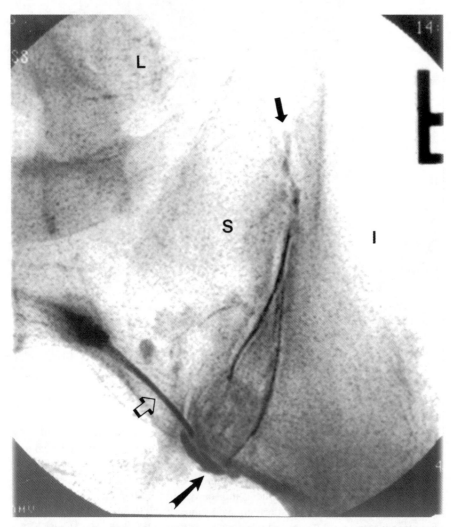

Figure 9.6 Fluoroscopy is essential to confirm intra-articular placement in sacroiliac joint injections. Needle entry into the joint is most readily achieved at its inferior aspect. A 22-g needle is used *(open arrow)*. (I = ilium; L = L5 segment; long closed arrow = inferior joint recess filled with contrast material; S = the sacrum; short closed arrow = superior joint recess.)

Sacrococcygeal Injections

The sacrococcygeal joint is a rudimentary intervertebral disk at the junction of the sacrum and coccyx. This region is covered by the sacrococcygeal ligaments, which may be another source of chronic coccygodynia. The rudimentary disk can be entered in the midline structures. The sacrococcygeal ligaments can be infiltrated with local anesthetic and corticosteroids in cases of refractory coccygeal pain.

Piriformis Syndrome

Sciatica due to piriformis syndrome may follow direct trauma to the buttock, such as a fall. The sciatic nerve passes in close contact and, at times, through the piriformis muscle. The piriformis muscle may also become secondarily irritated associated with SIJ pain. Physical findings supportive of piriformis syndrome include focal pain in the piriformis muscle and relief of sciatica with external rotation of the hip. Internal rotation of the hip with the knee extended often precipitates symptoms of sciatic nerve entrapment associated with piriformis syndrome. Treatment of piriformis syndrome may occasionally include local injection. Injection can be performed either in the lateral decubitus position with the asymptomatic side adjacent to the table, or in the prone position. Starting point is approximately 3 cm below the midpoint of a line connecting the greater trochanter and the posterior superior iliac spine. Fluoroscopy can be useful to ensure the medication is being injected at the appropriate depth. Contrast should flow in a diagonal pattern along the orientation of the muscle fibers. Contrast also confirms that there is no inadvertent vascular uptake. Typical injectants include 2–5 ml of lidocaine 1.0–1.5%, and some clinicians add 3–6 mg of betamethasone.[70,71]

Hardware

Placement of a local anesthetic block along orthopedic hardware, such as fusion plates and screws, provides selective blockade of nociception from a target area. Hardware blocks are used to determine if a piece of hardware that has migrated or loosened is responsible for the patient's pain. Local anesthetics applied around the hardware block nociception from that region. Voluminous injections should be avoided because injectant may spread to nearby structures and result in loss of specificity. The proposed site of pain is identified before the procedure. Fluoroscopic visualization of contrast and anesthetic spread can help to determine the specificity of the block.

Diskography

Diskography involves injecting the intervertebral disks to study their potential to cause pain while assessing their internal architecture. Lumbar diskography remains a controversial diagnostic procedure, but it is unique in its ability to assess symptomatology. Traditional imaging studies cannot reveal whether an anatomic lesion is painful, and computed tomography, bone scans, myelography, or radiographs cannot reliably identify symptomatic internal disk disruption. MRI may reveal degenerative disk changes, but such changes are common in the general population and not unique to painful disks.[1] Certain findings, such as a high-intensity zone on T2-weighted MRI scans or inflammatory end plate changes, signal a greater chance of diskogenic pain; however, diskography remains the gold standard physiologic test of the disk.[72] Diskography is often used to confirm abnormal internal disk architecture and the pain-producing status of a given disk. Typically diskography is performed as a surgical staging tool when fusion is being considered. At times, diskography may also be used to test a disk adjacent to a planned fusion for a structural abnormality. Additionally, diskography may be used before chemonucleolysis or newer radiofrequency or electrotherm interventions for internal disk-mediated pain.[73,74] Intradiskal corticosteroids have been shown in a randomized control not to be effective in single-level internal disk pain,[75] but may hold promise in an acute inflammatory anular tear as documented by a high-intensity zone in the posterior anulus.[76]

There has been concern over potential damage to normal disks, but animal studies have not demonstrated significant damage after diskography,[77] and human disks examined either after surgical removal or at post mortem do not show inflammation or other structural changes as a result of diskography. The risk of infection with diskography is 0.05–4.0% per disk injected[78–80] and may be higher than with other spinal injections. Strict adherence to aseptic technique is imperative to prevent diskitis. In addition, several studies suggest that prophylactic intravenous or intradiskal antibiotics may be of benefit.[79,81] Overall, the risk of disk space infection ranges from less than 0.5% to 2.7%. Skilled technique and slow advancement of the needle in the region of the nerve root help to avoid neural injury.

Diskography is performed in either a radiology suite or operating room under sterile conditions and light sedation. The patient must be conscious and able to communicate fully with the injectionist regarding his or her pain. A conscious patient can notify the injectionist of early radicular pain, allowing the needle to be redirected to avoid neural injury. The disks selected for the procedure are the suspected painful disk and adjacent control level(s). It is important to recognize any anomalous lumbosacral vertebrae, such as a lumbarized S1 segment, number them consistently with earlier studies, and identify the numbering scheme in the report.

A positive diskogram requires reproduction of the patient's usual pain and an abnormal nucleogram (Figure 9.7). Also, at least one additional control disk injection should be free of a concordant pain response. This control disk injection guards against false-positive responses, which are rare events when diskography is carefully performed by contemporary standards.[82]

Medications

Local anesthetics and corticosteroids are the most commonly used agents for spinal injections. Pharmacology texts provide a more comprehensive review of their mechanism of action, dosage, and potential adverse effects.

Local anesthetics inhibit transmission of pain through inhibition of nerve impulses by blocking the intracellular sodium channel and preventing nerve depolarization by binding within the sodium channels and impairing sodium influx. Lidocaine (Xylocaine) is the most versatile and widely used of the local anesthetic agents. It has a short onset of action (1–15 minutes) and a short duration of action (1–2 hours). Lidocaine has a high therapeutic index compared with other local anesthetic agents (i.e., the effective dose is well below the toxic dose). Typically,

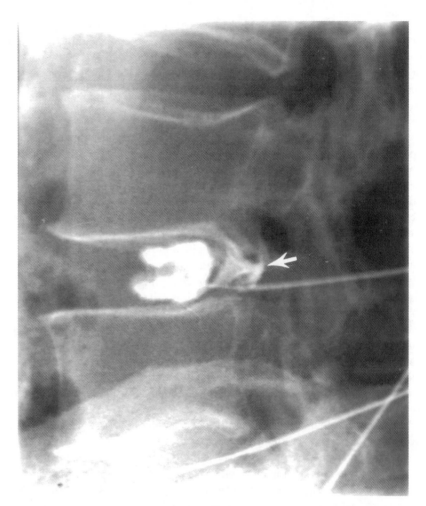

Figure 9.7 Lateral radiograph during an L3–L4 diskogram. Contrast is seen to extend through an anular tear into a posterior herniation *(arrow)*. This abnormal diskogram finding is then correlated to the patient's pain provocation.

concentrations of 0.5–2.0% are used for injection; recall 1 ml of 1% lidocaine equals 10 mg of lidocaine (1% lidocaine = 1 g/100 ml = 1,000 mg/100 ml). Quantities for intra-articular and selective spinal injections are far below the toxic dose of 400 mg lidocaine epidurally or 250 mg intravascularly.[83]

Bupivacaine (Bupivacaine) is another widely used local anesthetic. Compared to lidocaine, bupivacaine has a slower onset (5–20 minutes) and a longer duration of action (2–5 hours). Bupivacaine is commonly administered in concentrations of 0.125–0.75%. The higher concentrations have the shortest onset of action but are not recommended for epidural injections because of the risk of cardiac arrest. Bupivacaine is more cardiotoxic than lidocaine, and cardiotoxicity is exaggerated by accidental intravascular injection. Toxic doses are in the range of 100–200 mg, depending on the site of extravascular injection; 80 mg given intravascularly may be toxic.

Local anesthetics can cause confusion, convulsions, respiratory arrest, seizures, and even death if inadvertent intravascular injection occurs. These risks are greatest in the head and neck regions in which unintentional intra-arterial injection can reach the cerebral circulation. All local anesthetics have a cardiac depressant effect, and they have the potential to trigger malignant hyperthermia and hypersensitivity reactions, including anaphylaxis. Appropriate selection of agents and adjustments of dose are essential for patients with decreased renal or hepatic function, as well as for patients with reduced levels of plasma esterases. Local anesthetics used for epidural administration should be free of preservatives when used with betamethasone to prevent precipitation of the steroid.

Corticosteroids have a number of significant effects, the most important of which appears to be their potent anti-inflammatory activity.[84,85] Corticosteroids also suppress ectopic neural discharges that may cause pain and paresthesias.[21,22,86] Agents with prominent glucocorticoid (anti-inflammatory) actions and relatively low mineralocorticoid activity are typically chosen. Betamethasone sodium phosphate and betamethasone acetate (Celestone) are commonly used medications. Each ml of Celestone Soluspan combines 3 mg of betamethasone sodium phosphate, a highly soluble glucocorticoid with a rapid onset, with 3 mg of the relatively insoluble acetate salt for extended activity. It is approved for intra-articular or soft tissue injection to provide short-term adjuvant therapy in osteoarthritis, tenosynovitis, gouty arthritis, bursitis, epicondylitis, and rheumatoid arthritis. It is also commonly used in epidural administration.

Methylprednisolone acetate (Depo-Medrol) is a poorly soluble form of methylprednisolone that provides a sustained anti-inflammatory effect. This glucocorticoid is approved for intra-articular or soft tissue injection in short-term adjuvant therapy of osteoarthritis, tenosynovitis, gouty arthritis, bursitis, epicondylitis, and rheumatoid arthritis. It is also commonly used for epidural administration, but there is a potential for arachnoiditis from the preservative (polyethylene glycol) if the injection is inadvertently placed into the subarachnoid space. Depo-Medrol is also available in a preservative-free form.

Triamcinolone hexacetonide (Aristospan) is another insoluble glucocorticoid with a sustained anti-inflammatory effect that lasts several weeks. Indications for use are similar to the preceding two agents. Dermatologic side effects, such as fat atrophy and hypopigmentation, are reported more frequently with triamcinolone than with other long-acting corticosteroids.

Corticosteroids have many potential adverse effects. All intra-articular corticosteroid injections carry the risk of significant systemic absorption; repeat doses should be limited to avoid adrenal suppression and iatrogenic Cushing's syndrome.[29,87,88] No rigorous clinical trials have established the limit of frequency and number of injections. However, Raff et al. reported suppression of plasma cortisol levels and adrenocorticotropic hormone secretion for 3 months after patients received 80 mg of triamcinolone at weekly intervals for 3 weeks.[89] Nonetheless, most practitioners limit the number of injections to three per year at intervals of no more than every 2 weeks.

In general, short-term use of corticosteroids is associated with far fewer complications than long-term use. However, serious consequences, such as avascular necrosis of the hip, have been reported with single exposure to corticosteroids. Corticosteroids can also mask signs of infection or unmask a new infection. Because of their immunosuppressant effects, vaccination with live viruses should be avoided during corticosteroid use. Average to large doses can precipitate dangerous changes in fluid balance, electrolyte levels, and blood pressure in susceptible individuals.[90]

Although uncommon, corticosteroids may cause hypersensitivity reactions. An autoimmune response, called a *steroid flare*, sometimes occurs within 4–24 hours after injection. A steroid flare, which is thought to result from a local response to the steroid crystals, presents as a hot, red, and very painful joint almost immediately after the injection. This early onset helps to distinguish the steroid flare from an infected joint. Improved formulation of long-acting steroid preparations has generally decreased the incidence of steroid flare.

Especially at high doses, these drugs may precipitate or exacerbate peptic ulcer disease. Steroid-induced psychosis is dose related and is more common with doses that exceed 40 mg of prednisone or the equivalent. Similarly, the risk of osteoporosis increases with increased dose and duration of steroid use.

Local reactions to corticosteroids depend, in part, on the route of administration: repeated subcutaneous or intra-muscular injections of corticosteroids into the same sites can cause atrophy; dermal and subdermal injections can cause hypopigmentation; intra-articular injections cause both local and systemic effects.

SUMMARY

Selective spinal injections offer important information regarding the source of pain and play a complementary role to other diagnostic tests. They often provide dramatic analgesia for appropriately selected patients in the context of a comprehensive rehabilitation program. They are not a panacea for back pain. Due to their invasive nature, all injections carry some risk. Patient selection requires that the potential benefit of any injection exceed its potential risk. Sterile technique and a skilled injectionist familiar with the technical aspects of the procedure, the medications, and the patient reduce the incidence of complications.

REFERENCES

1. Boden SD, Davis DO, Dina TS, et al. Abnormal magnetic-resonance scans of the lumbar spine in asymptomatic subjects: a prospective investigation. J Bone Joint Surg Am 1990; 72A:403–408.
2. Green PW, Burke AJ, Weiss CA, et al. The role of epidural cortisone injection in the treatment of discogenic low back pain. Clin Orthop 1980;153:121–125.
3. Harley C. Epidural corticosteroid infiltration. A follow-up of 50 cases. Ann Phys Med 1967;9:22–28.
4. Lord SM, Barnsley L, Bogduk N. The utility of comparative local anesthetic blocks versus placebo-controlled blocks for the diagnosis of cervical zygapophysial joint pain. Clin J Pain 1995;11:208–213.
5. Saal JA, Herzog RJ, Saal JS. The natural history of lumbar intervertebral disc extrusions treated nonoperatively. Spine 1990;15:683–686.
6. Weinstein SM, Herring SA, Derby R. Contemporary concepts in spine care. Epidural steroid injections. [Review]. Spine 1995;20:1842–1846.
7. Bigos SJ, Bowyer O, Braen G, et al. Acute low back problems in adults. Clinical Practice Guideline No. 14, AHCPR Publication No. 95-0642. Rockville, Maryland: Agency for Health Care Policy and Research, Public Health Service, U.S. Dept. of Health and Human Services; 1994.
8. Kepes E, Duncalf D. Treatment of backache with spinal injections of local anesthetics, spinal and systemic steroids. A Review. Pain 1985;22:33–47.
9. Benzon HT. Epidural steroids for lumbosacral radiculopathy. Adv Pain Res Ther 1990;13:231.
10. Haddox JD. Lumbar and cervical epidural steroid therapy. Anesth Clin North Am 1992; 10:179–201.
11. Koes BW, Scholten RJ, Mens JM, Bouter LM. Efficacy of epidural steroid injections for low back pain and sciatica: a systematic review of randomized clinical trials. Pain 1995;63:279–288.

12. White AH, Derby R, Wynne G. Epidural injections for diagnosis and treatment of low-back pain. Spine 1980;5:78–86.
13. Carette S, Leclaire R, Marcoux S, et al. Epidural corticosteroid injections for sciatica due to herniated nucleus pulposus. N Engl J Med 1997;336(23):1634–1640.
14. Haselkorn JK, Rapp SE, Ciol M, et al. Epidural steroid injections in the management of sciatica: a meta-analysis. Arch Phys Med Rehabil 1995;(abst):1037.
15. Mary A, Schug SA, Rodgers A. Epidural steroid injections for sciatica and back pain; a meta-analysis of controlled clinical trials. Reg Anesth 1996;21:64.
16. Watts RW. A meta-analysis on the efficacy of epidural corticosteroids in the treatment of sciatica. Anesth Intensive Care 1995;23:564–569.
17. McCarron RF, Wimpee MW, Hudkins PG, Laros GS. The inflammatory effect of nucleus pulposus. A possible element in the pathogenesis of low back pain. Spine 1987;12:760–764.
18. Saal J, Franson R, Dobrow R, et al. High levels of inflammatory phospholipase A2 activity in lumbar disc herniations. Spine 1990;15:674–678.
19. Crock HV. Internal disc disruption: a challenge to disc prolapse fifty years on. Spine 1986;11650–11653.
20. Lindahl O, Rexed B. Histologic changes in spinal nerve roots of operated cases of sciatica. Acta Orthop Scand 1964;1114–1116.
21. Devor M, Govrin-Lippmann R, Raber P. Corticosteroids suppress ectopic neural discharge originating in experimental neuromas. Pain 1985;22:127–137.
22. Johansson A, Hao J, Sjoulund B. Local corticosteroid application blocks transmission in normal nociceptive C-fibres. Acta Anaesthesiol Scand 1990;34:335–338.
23. El-Khoury G, Ehara S, Weinstein JN, et al. Epidural steroid injection: a procedure ideally performed with fluoroscopic control. Radiology 1988;168:554–557.
24. Holubec J, Holubec D. Evaluation of fluoroscopy in caudal epidural steroid injections. San Diego, CA. Paper presentation at North American Spine Society Annual Scientific Meeting, 1993.
25. Kraemer J, Ludwig J, Bickert U, et al. Lumbar perineural injection: a new technique. Eur Spine J 1997;6:357–361.
26. Derby R, Bogduk N, Kine G. Precision percutaneous blocking procedures for localizing spinal pain. Part 2. Lumbar neuroaxial compartment. Pain Digest 1993;3:175–188.
27. Weiner BK, Fraser RE. Foraminal injection for lateral lumbar disc herniation. J Bone Joint Surg Br 1994;79B:804–807.
28. Lutz G. Transforaminal lumbar epidural steroids. Vancouver, British Columbia, Canada: Paper presentation at North American Spine Society Annual Scientific Meeting, 1996.
29. Woodard JL, Herring SA, Windsor RE, et al. Epidural Procedures in Spine Pain Management. In TA Lennard (ed), Physiatric Procedures in Clinical Practice. Philadelphia: Hanley and Belfus, 1995;260–291.
30. Mehta M, Salmon N. Extradural block. Confirmation of the injection site by x-ray monitoring. Anaesthesia 1985;40:1009–1012.
31. Renfrew DL, Moore TE, Kathol MH, et al. Correct placement of epidural steroid injections: fluoroscopic guidance and contrast administration. Am J Neuroradiol 1991;12:1003–1007.
32. Nishimura N, Kitahara T, Kusakabe T. The spread of lidocaine in I-131 solution in the epidural space. Anesthesiology 1959;20:75.
33. Cousins MJ, Bromage PR. Epidural Neural Blockage. In MJ Cousins, PO Bridenbaugh (eds), Neural Blockage in Clinical Anesthesia and Management of Pain (2nd ed). Philadelphia: JB Lippincott, 1988;253–360.
34. Slipman CW. Diagnostic Nerve Root Blocks. In EG Gonzalez, RS Materson (eds), The Nonsurgical Management of Acute Low Back Pain. New York: Demos Vermande, 1997; 115–122.
35. Derby R, Kine G, Saal J, et al. Response to steroid and duration of radicular pain as predictors of surgical outcome. Spine 1992;17[Suppl]:S176–S183.
36. Dreyfuss PH, Dreyer SJ, Herring SA. Contemporary concepts in spine care: lumbar zygapophysial (facet) joint injections. Spine 1995;20:2040–2047.
37. Dreyer SJ, Dreyfuss PH. Low back pain and the zygapophysial (facet) joints. Arch Phys Med Rehabil 1996;77:290–300.
38. Dreyfuss P, Dreyer S. Lumbar Facet Joint. In EG Gonzalez, RS Materson (eds), The Nonsurgical Management of Acute Low Back Pain. New York: Demos Vermande, 1997;123–136.

39. Dreyer SJ, Dreyfuss P, Cole AJ. Zygapophysial (facet) joint injections: intra-articular and medial branch block techniques. Phys Med Rehabil Clin N Am 1995;6:715–741.

40. Schwarzer AC, Wang SC, Bogduk N, et al. Prevalence and clinical features of lumbar zygapophyseal joint pain: a study in an Australian population with chronic low back pain. Ann Rheum Dis 1995;54:100–106.

41. Schwarzer AC, Aprill CN, Derby R, et al. Clinical features of patients with pain stemming from the lumbar zygapophysial joints. Is the lumbar facet syndrome a clinical entity? Spine 1994;19:1132–1137.

42. Schwarzer AC, Scott AM, Wang S, et al. The role of bone scintigraphy in chronic low back pain: comparison of SPECT and planar images and zygapophyseal joint injection. Aust N Z J Med 1992;(abst):185.

43. Schwarzer AC, Wang SC, O'Driscoll D, et al. The ability of computed tomography to identify a painful zygapophysial joint in patients with chronic low back pain. Spine 1995;20:907–912.

44. Carette S, Marcoux S, Truchon R, et al. A controlled trial of corticosteroid injections into facet joints for chronic low back pain. N Engl J Med 1991;325:1002–1007.

45. Marks R, Houston T. Facet joint injection in facet nerve block: a randomized comparison in 86 patients. Pain 1992;49:325–328.

46. Nash TP. Facet joints: intra-articular steroids or nerve block? Pain Clinic 1990;3:563–564.

47. Dreyfuss P, Halbrook B, Bauza K, et al. Lumbar percutaneous medial branch neurotomy for chronic zygapophyseal joint pain: a pilot study. Denver, CO: Presented at International Spinal Injection Society Annual Scientific Meeting, 1997.

48. Gallagher J, Petriccione di Vadi P, Wedley J, et al. Radiofrequency of facet joint denervation in the treatment of low back pain: a prospective led, double blind study to assess its efficacy. Pain Clinic 1994;7:193–198.

49. North RB, Han M, Zahurak M, Kidd DH. Radiofrequency lumbar facet denervation: analysis of prognostic factors. Pain 1994;57:77–83.

50. Oudenhoven RC. Paraspinal electromyography following facet rhizotomy. Spine 1977;2:299–304.

51. Goldstone JC, Pennet JH. Spinal anesthesia and anesthesia following facet joint injections. Anaesthesia 1987;42:754–756.

52. Thomson SJ, Lomax DM, Collett BJ. Chemical meningism after lumbar facet joint block with local anaesthetic and steroids. Anaesthesia 1987;46:563.

53. Dreyfuss P, Schwarzer AC, Lau P, Bogduk N. Target specificity of lumbar medial branch and L5 dorsal ramus blocks: a CT study. Spine 1997;22:825–902.

54. Barnsley L, Bogduk N. Medial branch blocks are specific for the diagnosis of cervical zygapophyseal joint pain. Reg Anesth 1993;18:343–350.

55. Kaplan N, Dreyfuss P, Bogduk N. Lumbar medial branch blocks: a challenge of their effectiveness. Arch Phys Med Rehabil 1997;(abst):1024.

56. Kaplan M, Dreyfuss P, Bogduk N. The ability of lumbar medial branch blocks to anesthetize the zygapophysial joint: a physiologic challenge. Spine 1998;23:1847–1852.

57. Derby R. Diagnostic block procedures: use in pain localization. Spine State of the Art Reviews 1986;1:47–64.

58. Rashbaum RF. Radiofrequency facet denervation: a treatment alternative in refractory low back pain with or without leg pain. Orthop Clin North Am 1983;14:569–574.

59. Silvers R. Lumbar percutaneous facet rhizotomy. Spine 1990;15:36–40.

60. Schwarzer AC, Aprill CN, Derby R, et al. The false positive rate of uncontrolled diagnostic blocks of the lumbar zygapophysial joints. Pain 1994;58:195–200.

61. Dreyfuss P, Cole AJ, Pauza K. Sacroiliac Joint Injection Techniques. In SM Weinstein (ed), Injection Techniques: Principles and Practice. Philadelphia: Saunders, 1995;785–813.

62. Mainge JY, Aivalikilis A, Pfefer F. Results of sacroiliac joint double block and value of sacroiliac pain provocation tests in 54 patients with low back pain. Spine 1996;21:1889–1892.

63. Schwarzer AC, Aprill CN, Bogduk N. The sacroiliac joint in chronic low back pain. Spine 1995;20:31–37.

64. Dreyfuss P, Michaelsen M, Pauza K, et al. The value of medical history and physical examination in diagnosing sacroiliac joint pain. Spine 1996;21:2594–2602.

65. Dreyfuss P, Dreyer S, Griffin J, et al. Positive sacroiliac screening tests in asymptomatic adults. Spine 1994;19:1138–1143.

66. Slipman CW, Sterenfeld EB, Chou LH, et al. The predictive value of provocative sacroiliac stress maneuvers in the diagnosis of sacroiliac joint syndrome. Arch Phys Med Rehabil 1998;79:288–292.

67. Slipman CW, Sterenfeld EB, Chou LH, et al. The value of radionuclide imaging in the diagnosis of sacroiliac joint syndrome. Spine 1996;21:2251–2254.

68. Fortin JD. Sacroiliac joint dysfunction: a new perspective. J Back Musculo Rehab 1993;3:31–43.

69. Maugars Y, Mathis C, Berthelot JN, et al. Assessment of efficacy of sacroiliac corticosteroid injections in spondyloarthropathies: a double blind study. Br J Rheumatol 1996;35:767–770.

70. Barton PM. Piriformis syndrome: a rational approach to management. Pain 1991;47:345–352.

71. Durani Z, Winnie AP. Piriformis muscle syndrome: an underdiagnosed cause of sciatica. J Pain Symptom Manage 1991;6:374–379.

72. Ito M, Incorvaia K, Yu SF, et al. Predictive signs of discogenic lumbar pain on magnetic resonance imaging with discography correlation. Spine 1998;23:1252–1259.

73. Van Kleef M, Barendse GAM, Wilmik JT, et al. Percutaneous intradiscal radiofrequency thermocoagulation and chronic nonspecific low back pain. Pain Clinic 1996;(abst):268.

74. Saal JS, Saal JA. Percutaneous treatment of painful lumbar discs derangement with a navigable intradiscal thermal catheter: a pilot study. Charleston, SC: Paper presented at North American Spine Society—American Pain Society First Joint Meeting, 1998.

75. Simmons JW, McMillin JN, Emery SF, Kimmich SJ. Intradiscal steroids: a prospective double blind trial. Spine 1992;17:S172–S175.

76. Schellhas KP, et al. Lumbar disc high intensity zone: pain management with intradiscal steroids. New Orleans, Louisiana: Presented at the International Spinal Injection Society Third Annual Scientific Meeting, 1995.

77. Kahanovitz N, Arnocky SP, Sissons HA. The effect of discography on canine intervertebral discs. Spine 1985;10:26–27.

78. Fraser RD, Osti OL, Vernon-Roberts B. Discitis after discography. J Bone Joint Surg Br 1987;69:26–35.

79. Osti OL, Fraser RD, Vernon-Roberts B. Discitis after discography: the role of prophylactic antibiotics. J Bone Joint Surg Br 1990;72:271–274.

80. Guyer RD, Collier R, Stith WJ, et al. Discitis after discography. Spine 1988;13:1352–1354.

81. Fraser RD, Osti OL, Vernon-Roberts B. Iatrogenic discitis: the role of intravenous antibiotics in prevention and treatment. Spine 1989;14:1025–1032.

82. Walsh TR, Weinstein JN, Sprat KF. Lumbar discography in normal subjects. J Bone Joint Surg Am 1990;72A:1081–1088.

83. Scott DB. Introduction to Regional Anesthesia. [Anonymous] East Norwalk, Connecticut: Appleton & Lange, 1989.

84. Robinson JP, Brown PB, Fisk JD. Pathophysiology of Lumbar Radiculopathies and the Pharmacology of Epidural Corticosteroids and Local Anesthetics. In SM Weinstein (ed), Injection Techniques: Principles and Practice. Philadelphia: Saunders, 1995;671–690.

85. Flower RJ, Blackwell GJ. Anti-inflammatory steroids induce biosynthesis of aphospholipase A2 inhibitor which prevents prostaglandin generation. Nature 1979;278:554–557.

86. Weinstein JN. Mechanisms of spinal pain: the dorsal root ganglion and its role as a mediator of low back pain. Spine 1986;11:999–1001.

87. Tuel SM, Meythaler JM, Cross LL. Cushing's syndrome from epidural methylprednisolone. Pain 1990;40:81–84.

88. Knight CL, Burnell JC. Systemic side effects of extradural steroids. Anesthesia 1980;35:593–594.

89. Raff H, Nelson DK, Finding JW, et al. Acute and chronic suppression of ACTH and cortisol after epidural steroid administration in humans. Washington, DC: Program of the 73rd annual meeting of the Endocrine Society, 1991;(abst).

90. Goebert HW, Jallo SJ, Gardner WJ, Wasmuth CE. Painful radiculopathy treated with epidural injections of procaine and hydrocortisone acetate: results in 113 patients. Anesth Analg 1961;140:130–134.

Chapter 10
Modern Advances in Lumbar Surgery

Paul A. Anderson

Advances in technology, such as fiberoptic imaging, new materials (e.g., carbon fiber and titanium), improved diagnostic imaging, and the development of increasing numbers of highly skilled surgeons have led to the development of minimally invasive spinal procedures to relieve nerve compression and perform fusion. These advances correspond to similar advances in arthroscopic knee surgery, abdominal laparoscopy, and trauma care.

This chapter examines minimally invasive techniques for management of radicular pain secondary to a herniated disk with comparison of those results to standard open and microsurgical techniques. Finally, the role of lumbar fusion in the management of low back pain and the use of interbody cage techniques is discussed.

MANAGEMENT OF LUMBAR RADICULOPATHY
SECONDARY TO HERNIATED DISK

Patients with lumbar radiculopathy secondary to herniated disks or foraminal stenosis, or a combination thereof, are usually managed nonoperatively, including the use of rest for 1–2 days, nonsteroidal anti-inflammatory drugs, physical therapy modalities and postural exercises, and the administration of glucocorticoids, either orally or via epidural routes. Only after 6–8 weeks of symptoms should the patient be advised to consider surgery, unless there is progressive neurologic deficit or cauda equina syndrome. In addition to a neurologic examination and testing of root tension signs, a spinal imaging study should be obtained. Magnetic resonance imaging (MRI), being noninvasive, is preferred over computed tomography-myelography. To have a successful surgical outcome, the patient's pattern of leg pain and neurologic changes should correlate with the findings on MRI. Symptoms that do not match abnormalities on imaging rarely improve with surgical treatment.

Techniques have been developed to surgically treat patients with herniated lumbar intervertebral disks. The indications for all surgical modalities, whether open or percutaneous, are the same: unremitting leg pain in specific nerve root distribution, corresponding neurologic findings, and confirmatory neuroimaging. However, a tendency to use these less invasive techniques outside these indications has led to poor outcomes and loss of favor of a potentially useful technique.

Table 10.1 Treatment of Lumbar Radiculopathy

Percutaneous techniques
    Chemonucleolysis
    Percutaneous nucleotomy
    Automated percutaneous diskectomy
    Arthroscopic microdiskectomy
    Spinal endoscopy
Open techniques
    Microdiskectomy
    Open laminectomy/diskectomy

This chapter describes techniques that are percutaneous and performed with either a needle or small stab incision and minimally invasive open techniques that require a somewhat larger incision, but are thought to be associated with less morbidity than the open laminectomy and diskectomy originally described by Mixter and Barr (Table 10.1).[1]

Chemonucleolysis

Chymopapain is a proteolytic enzyme extracted from crude papain derived from the leaves of the Carica papaya. Lyman Smith recognized the possible usefulness of this enzyme and tested it on rabbit disks in which he was able to remove the nucleus pulposus without injury to the annulus fibrosis.[2] Animal studies continued, and its efficiency was established in dachshunds, of whom 86% recovered from nerve compression treated by intradiskal chymopapain injection.

Chymopapain acts to hydrolyze peptide bonds of the proteoglycan molecule. This releases polysaccharide (glycosamine glycans) side chains that diffuse out of the disk. Loss of the glycosamine glycans reduces the capacity to bind water and decreases intradiskal pressure. Chymopapain is rapidly deactivated by $alpha_2$-macroglobulin, cathepsin, and specific enzymes. The major adverse effect of chymopapain is its ability to rupture capillaries, leading to central nervous system hemorrhage. The dura, peripheral nerves, collagen, and clotting factors are not affected by chymopapain.[3]

The mode of action to relieve sciatic pain is unknown. Possible mechanisms include reduction of size of the disk prolapse, a reduction of the pressure head of the extruded disk, an unknown effect on the inflammatory process, or a direct effect on the nerve root. Radiographically, disk space narrowing is observed after chemonucleolysis. Several studies have correlated a large reduction in the size of disk height and clinical outcome.[4] Although regeneration of some nuclear material has been demonstrated in animals, postinjection MRI in humans shows permanent decreased signals.[5]

Indications for Chemonucleolysis

Chymopapain is indicated for the patient with sciatic pain from a herniated disk who has had 6–8 weeks of unsuccessful medical therapy. Successful results in juveniles ages 13–18 years and senior patients older than age 60 years have been reported.[6,7] In the latter group, some authors believe that the spinal stenosis could develop with loss of disk height and, therefore, chymopapain should not be used.

Contraindications include patients with obvious sequestered disk fragment, patients with prior injection of chymopapain, pregnancy, cauda equina syndrome, or allergy to iodine compounds.

Outcomes

Nordby reported a minimum 8-year follow-up of 739 patients evaluated by questionnaire.[8] Fifty-one percent had excellent results (85–100% pain relief), 16% had good results (50–85%), 9% fair results (25–50%), and 24% unsatisfactory results (<25%).

The Adelaide double-blind study compared chymopapain to placebo at 10 years.[9] Eighty percent of patients treated by chymopapain considered the injection successful compared to only 34% for the placebo group. Overall, success was rated independently as 77% versus 38%.

Alexander performed a randomized study comparing chymopapain to open diskectomy in a military population.[10] Overall, satisfactory results were seen in 78% compared to 80% of patients, respectively. Similarly, Muralikuttan, in another randomized study, found no difference at 1 year, but that the open diskectomy had better earlier results at 6 and 12 months.[11]

Complications

Despite these and other studies documenting successful results, chymopapain has fallen from favor and is rarely performed today because of the rare, but catastrophic, complications that were reported in the first 2 years after general release of the technique by the U.S. Food and Drug Administration (FDA) in 1982. Of approximately 135,000 patients treated between 1982 and 1991, 32 patients had hemorrhagic events in the central nervous system.[3] The hemorrhagic complications were thought to be secondary to intrathecal administration of the enzyme, causing breakdown of capillaries. Another 32 patients had nonhemorrhagic neurologic deficits, including transverse myelitis. However, mortality was much lower with chymopapain than standard open laminectomy (0.02% compared to 0.05%).[3]

Another significant complication of chymopapain results is anaphylactic shock. Anaphylactic shock occurs in approximately 1% of patients and can be reduced to 0.3% by preoperative serum sensitivity and skin testing. Women and blacks have a significantly higher incidence of this reaction. Emergency treatment must be readily available before injection, and includes large bore intravenous access, epinephrine, and oxygen.

Conclusion

Chymopapain is an effective percutaneous technique for the management of lumbar radiculopathy secondary to herniated nucleus pulposus. Good results can be expected in 70–80% of selected cases. Risks, however, are significant, which has limited its use in the 1990s.

Percutaneous Nucleotomy

The concept of decompressing the nucleus is a natural outgrowth of the experience of chymopapain. Therefore, it is theorized that removal of a substantial part of the

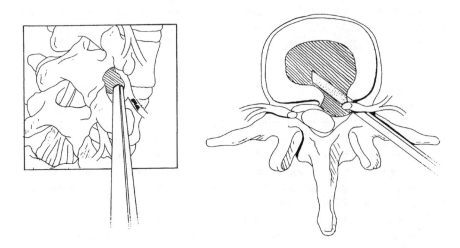

Figure 10.1 Posterolateral approach for uniportal percutaneous nucleotomy. (Reprinted with permission from HH Mathews, BE Mathern. Percutaneous Procedures in the Lumbar Spine. In HS An [ed], Principles and Techniques of Spine Surgery. Baltimore: Williams & Wilkins, 1998;735.)

nucleus without removal of the offending fragment could lead to a decrease of root tension and possibly removal of the inflammatory agents. Hoppenfeld and Hijikata simultaneously developed the technique of uniportal nucleotomy.[12,13] In this technique, the disk space is entered posterolaterally through a series of cannulae (Figure 10.1). Through the cannula, special instruments can be inserted to remove the nuclear material. Hijikata reported 72% excellent or good results with 19% of patients going on to have open surgery.[13] He was able to remove between 1 g and 3 g of tissue. Hoppenfeld similarly reported 43 of 50 patients had relief of their sciatic pain; however, only one of eight patients with motor weakness recovered.[12] Kambin used a similar technique with improved instruments and reported that 61 of 93 patients experienced immediate pain relief.[14] Long term, 51 patients were cured, whereas 33 were helped but not cured.

To simplify the procedure, Onik developed a nucleotome that simultaneously aspirated and sectioned disk material by means of a rotating blade.[15] The instrument is similar to that developed for arthroscopic knee surgery. This automated percutaneous procedure takes between 20 to 30 minutes and aspirates up to 5–7 g of disk material. The inner rotating blade cycles at a rate of 180 Hz, and 600 mm Hg of suction is applied. A special curved cannula is available for insertion into the L5–S1 disk space. Overall, results of automated percutaneous nucleotomy have been disappointing. Goldstein reported only 9 of 17 patients had successful outcomes.[16]

A multicenter study of the efficacy of automated percutaneous diskectomy was reported by Onik.[15] One-third of patients enrolled in the study did not meet the inclusion criteria (treatment of sciatica secondary to herniated nucleus pulposus). Patients who were in-protocol demonstrated a 75% success rate versus only 49% for out-of-protocol patients. Revel performed a randomized study comparing chymopapain to automated percutaneous diskectomy.[17] Excellent or good results were seen in 66% of chymopapain patients and only 37% with automated diskectomy. Kahanovitz also reported poor results in automated percutaneous diskectomy.[18] Only 21 of 39 patients were able to return to work within 17 months of the procedure.

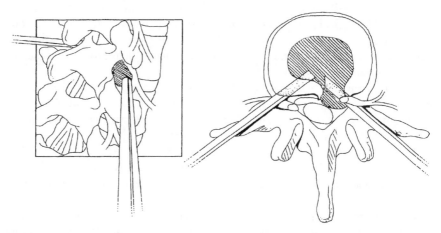

Figure 10.2 Biportal approach for arthroscopic nucleotomy. (Reprinted with permission from HH Mathews, BE Mathern. Percutaneous Procedures in the Lumbar Spine. In HS An [ed], Principles and Techniques of Spine Surgery. Baltimore: Williams & Wilkins, 1998;735.)

Chatterjee performed a controlled randomized study comparing microdiskectomy to automated percutaneous diskectomy.[19] Eighty percent of patients with microdiskectomy had satisfactory results compared to only 71% in the percutaneous group. Twenty of 22 patients with unsuccessful automated percutaneous diskectomy went on to have open surgery. Only 65% of these patients had successful outcome.

Complications

Complications related to percutaneous nucleotomy are surprisingly few. Infections are seen in fewer than 1% of cases. Inadvertent bowel perforation from insertion of cannulae has been reported. Neurologic deficits are rare.

Conclusion

Percutaneous diskectomy or nucleotomy without direct removal of the herniated fragment has a lower success rate than either chymopapain or microdiskectomy. Although the procedure is safe, unsuccessful procedures have poorer outcomes if additional surgery is ultimately required.

Arthroscopic Microdiskectomy

The preceding procedures are aimed to decrease the amount of nuclear material and do not directly remove the herniated fragment. For safety of the neural structures, removal of disk fragments in close proximity requires some visualization. Advances in fiberoptics and the design of special instruments allow intradiskal visualization while instruments can be used to extract herniated disk fragments.

Schreiber described the use of bilateral portals inserted posterolaterally.[20] Through one cannula, a standard arthroscope tool is placed and through the opposite portal instruments can be inserted (Figure 10.2). Arthroscopes of varying angles are required to allow complete visualization. Irrigation and suction are also essential. The surgical techniques based on triangulation are similar to arthroscopic surgery. Kambin developed a specialized microdiskoscope that allows inflow and outflow through a single portal.[21] The approach of using an arthroscope in the disk space has been termed *diskoscopy.*

Schreiber reported outcomes of 109 patients treated by arthroscopic microdiskectomy.[20] Twenty-two patients had excellent results, 45 had good results, 12 had fair results, and 30 had poor results. Transient neurologic deficits occurred in two patients, and spondylodiskitis occurred in eight patients.

Kambin reported 200 patients treated by arthroscopic-aided diskectomy with an 87% success rate.[22] Complications were few, including two patients with psoas hematomas and one postoperative wound infection. No patient had a neurovascular injury.

Casey compared prearthroscopy and postarthroscopy diskectomy computed tomography scans.[23] He found between 75% and 100% canal clearance in herniations that were classified as subligamentous and nonmigrated extraligamentous. Less change was seen in those that were intraforamenal or extraforamenal.

Conclusion

Arthroscopic microdiskectomy allows direct visualization through the disk space of extruded disk fragments with the possibility of direct removal. Postoperative imaging demonstrates that this occurs in the majority of cases, but depends on the location of disk herniation and its size. The procedure has a low complication rate and morbidity with rapid return to function. Unsuccessful procedures appear to be salvageable with standard open techniques.

Arthroscopic microdiskectomy has not been enthusiastically embraced by most surgeons because of the steep learning curve to safely perform the procedure. A major concern is the risk of injury to the cauda equina when using triangulation surgical techniques.

Spinal Endoscopy

Spinal endoscopy is the inspection of the contents of the spinal canal using a magnifying scope inserted into the epidural space translaminarly or transforamenally. Myeloscopy had been performed even before myelography by Burman in 1934.[24] Pool used a large bore rod lens myeloscope and reported findings in 400 cases in 1942.[25]

In 1989, Stoll used a small fiberoptic epiduraloscope as an adjunct to open surgery to assess adequacy of root decompression.[26] Based on a multicenter study that documented no complications, the scope was released for use in 1991 by the FDA. Mathews developed a 4.5 mm steerable scope with a 2.5 mm working channel that allows not only inspection, but also removal of pathologic tissue under direct visualization (Figure 10.3).[27]

In addition to navigable small fiberoptic scopes, adjuncts such as C-arm fluoroscopy are essential to safely enter the epidural space. The use of two channels placed on opposite sides allows for some retraction and the use of working instruments. The endoscopes can be inserted into the epidural space dorsally between the lamina or through the foramen. The translaminar approach allows limited visualization of the disk, and, therefore, the transforamenal approach is preferred.

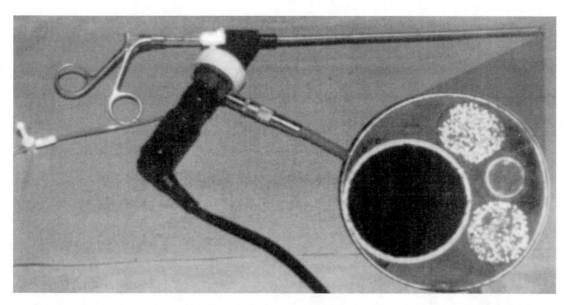

Figure 10.3 4.5 mm steerable scope with 2.5 mm working channel. Two fiberoptic bundles provide light source. (Reprinted with permission from HH Mathews, BE Mathern. Percutaneous Procedures in the Lumbar Spine. In HS An [ed], Principles and Techniques of Spine Surgery. Baltimore: Williams & Wilkins, 1998;736.)

The transforamenal approach has led to the development of the foramenal epidural endoscopic surgery.[28] The endoscope is inserted from 10 cm to 13 cm laterally passing below the pars interarticularis, and then docked down onto the disk (Figure 10.4). A safe triangular working zone is established between the exiting nerve root, the traversing nerve root, and the disk. Through this approach, herniated disks that are posterolateral, transforamenal, or far lateral can be decompressed (Figure 10.5). The process requires a high flow irrigant to wash away debris, maintain hemostasis, and help with dissection.

Indications

Indications for transforamenal spinal endoscopy include patients with unremitting radicular pain at a nonoperated level with a contained herniated disk that is posterolateral, foramenal, or extraforamenal and is less than 50% canal diameter in size.

Results

Mathews reported outcomes of 75 patients.[27] Sixty-eight patients (88%) had relief of their radicular pain, and seven were deemed unsuccessful. The procedure was done while the patient was awake with sedation and as an outpatient.

Complications

Fewer complications are seen with spinal endoscopy compared to open surgical techniques. The most common difficulty is that the L5–S1 disk space cannot be cannulated secondary to the iliac crest.

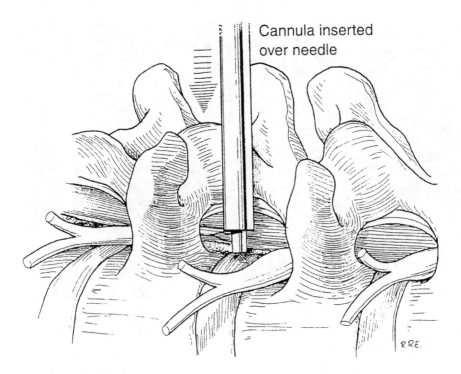

Figure 10.4 The placement of the scope into the neuroforamena. A triangular working zone is present between the traversing root, exiting root, and pedicle. The roof of the neuroforamena is the pars interarticularis. The probe is docked onto the disk. (Reprinted with permission from HH Mathews, BE Mathern. Percutaneous Procedures in the Lumbar Spine. In HS An [ed], Principles and Techniques of Spine Surgery. Baltimore: Williams & Wilkins, 1998;739.)

Conclusion

The technique of spinal endoscopy is evolving as technologic improvements occur in optical devices and instruments. The transforaminal approach is appealing for the more lateral disk herniation that can be difficult to approach using an open technique. However, there is a steep learning curve with these techniques, and only a few surgeons are adequately trained in their use. These approaches have yet to show convincing evidence that they have better outcomes than standard open microdiskectomy.

Open Techniques for Management of Lumbar Disk Herniation

The open techniques, as initially described by Mixter and Barr, have well-established outcomes and serve as a gold standard in comparison to newer techniques.[1] In the open techniques, the ipsilateral paraspinal musculature is stripped off the adjacent lamina and retracted laterally. Varying amounts of the cranial and caudal lamina are removed, exposing the ligamentum flavum. The ligamentum flavum is split and then removed, exposing the epidural space. Laterally, the overhanging superior facets are resected to allow improved visualization. The nerve root is identified, and, by dissection vertically along the root, it is mobilized and retracted

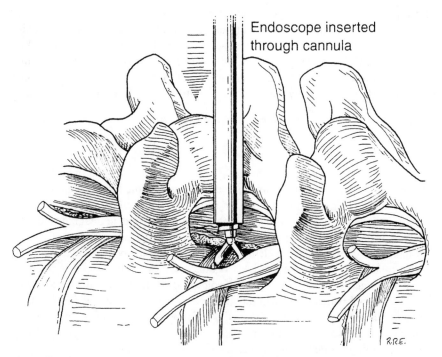

Endoscope inserted
through cannula

Figure 10.5 Application of small rongeur to remove disk material. (Reprinted with permission from HH Mathews, BE Mathern. Percutaneous Procedures in the Lumbar Spine. In HS An [ed], Principles and Techniques of Spine Surgery. Baltimore: Williams & Wilkins, 1998;739.)

medially over the herniated disk. If necessary, the membrane over the disk is incised, and the extruded disk is removed. The amount of disk that should be removed has been controversial. Spengler performed a randomized study comparing radical disk removal to the partial diskectomy.[29] He found improved results and lower recurrence when only the extruded fragment and adjacent loose disk material was removed.

Surgeons performing standard laminectomy and diskectomy are usually using loupe magnification and head lamp illumination. The use of the operating microscope fosters shortening the incision, lessening the muscle dissection, and allowing for a smaller fenestration between lamina. Additionally, epidural veins can be more easily visualized and coagulated, leading to less epidural scarring. These advantages are largely due to direct versus para-axial illumination, maintenance of three-dimensional vision, and the ability to angle the scope in different directions.[30] Another advantage to the surgeon is ergonomics, because the surgeon looks directly forward rather than bending over.

In performing microdiskectomy, a localized 1 1/2 in. incision is made between the spinous processes. The ipsilateral paraspinal muscles are subperiosteally elevated and retracted laterally, exposing the interlaminal space and facet capsule. A small amount of cranial and caudal lamina is resected, exposing the ligamentum flavum. The ligamentum flavum is mobilized and detached inferiorly and laterally. Delamarter recommends creating a flap of the ligamentum and retracting it medially, thereby preserving it.[30] Once the epidural space is entered, the caudal pedicle is identified. This is the key to safe navigation in the epidural space. The disk space is located just cranially to the pedicle, and the traversing nerve root is always along its medial border. By beginning dissection just medial to the pedicle and proceeding cranially, one is always assured of having control of the root. Using microdiskectomy instruments, such as the ball-tipped dissector, the root is elevated over the disk and retracted medially. Disk removal is carried out in the same manner as the open technique. After diskectomy, the mobility of the nerve is checked, as well as patency of the neuroforamina.

Results

The long-term results of open techniques depend primarily on the indications for surgery. Classically, the best results are in patients with radicular leg pain who have a corresponding neurologic sign, such as absent reflex, motor weakness, or paresthesia, a positive straight leg raising or other tension sign, and an imaging study that corresponds to the pattern of radicular pain and neurologic signs.

Kahanovitz compared 34 patients treated by limited open diskectomy to 30 patients treated by microdiskectomy.[31] No substantial difference was found regarding outcomes at 18 months between the two groups. Pain levels in the back and leg were low, and all patients returned to work except one patient in each group. Only one patient in the limited open group had to be reoperated. The only statistical difference was increased length of hospital stay for the open diskectomy group. Today, microdiskectomy is often performed as an outpatient procedure.

Barrios retrospectively compared 75 patients who had open diskectomy with 75 patients who had microdiskectomy.[32] He found no significant difference in operative time, infection rate, or residual pain. Patients in the microscopic group returned to activities at one-half the time and were released earlier from the hospital.

Tullberg prospectively randomized patients into either a microsurgical or an open laminectomy group.[33] Patients were followed for 1 year. Overall, success was seen in 85% of patients in each group. No difference was seen in patient length of stay, time to return to work, complication rate, or residual symptoms. He concluded that no benefit was received using the microscope and that the decision to use a microscope should be left to the surgeon.

Silvers compared consecutive series of 270 patients treated by open laminectomy and 270 patients treated by microdiskectomy.[34] The laminectomy group had 88.5% excellent results and 6.7% good results compared to 95.5% excellent results and 3% good results in the microdiskectomy group. No differences were seen regarding reoperation or recurrence. Length of stay was prolonged an average of 7 days versus 3 days in the open and microsurgical groups, respectively. Return to work was 10 weeks versus 13 weeks, favoring microdiskectomy.

These studies and others demonstrate the effectiveness of either technique in relieving leg and, in the majority of cases, back pain. Overall, successful results in properly selected patients are between 85% and 95%. Microscopic diskectomy may decrease length of stay and promote slightly earlier return to work or function, but has little extra benefit at 1-year follow-up over limited open laminectomy. Hanley has shown that the costs of open diskectomy and microdiskectomy are similar, and, therefore, the decision of which technique to use should be left to the surgeon (Hanley EN. Personal communication, 1998).

The microscopic technique requires thorough preoperative planning. The type of disk herniation and location are especially important. Delamarter has proposed localizing the disk pathology vertically in a three-story house (Figure 10.6).[30] The

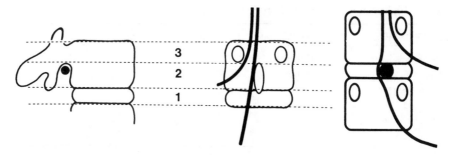

Figure 10.6 The disk and vertebral body can be thought of as a three-story house. Preoperatively, disk herniations are localized in the first story if they are directly opposite the disk. If they have migrated cranially between the pedicle and disk, they are in the second story. Disks localized medial to the cranial pedicle are in the third story. Occasionally, they may migrate caudally and are localized in the next caudal house's third story. When using minimally invasive techniques, accurate localization using this type of analysis is essential. (Reprinted with permission from JM Frymoyer [ed], The Adult Spine: Principles and Practice [2nd ed]. Philadelphia: Lippincott–Raven, 1997;1966.)

first story is the disk level, the second story is below the cranial pedicle, and the third story is at the superior pedicle. In some cases, the disk will be at the third story of the house below (i.e., opposite the caudal pedicle). By noting the exact position of the disk herniation preoperatively, the surgeon can remove the correct amount of lamina cranially and caudally and be prepared for identification of a displaced root that could otherwise be harmed.

Disk herniations may be classified as central, posterolateral, foramenal, or far lateral. Symptoms vary according to location, as do treatment methods and outcomes. The posterolateral is the most common and easily treated with microdiskectomy. Approaching the foramenal and extraforamenal herniation, one must remember that it is the root exiting above the disk that is compressed. The foramenal disk is always difficult to access surgically and may require sacrifice of a significant portion of the facet articulation. In some cases, the foramen is approached medially from the spinal canal and from the outside of the foramen to assure decompression. The far lateral disk herniation is often missed preoperatively. It is approached using microscopic techniques through the intertransverse membrane. These latter two disk ruptures may be better handled by endoscopic approaches, as described by Mathews. The central disk herniation is a failure of a large segment of the posterior annulus. This often occurs at L4–L5 and results in buttock and proximal bilateral leg pain. In some cases, spinal stenosis may be present. In other patients, significant loss of disk height is seen. The treatment of the central disk herniation is not well defined because of poor prognosis, despite a variety of treatments. If the patient has primarily radicular leg pain, then decompression with or without diskectomy can be attempted. Patients with primary low back pain can be considered candidates for fusion with interbody cages, as described in the section Results of Anterior Lumbar Interbody Fusion Using the Bagby-Kuslich Device, if they do not respond to medical management.

Complications

A list of complications and frequency is given in Table 10.2. As the techniques become less invasive, the chance of operating at the wrong level increases. Operating

Table 10.2 Complications of Microdiskectomy

Complication	Occurrence (%)
Wrong level	Unknown
Vascular	<0.05
Neurologic	1–3
Infection	0.5–2.0
Reoccurrence	5–7
Dural tears	1–3

at the wrong level can be avoided by obtaining high-quality intraoperative radiographs with markers placed at the exposed interspace and correlating the level with preoperative imaging studies.

Recurrence of symptoms secondary to reherniation occurs in 5–7% of cases. Chances of recurrence is not related to the postoperative course of rehabilitation or time to return to work. The rate of recurrence is probably more influenced by residual disk height and body mechanics.

Postoperative infection can be seen in the wound or in the intervertebral disks. Disk space infection often appears several months later without any drainage. The condition can be diagnosed with MRI, and the disk space should be biopsied to obtain an organism. Erythrocyte sedimentation rate, c-reactive protein, and white blood cells may be elevated. If antibiotics do not control symptoms, patients with diskitis are best treated with anterior interbody fusion.

Neural injury is being seen less frequently. Before disk removal, the medial edge of the exiting root must be identified and protected. Rarely, it is not possible to retract the root over the disk, and the disk is lying in the axilla between the lateral edge of the dura and the medial edge of the root. In this case, the neural tissues on both sides must be protected.

Vascular or other intra-abdominal injuries occur at a rate of 0.05% or less and are secondary to inadvertent passage of instruments out of the anterior annulus. Most common are injuries to the common iliac artery or vein, or both. Bleeding may be noted and is associated with a rapid loss of blood pressure. If this occurs, the patient should immediately be turned supine and undergo laparotomy. In more than 30% of cases, no bleeding is observed at the time of surgery. Increasing abdominal girth, low blood pressure, and a falling hematocrit are hallmarks of occult vascular injuries.

Conclusion

The results of open and microdiskectomy in properly selected patients are 85–95% good and excellent. Minimally invasive procedures have not shown better results and are associated with more complications, especially during the physician's learning curve. Microdiskectomy is cost effective and has been associated with decreased hospitalization times and earlier return to work. In a majority of centers, microdiskectomy is performed as an outpatient procedure. Postoperative early return to work and activities does not appear to increase the chance of recurrence or reduce overall results.

ADVANCES IN THE MANAGEMENT OF
CHRONIC DISKOGENIC LOW BACK PAIN

Episodes of acute low back pain resolve in the majority of patients, allowing them to regain full function; however, persistent pain and disability may last longer than 6 months. This chronic pain group contributes greatly to the escalating cost of back health care: up to $25 billion of direct medical costs and $75–$100 billion of indirect costs.[35] Despite this level of expenditure, the cause of chronic pain frequently eludes both the patient and physician. Advances in basic science, including the understanding of the neurophysiologic basis of pain, the distribution of nociceptors, histochemical markers of inflammation identified in the disk annulus and dorsal root ganglion, and newer modalities of imaging, such as MRI, have provided physicians with a greater ability to identify spinal pathology. Once identified, however, it is still uncertain if there is any surgical procedure that provides long-term, satisfactory outcome of the treatment of low back pain.

The majority of spine surgeons treat chronic low back pain nonoperatively. This is a consequence of the inability to determine the exact location of the pain generator, observed poor results from attempted surgery, high pseudarthrosis rates, and inappropriate surgical techniques. Even with pedicle screw instrumentation, in which a higher rate of successful lumbar fusion is obtained, the outcomes following lumbar fusion in chronic low back pain are still relatively poor. One explanation may be that the disk annulus is the most important pathologic feature of chronic low back pain, and, therefore, posterior surgery without directly treating the disk and annulus is not appropriate. The early success of interbody cage devices has reaffirmed the importance of the disk annulus as the source of the pain. Also, physicians are becoming more aware of the psychosocial aspects of chronic low back pain and disability and barriers to recovery. The use of psychometric testing and consultations with mental health providers can frequently identify patients who are unlikely to improve with surgery. The purpose of this section of the chapter is to promote the idea that there is a condition of diskogenic low back pain that can be treated surgically using interbody cage devices, with or without supplemental posterior fusion instrumentation.

Model for Diskogenic Low Back Pain

The intervertebral disk is a complex structure consisting of an inner nucleus and a surrounding annulus. The inner core or nucleus is made up of mucopolysaccharides, and the outer annulus is largely multilayers of collagen fibers oriented 30 degrees from the vertebral end plates. Few chondrocyte cells are present in the nucleus or annulus, and there is no obvious blood supply. Nutrients must diffuse through the vertebral end plates. Therefore, when injured, the disk annulus has a limited ability to heal.

In the normal state, nuclear pressure increases when loads are applied to the vertebral column, causing deflection of the vertebral end plates and transmission of forces through the vertebral bodies. With loss of nuclear mucopolysaccharides, the forces are transmitted peripherally onto the annulus. With repetitive overload, the disk annulus fragments and fissures with subsequent loss of disk height. As the degenerative process continues, stiffness develops in the vertebral end plate. Pain may be generated when the annulus sustains full thickness cleavages or fragmentation. Neuroanatomic and histologic studies of the disk reveal only the outer annulus to have nociceptors; therefore, the process of diskogenic pain must have disease extending to the outer annulus.[36] The highest concentration of nociceptors are in the posterior annulus in which the majority of annular injures are clinically observed.

Kuslich has reported observations that are consistent with the preceding noted mechanism of pain.[37] In awake patients undergoing lumbar diskectomy, he determined whether structures were painful to touch or pinching. The most painful structure is an inflamed nerve root, whereas a noninflamed nerve root is not associated with pain, even secondary to retraction or pinching. The second most painful structure in a normal disk is the posterior midline annulus. The facet capsules and the vertebral end plates have a moderate degree of pain when stimulated. MRI findings that demonstrate annular tears also help to confirm the concept of diskogenic pain.[38] In these cases, a high-intensity zone lesion is seen at the posterior annulus. During provocative diskography, dye is seen to exit the disk into the spinal canal through this annular disruption and is associated with pain provocation in more than 90% of cases. Finally, histochemical markers of inflammation have been identified at the sites of annular disruption and at the dorsal root ganglion, which is afferent to the annular nociceptors.[36]

Thus, there appears to be strong evidence for a source of pain caused from disk derangement involving the annulus. Two large groups of patients may be observed. First are those patients with nearly normal disk heights, but who have an annular tear. These patients are frequently workers who have been lifting and heard a pop or tear in their backs and developed sudden acute low back pain. Second is a group of patients with obvious degenerative disk disease as manifested by disk space narrowing, bony sclerosis, and, often, osteophytes.

Patient Evaluation

Careful patient evaluation is required to determine the source of the pain and whether a patient may benefit from surgical intervention. An understanding of the duration of pain and its effect on function is important. In general, patients who have long-term pain and disability for longer than 2–3 years rarely benefit from a surgical procedure. The type and character of the pain is significant. Most patients with diskogenic low back pain have mechanical-type symptoms (i.e., the pain is worse when they are up and active on their feet and better in a recumbent position). In general, these patients may be able to flex forward, but have difficulty returning to a standing position. In many cases, the patients have a history of radiculopathy that has either resolved or has been treated surgically and are now left with chronic low back pain of disk origin. The degree of pain should be measured using the visual analog scale. Pain diagrams are also useful in identifying patients who may have a nonanatomic distribution of pain and who would not be considered candidates for surgical treatment. An index of disability, such as the Roland's Index or Oswestry, should be obtained to objectively determine levels of disability.

The physical examination is often nonspecific. Patients may have limited and painful range of motion and paraspinal muscle spasms. Tenderness over specific spinous processes should be elicited because this may help to determine the segmental level of the pain generator. More important, nonorganic physical findings should be assessed using the Waddell's technique.[39] Patients with more than two Waddell's findings are not likely to benefit from surgical treatment. Patients with residual foramenal stenosis or disk herniation may manifest straight leg raising and objective neurologic findings, but these are usually negative in patients with only diskogenic pain.

Plain Radiographs

In assessing patients for diskogenic low back pain, four views of the lumbar spine are obtained: standing anteroposterior, standing lateral, and lateral flexion and extension. Although radiographic findings are well known to be nonspecific, certain findings may help identify the source of pain. Important or suspicious findings include mild degrees of instability, such as 3–4 mm of retrolisthesis often seen at L5–S1, increased angulation between vertebrae greater than 11 degrees, isolated disk space narrowing, peri–end plate sclerosis, bone on bone deformity, or nitrogen gas appearing in the intervertebral disk. Plain radiographs also help exclude other pathologic entities, such as isthmic spondylolisthesis, lumbar scoliosis, or fractures.

Magnetic Resonance Imaging

MRI not only allows physicians to identify anatomic lesions, but also gives evidence of physiologic dysfunction. For instance, the hydration of the disks as previously outlined is essential to their normal biomechanical function. When disks lose their hydration, a loss of signal on T2-weighted images is observed. This has been called *black disk disease*, and may be associated with chronic low back pain. The annular wall can be visualized, and abnormalities, such as a large central disk herniation, indicate a potential source of pain. Signal changes in the end plates and peri–end plate marrow spaces have been described as *Modic type I* and *type II*.[40] In Modic I changes, there is decreased signal in T1 and increased signal in T2. Histologically, this represents disruptive fissuring of the end plate and vascularized fibrous tissue within the marrow space. Type II changes show increased signal on T1 and isointense on T2. Histologically, these changes are associated with increased lipid content within the marrow space, possibly secondary to inflammation. Plain radiographs often demonstrate degenerative disk disease at this location. Other important findings are loss of disk space height, subluxation, disk herniation, foramenal stenosis, and epidural fibrosis. In patients who have had previous surgery, gadolinium enhancement is indicated.

One of the most significant lesions that is occasionally observed is the high-intensity zone lesion.[38] This lesion is seen on T2-weighted images as a small, round area of high-intensity signal at the posterior annulus, usually at the junction of the disk and caudal end plate. It is most often directly in the midline. High-intensity zone lesions strongly correlate with leakage of dye into the annulus secondary to annular disruption on provocative diskography and reproduction of concordant pain in more than 90% of cases.[38] The associated disk is usually desiccated, although it may still have a well-maintained disk height.

Psychometric Evaluation

A large majority of patients with low back pain and disability have or will develop psychosocial dysfunction. Anxiety, depression, and anger are common, especially in patients with third-party payors, such as workers' compensation or personal injury. The divisiveness introduced by the workers' compensation system, which has different goals than the patient and physician, leads to stress and financial difficulties for the patient. Many of these psychosocial factors can become barriers to successful outcomes of surgery. There should be particular emphasis on identifying drug, alcohol, and tobacco abusers. Patients who are polydrug abusers or are addicted to narcotic pain medications rarely benefit from surgery unless they voluntarily enter a drug treatment program. Similarly, patients with alcoholism tend to have poor outcomes. Finally, tobacco abuse appears to interfere significantly with the chance of fusion success. In our practice, all patients must quit smoking cigarettes before lumbar spinal fusion. Urine nicotine levels are checked randomly before surgery. If found positive, surgery is canceled and the patient is referred for further psychological management to deal with his or her tobacco addiction.

Standard psychometric tests, such as Minnesota Multiphasic Personality Inventory II and Beck Depression Index, are used to assess personality factors such as hypochondriasis, depression, and hysteria. If these scales are high, patients are not candidates for surgery. Depression, if severe and associated with more than three vegetative symptoms, should be treated with antidepressant medication and psychiatric consultation. Finally, the psychologist can help to clarify the patient's expectations, lowering them to reality before surgery. It is our practice before lumbar fusion to refer all patients for psychological consultation with a practitioner who specializes in chronic pain.

Confirmation of Pain Generator—Lumbar Diskography

After the history, physical examination, and radiographic review, one should have a reasonable idea of the source of pain or the pain generator. Several diagnostic categories are present and include internal disk derangement, high-intensity zone lesion, degenerative disk disease, unsuccessful diskectomy, mild instability syndrome, spondylolisthesis, and foramenal stenosis in conjunction with severe disk space narrowing (Table 10.3). All of these lesions may be associated with development of back pain and, possibly, referred pain into the lower extremities. Before surgery, however, it is incumbent that the anatomic level be confirmed using a provocative test. The hallmark of all of these conditions is that they affect the disk annulus, and, therefore, lumbar diskography can be used to generate pain, confirming the location of the pain generator.

Lumbar diskography is highly controversial. It was initially developed in an effort to avoid painful air-contrast myelography to diagnose herniated disks. Steindler observed that some patients without a mass lesion compressing a nerve root actually exhibited radicular leg pain from dye that leaked out of the disk during diskography.[41] Also, sciatic leg pain could be eliminated by installation of local analgesic. Smith used diskography to accurately diagnose the level of the herniated disk and proposed treatment with chemonucleolysis.[42]

Table 10.3 Etiology of Diskogenic Pain Syndromes

Internal disk derangement
High-intensity zone lesion
Degenerative disk disease
Unsuccessful diskectomy
Mild instability
Spondylolisthesis
Foramenal narrowing in conjunction with narrow disk space

Lumbar diskography, however, was largely discredited by Holt, who performed diskography at the bottom three disk levels on 30 asymptomatic prisoners in Illinois.[43] The injections were done transdurally with a 24-g needle, and 1–2 ml of 50% Hypaque was instilled in the disk. The patients were asked to respond to the pain during injection and were also studied morphologically. Seventy-two disks were injected, whereas 18 were unsuccessful. At L3–L4, there were 21 normal disks, four disks appeared to be degenerative, and two had associated herniated disks. At L4–L5, there were 14 normals, one degenerative, and eight with herniated disks. At L5–S1, there were 10 normals, six degenerative, and four with herniated disks. The pain response, however, showed no pain in all 45 disks that had normal morphology. Eleven disks were associated with complaints of low back pain, and all had degeneration. Sixteen disks had low back and leg pain after injection. All of these disks had an associated annular disruption. Overall, there was a 37% false-positive rate. Holt concluded from the study that provocative diskography had no value as a diagnostic test.

Many other authors have reviewed the study and identified several important limitations. Simmons reviewed the Holt study and noted that there was a high nonsuccess rate due to the needles not being placed under fluoroscopic control.[44] Therefore, there was a possibility that the needles were inaccurately placed into the annulus rather than into the nucleus. They questioned the sincerity of volunteers from a prison population and noted that there are numerous inaccuracies between the results given by Holt and the tables produced in his text. Hypaque is well known to be a toxic and irritating iodinated contrast material that can cause pain. Finally, transdural injections clearly could be associated with false-positives due to leakage of dye into the spinal fluid.

Walsh performed diskography at the lower three levels of 10 asymptomatic volunteers and seven patients with chronic low back pain.[45] None of the asymptomatic volunteers had any pain provocation; however, 17% of the disks injected had morphologic abnormalities, such as degeneration. In the patients with low back pain, 65% of the disks were painful and correlated with the patient's usual and customary pain. There was at least one abnormal disk in all of the patients morphologically. The conclusion from this study is that diskography is a specific test in determining if a disk is painful.

Moneta reviewed 833 diskograms in 306 symptomatic patients who were considered candidates for surgery.[46] He assessed the degree of annular disruption and degeneration on scales from zero to three. He found a strong correlation between the annular disruption and pain generation, whereas degenerative disk disease did not correlate with pain generation. Schwarzer investigated 92 patients who had 255 disks injected.[47] Pain was assessed and did not correlate to morphology of the disk, but did correlate if there was dye extravasation through an annular tear. There was also no correlation between any physical findings and patterns of pain. Several authors have investigated the effectiveness of using provocative diskography in determining surgical outcome. Colhoun operated on 137 patients with positive pain response and 25 patients who had no pain but abnormal morphology.[48] In the pain group, 89% of patients had good outcome; in the group with no pain, only 52% had good outcome. Gill and Blumenthal performed a single-level anteroposterior fusion at L5–S1 based on results of diskography.[49] In those patients with an outer annular tear, 75% had good outcome, whereas only 50% of patients had good outcome if there was only degeneration without leakage of dye.

Lumbar diskography is associated with few complications. There is increased pain for 1–2 weeks after diskography in some cases. Diskitis occurs in less than 1%

Table 10.4 Criteria for Positive Diskogram

Normal control
Concordant pain response
Dye extravasation out of outer annulus

of cases, and this decreases with the use of a double-needle technique. There appears to be no long-term effect from undergoing diskography or having installation of contrast material. This conclusion is confirmed in animal studies and clinical studies by Johnson and Flanagan. These authors studied patients who underwent a second diskography up to 10 years after the initial examination. No obvious significant deterioration was noted.[50,51]

Diskography is a highly technical test that should be performed and interpreted in a meticulous manner. It is usually performed with a lateral technique using two needles. An outer needle engages the annulus and an inner needle is then positioned in the center of the disk. This should be done in at least two or three levels and in a blinded fashion. Once all needles are properly positioned into the center of the disk, pressurization ensues in a blinded fashion. During the procedure, the patient is continually asked what he or she is feeling and whether any discomfort is concordant or nonconcordant with his or her customary back or leg pain, or both. Pressurization is performed with a 3-ml syringe at a slow flow rate of 1–2 ml per minute. The morphology of the disk and whether there is any leakage is noted under fluoroscopy. A computed tomography scan is then performed of abnormal disk levels. Additional information may be obtained by manometric measurements and pain responses. It is thought that there are two types of diskogenic pain syndromes: one that is chemically irritating in which pain is associated with low pressures, and a second type that requires high levels of pressure to generate pain. The significance of these two types of pain provocation is still uncertain.

The accepted criteria for a positive diskography are that the patient has a nonpainful control level, pain is produced in the patient's usual and customary location, and there is leakage of contrast out of the outer annulus (Table 10.4). It is essential that all three parts of this criteria be met before the diskogram is considered positive (Figure 10.7).

In summary, diskography is a highly technical procedure that is specific in identifying a source of pain generation. It is most commonly associated with annular disruption. When done properly, diskography appears to be a safe diagnostic test. Typically, diskography is used as a preoperative test to confirm the painful level. Occasionally, diskography may be indicated to prove to the patient, physician, or third party that a pathologic entity exists. Even though the test is painful, many patients have expressed gratitude that a test was ordered that could identify a pain-generating condition.

Surgical Indications for Chronic Diskogenic Low Back Pain

The indications for surgical treatment of patients with diskogenic pain are patients with disabling pain lasting longer than 6 months, who have had unsuccessful non-operative management, who have a positive diskogram at one or two adjacent motion segments, who have back pain greater than leg pain, and who are without

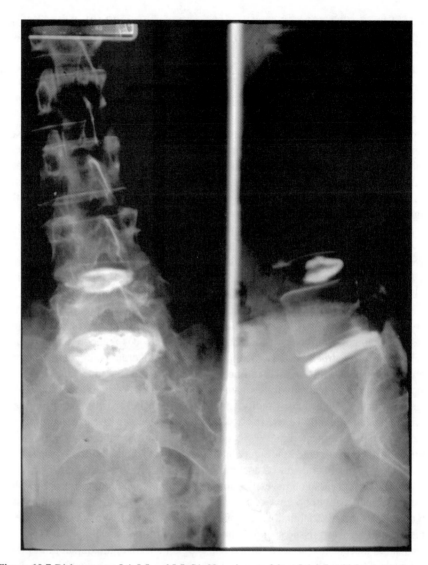

Figure 10.7 Diskogram at L4–L5 and L5–S1. No pain was felt at L4–L5, which appeared morphologically normal. At L5–S1, when the dye leaked into the epidural space, intense concordant pain was felt. The patient underwent successful anterior fusion with a cage, which relieved her back and leg pain.

significant disk herniation or stenosis. Patients should be without significant psychosocial factors that could affect recovery.

Before surgery, all patients should have had a trial of nonsteroidal anti-inflammatory agents, acetaminophen compounds, and active physical therapy. The rehabilitative techniques, as described by Saal, emphasizing reconditioning of back muscles starting gently and then advancing to more vigorous states are recommended.[52] Physical therapy using modalities and other passive techniques should be stopped and changed to active, strength-building techniques. In the early phases, aquatic training may be useful. Only after a patient is unresponsive to a concerted effort should he or she be considered for surgical treatment of his or her diskogenic disease. The location of the disease is determined initially by plain radiographs and MRI, then confirmed with lumbar diskography as described in the section Confirmation of Pain Generator—Lumbar Diskography. Based on poor outcomes, there seems to be little role for fusions involving three or more levels. Additionally, skip lesions (in which there is an intervening normal disk space) are best treated nonsurgically.

The rationale for the current treatment of diskogenic pain is to remove the disk, re-establish normal tension in the annulus by re-establishing disk height, increasing lumbar lordosis, indirectly opening neuroforamina, and stabilizing the motion segment. Historically, the treatment of chronic diskogenic pain was largely inadequate. This was because most patients were treated with posterior fusions that did not adequately address the disk pathology and did not correct many of the anatomic abnormalities. Even when anterior fusions were attempted, they were associated with a high pseudarthrosis rate unless they were combined with posterior stabilization.

Bagby developed the interbody cage for treatment of wobbler's disease in thoroughbred race horses. As the horse runs, it develops a cervical subluxation and a progressive myelopathy with ataxia. Bagby treated these animals by anterior cervical fusion using stainless steel cylindric baskets placed in the disk space. Bagby's clinical results were excellent in approximately 90% of horses, many of which returned to racing and won stakes races.[53] The Bagby baskets have been modified by adding threads, changing sizes to fit the human cervical and lumbar spines, and are now made of titanium. Interbody fusion with these cage devices is theoretically ideal in that they allow distraction of the disk space, provide inherent stabilization, act as a reservoir for bone grafting, and can be placed from either the anterior or posterior approach.[54] Biomechanical studies have confirmed that the Bagby-Kuslich (BAK) interbody cage devices have rigidity equal to pedicle screw instrumentation; therefore, they can frequently be used as a stand-alone device and do not require supplemental spinal instrumentation.[55,56] Seven different animal studies, including two in primates, have documented the safety and efficacy of threaded interbody cages.

Lumbar spinal fusion can be accomplished either through an anterior or posterior approach, or, in some cases, a combined technique. The anterior approach is becoming increasingly popular because it is not associated with the morbidity seen in posterior surgery. Zdeblick has termed this *morbidity fusion disease* and believes it is secondary to soft tissue stripping and retraction of the paraspinal muscles. This can lead to muscle atrophy and subsequent fatigability. Also, the dorsal rami plexus is stretched or directly injured with consequences of a feeling of numbness in the back by the patients and further weakness of the paraspinal musculature. Epidural scarring and interference with the adjacent motion segment are also avoided by performing anterior fusion. Disadvantages of the anterior approach are potential for massive blood loss, retrograde ejaculation in males, and lower fusion rates until the development of cage devices.

Anterior Approach

The anterior approach to the lumbar spine affords excellent access to the intervertebral disk. Extension of the patient on the operating table over a bolster opens the disk space. During surgery, the disk space can be distracted further, if desired. A diskectomy is performed by incising the anterior annulus and completely removing the disk back to the posterior annulus. Once the diskectomy is performed, reconstruction is carried out. Before cages, this procedure was performed by bone dowels or various allografts, such as femoral rings. The femoral rings can be stabilized with interference screws or plates. However, a high pseudarthrosis rate occurs unless the patient is treated concomitantly with a posterior instrumentation.

The development of the interbody cages has been an important innovation in the care of patients with diskogenic low back pain. Threaded interbody cages, such as the BAK or Ray cage, can be inserted either through an open or laparoscopic technique. The open technique is performed through a ventral incision with retroperitoneal dissection. At L5–S1, the cages are inserted between the right and left common iliac artery and veins. Once the middle sacral artery is identified and ligated, blunt dissection laterally allows easy retraction of the iliac vessels to allow access to the disk. At the L4–L5 or higher levels, the dissection occurs to the left of the aorta where segmental vessels and the recurrent iliolumbar vein are identified and ligated. The aorta, vena cava, and left iliac vessels are then mobilized along their left side and retracted to the patient's right side. Occasionally, inadequate exposure at L4–L5 prevents the placement of two interbody cages.

The laparoscopic technique is done through four portals.[57] In most cases, the camera is placed in an umbilical portal and looks down onto the sacral promontory. Two 5-mm lateral portals are used to insert instruments to retract soft tissues and vessels. A suprapubic portal is used for insertion of the drill tube to allow reaming and then subsequent insertion of cages. The laparoscopic technique takes approximately twice the operative time as the open technique, but does shorten the hospital stay. It is well received by the public, although no long-term benefits have been observed over the open technique.

The BAK device, which was the modification of the Bagby basket, was the first intervertebral device to be approved by the FDA. Subsequently, the Ray cage and Danek cage have been approved for use in the lumbar spine. A number of other manufacturers have ongoing investigations using their proprietary devices. Threaded cortical dowels, which look similar to the cages, have been introduced and appear to have a high rate of success, although published results are lacking.

Results of Anterior Lumbar Interbody Fusion Using the Bagby-Kuslich Device. Kuslich reported the results of 947 patients treated by the BAK device under an FDA-monitored multicenter study.[54] Five hundred and ninety-one patients had the cages placed through the anterior approach. Major complications occurred in 2% of the patients, including vascular injuries, retrograde ejaculation, implant migration, or sacral fractures. Overall, 4.5% of patients required reoperation. Fusion success of one-level fusions was 92% and 98% at 1 and 2 years, respectively. Two-level fusions did not fair as well, with success at 78% and 80% at 1 and 2 years, respectively. Return to work was seen in 48% of disabled patients by 2 years. Of those working or eligible to work at the time of surgery, 78% were working at 2 years. Pain was scored by a visual analog scale of 0–6. Pain averaged 5.0 before surgery and 2.9 2 years later. Eighty-five percent of patients noted improvement. Similarly, dysfunction was measured on a scale of 0–32. This index improved from 19 to 10 at 2 years. A case example is given in Figure 10.8.

Posterior Approach

Standard posterior and posterolateral fusions without instrumentation have had relatively poor outcomes in management of patients with diskogenic diseases.[58] Results of only 50–80% good to excellent have been reported. The posterior lumbar interbody fusion, as proposed by Cloward, has the theoretic advantages of removal of the

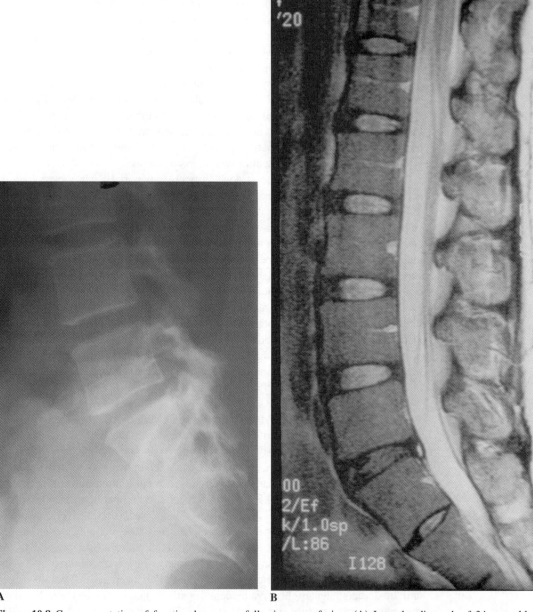

A   B

Figure 10.8 Case presentation of functional recovery following cage fusion. **(A)** Lateral radiograph of 34-year-old woman with severe low back pain after a lifting injury. Unable to work, she lost her home, was separated from her children, and was living in her van. Social services was consulted and found her a home and medical insurance. Psychometric testing was negative. **(B)** Sagittal T2-weighted magnetic resonance imaging shows normal disk hydration, except at L5–S1, which is desiccated. A high-intensity lesion is seen at posterior margin of L5–S1 annulus. **(C)** Axial T2-weighted image at L5–S1 showing the high-intensity lesion at the center of the posterior annulus. **(D)** The patient had a positive diskogram at L5–S1 and negative L4–L5. She underwent laparoscopic L5–S1 Bagby-Kuslich cage fusion with autograft. Postoperative lateral radiographs 12 months later show good position of cages. The fusion cannot be visualized.

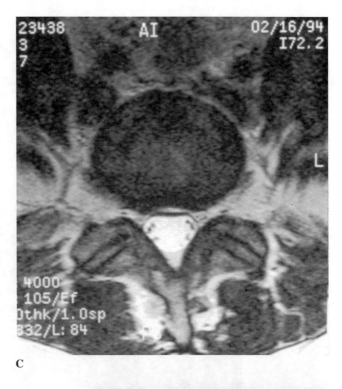

C

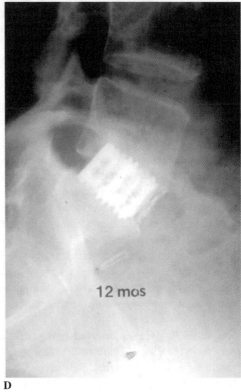

12 mos

D

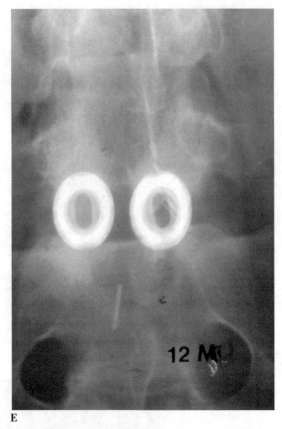

E

Figure 10.8 *(continued)* **(E)** Postoperative anteroposterior radiographs at 12-month follow-up. The patient had no pain, was working two jobs, and had re-established her family.

disk, thereby removing the painful nidus, anterior column support, and correction and maintenance of lordosis.[59] However, results were disappointing secondary to a high pseudarthrosis rate and chronic leg pain, which occurred in many patients, secondary to excessive root retraction required during insertion of the bone grafts. Cylindrical, threaded intervertebral cages, similar to those discussed in the anterior approach, have been developed for posterior lumbar interbody fusion. Although the instrumentation is an improvement over Cloward's technique, a significant amount of retraction still exists, which occurs during insertion, with the possibility of patients developing postoperative neurologic deficits. However, early results of intervertebral cages placed with a posterior lumbar approach appear satisfactory.

Results of Ray Cages Inserted Using a Posterior Lumbar Interbody Technique.
Ray reported the outcome of a multicenter FDA-monitored study of Ray cages inserted through a posterior lumbar interbody fusion approach.[60] No supplemental fixation was used. Two hundred thirty-six patients were enrolled and 211 were reported at 2-year follow-up. Fusion was seen in 98% of patients. Pain relief was good or excellent in 65% of patients. Functional improvement, as determined by

the Prolo method, was poor in only 14% of patients. Infection was seen in 3% of patients. Up to 10% of patients had temporary foot weakness or numbness, which resolved in all but two patients.

Another technique, approved by the FDA, is the Brantigan cage.[61] This is a rectangular-shaped, carbon fiber cage, which is available in sizes 9–13 mm tall and 25 mm long. It is placed into the intervertebral disk space after diskectomy and disk distraction. The advantage of this cage is that less retraction of the roots and dura is needed because it is narrower than the cylindric cages. This cage is not a stand-alone device, however, and it requires the augmentation of pedicle screw instrumentation. Tullberg reported successful fusion in 89% of levels treated by the Brantigan cage with supplemental pedicle screws.[62] Other products, such as cortical rectangular-shaped bone grafts, have been developed for posterior lumbar interbody fusions.

The use of posterior lumbar interbody fusion device with posterior pedicle screw instrumentation increases the biomechanical rigidity and appears to increase the fusion success. This approach is especially indicated when there is ipsilateral collapse with narrowing of the neuroforamena, lateral translocation, isolated kyphoscoliosis, or severe foramenal stenosis due to loss of disk height. The disadvantages of the posterior lumbar interbody fusion plus pedicle screw approach are increased instrument costs and the possibility of neurologic injury due to retraction.

Combined Anteroposterior Surgery

Patients treated for diskogenic pain are often complex and often have difficulty recovering and returning to work. Lack of success of both nonoperative and operative treatment modalities leads to prolongation of pain and disability, with progressive loss of faith in the medical system by both the patient and family. The time off work raises both the medical and indirect costs. Increased pressure is exerted by vocational counselors and industrial insurance claims managers, leading to anxiety and divisiveness in the patient's overall care. Therefore, it may be justified to perform as aggressive a surgery as necessary to give the earliest and greatest chance of success. Biomechanical studies indicate insertion of interbody devices, along with pedicle screw instrumentation, leads to the stiffest motion segment. Animal studies show that combined approaches result in earlier healing and higher rates of healing. Clinically, higher fusion rates are observed. The disadvantages are the added surgical time, costs, and slower rehabilitation. With improvements in surgical techniques, including minimally invasive surgical technologies, and as more skilled surgeons perform these operations, the combined anteroposterior approach may become cost justified.

Results of the combined anteroposterior surgical approach are excellent, even in a workers' compensation population.[63] Hinkley reported 81 patients with positive diskograms and evidence of posterior column pathology treated by anterior interbody fusion with allograft and posterolateral fusion with pedicular instrumentation. Twelve patients who had the same preoperative testing results, but who did not have surgery, acted as controls. Overall, pain reduction and improved function were seen in 91% of the surgical group, whereas the control group had increased pain and decreased function. Fusion success was 100% for one-level fusion, 95% for two-level fusion, and 92% for three-level fusion. Given the catastrophic results of unsuccessful fusion, especially in workers' compensation, I wonder if an anteroposterior surgery should always be performed to yield the highest chance of success the first time.

SUMMARY

Less invasive techniques of treating lumbar spine conditions are available that decrease morbidity and allow earlier return to function. However, their results in the management of radiculopathy have not been shown to be better than accepted techniques and are more related to patient selection than the specific technique. For patients with radiculopathy, surgical indications include no response after 6 weeks of conservative care, leg pain in a specific distribution confirmed by a neuroimaging study, and associated neurologic signs. Patients with these findings should have an 85–95% chance of successful outcome from a surgical procedure.

For patients with chronic diskogenic low back pain, interbody fusion with cage devices may be appropriate. Before surgery, patients should have the painful level confirmed by diskography and should have been evaluated by psychometric testing. Use of tobacco products must be discontinued for 6 weeks before surgery. My preferred approach is to perform anterior lumbar interbody fusion with threaded cages. Long-term studies are needed to determine true rates of fusion and establish efficacy.

REFERENCES

1. Mixter WJ, Barr JS. Rupture of the intervertebral disc with involvement of the spinal canal. N Engl J Med 1934;211:210–215.
2. Smith L, Garvin PJ, Jennings RB, Gesler RM. Enzyme dissolution of the nucleus pulposus. Nature 1963;198:1311–1312.
3. Nordby EJ, Fraser RD. Chemonucleolysis. In JW Frymoyer (ed), The Adult Spine: Principles and Practice. Philadelphia: Lippincott–Raven 1997;1989–2008.
4. Konings JG, Williams FJ, Deutman R. The effects of chemonucleolysis as demonstrated by computerised tomography. J Bone Joint Surg Br 1985;66B:417–421.
5. Kato F, Mimatsu K, Kawakami N, et al. Serial changes observed by magnetic resonance imaging in the intervertebral disc after chemonucleolysis. A consideration of the mechanism of chemonucleolysis. Spine 1992;17:934–939.
6. Lorenz M, McCulloch J. Chemonucleolysis for herniated nucleus pulposus in adolescents. J Bone Joint Surg Am 1985;67:1402–1404.
7. Benoist M, Bouillet R, Mulholland R. Chemonucleolysis. Results of a European survey. Acta Orthop Belg 1983;49:32–47.
8. Nordby EJ. Eight- to 13-year follow-up evaluation of chemonucleolysis patients. Clin Orthop 1986;206:18–23.
9. Gogan WJ, Fraser RD. Chymopapain. A 10-year double-blind study. Spine 1992;17:388–394.
10. Alexander AH, Burkus JK, Mitchell JB, Ayers WV. Chymopapain chemonucleolysis versus surgical discectomy in a military population. Clin Orthop 1989;244:158–165.
11. Muralikuttan KP, Hamilton A, Kernohan WG, et al. A prospective randomized trial of chemonucleolysis and conventional disc surgery in single level lumbar disc herniation. Spine 1992;17:381–387.
12. Hoppenfeld S. Percutaneous removal of herniated lumbar discs: 50 cases with ten-year follow-up periods. Clin Orthop 1989;207:92–97.
13. Hijikata S, Yamagishi M, Nakayama T, et al. Percutaneous discectomy: a new treatment method for lumbar disc herniation. J Toden Hosp 1975;5:5–13.
14. Kambin P, Sampson S. Posterolateral percutaneous suction-excision of herniated lumbar intervertebral discs. Clin Orthop 1986;207:37–43.
15. Onik G, Helms C, Ginsburg I, et al. Percutaneous lumbar discectomy using a new aspiration probe. AJNR Am J Neuroradiol 1985;6:290.
16. Goldstein TB, Mink JH, Dawson EG. Early experience with automated percutaneous lumbar discectomy in the treatment of lumbar disc herniation. Clin Orthop 1989;238:77–82.

17. Revel N, Payan C, Vallee C, et al. Automated percutaneous lumbar discectomy versus chemo-nucleolysis in the treatment of sciatica: a randomized multicenter trial. Spine 1993;18:1–17.
18. Kahanovitz N, Viola K, Goldstein T, et al. A multicenter analysis of percutaneous discectomy. Spine 1990;15:713–715.
19. Chatterjee S, Foy PM, Findlay GF. Report of a controlled clinical trial comparing automated percutaneous lumbar discectomy and microdiscectomy in the treatment of contained lumbar disc herniation. Spine 1995;20:734–738.
20. Schreiber A, Suezawa Y, Leu HJ. Does percutaneous nucleotomy with discoscopy replace conventional discectomy? Eight years of experience and results in treatment of herniated lumbar disc. Clin Orthop 1989;238:35–42.
21. Kambin P, Schaffer J. Percutaneous lumbar discectomy: prospective review of 100 patients. Clin Orthop 1989;238:24–34.
22. Kambin P. Arthroscopic microdiscectomy. Arthroscopy 1992;8:287–295.
23. Casey KF, Chang MK, O'Brien ED, et al. Arthroscopic microdiscectomy: comparison of preoperative and postoperative imaging studies. Arthroscopy 1997;13:438–445.
24. Burman MS. Myeloscopy or the direct visualization of spinal cord. Am J Bone Joint Surg 1931;13:395.
25. Pool JL. Direct visualization of dorsal nerve roots of the cauda equina by means of the myeloscope. Arch Neurol Psychiat 1938;39:1308.
26. Stoll JE. Endoscopic spatial orientation and surgical approaches in the epidural space. Williamsburg, VA: Current Concepts in Spinal Endoscopy Symposium, 1993.
27. Mathews HH, Stoll JE. Palm Springs, CA: Current Concepts in Spinal Endoscopy Symposium, 1994.
28. Mathews HH. Spinal Endoscopy: Evolution, Foundations and Applications. In KH Bridwell, RL DeWald (eds), The Textbook of Spinal Surgery (2nd ed). Philadelphia: Lippincott–Raven, 1997;2297–2311.
29. Spengler DM. Lumbar discectomy. Results with limited disc excision and selective foraminotomy. Spine 1982;7:604–607.
30. Delamarter RD, McCulloch JA. Microdiscectomy and Microsurgical Spinal Laminotomies. In JW Frymoyer (ed), The Adult Spine: Principles and Practice (2nd ed). Philadelphia: Lippincott–Raven, 1997;1961–1988.
31. Kahanovitz N, Viola K, McCulloch J. Limited surgical discectomy and microdiscectomy: a clinical comparison. Spine 1989;14:79–81.
32. Barrios C, Ahmed M, Arrotequi J, et al. Microsurgical versus standard removal of the herniated lumbar disc. Acta Orthop Scand 1990;61:399–402.
33. Tullberg T, Isacson J, Weidenhielm L. Does microscopic removal of lumbar disc herniation lead to better results than standard procedure? Spine 1993;18:24–27.
34. Silvers HR. Microsurgical versus standard lumbar discectomy. Neurosurgery 1998;22:837–841.
35. Pope MH. Occupational Hazards for Low Back Pain. In JN Weinstein, SL Gordon (eds), Low Back Pain: A Scientific and Clinical Overview. Rosemont, IL: American Academy of Orthopedic Surgery, 1996;33.
36. Cavanaugh JM. Neural Mechanisms of Idiopathic Low Back Pain. In JN Weinstein, SL Gordon (eds), Low Back Pain: A Scientific and Clinical Overview. Rosemont, IL: American Academy of Orthopedic Surgery, 1996;583–605.
37. Kuslich SD, Ulstrom CL, Michael CJ. The tissue origin of low back pain and sciatica: a report of pain response to tissue stimulation during operations on the lumbar spine using local anesthesia. Orthop Clin North Am 1991;22:181–187.
38. Aprill CN, Bogduk N. High intensity zone: a diagnostic sign of painful lumbar disc on magnetic resonance imaging. Br J Radiol 1992;65:361–369.
39. Waddell G, McCulloch JA, Kummel E, Venner RM. Nonorganic physical signs in low-back pain. Spine 1980;5:117–125.
40. Ross JS, Modic MT. Current assessment of spinal degenerative disease with magnetic resonance imaging. Clin Orthop 1992;279:68–81.
41. Steindler A, Luck J. Differential diagnosis of pain low in the back: allocation of the source of pain by procaine hydrochloride method. JAMA 1938;110:106–113.
42. Smith L, Brown JE. Treatment of lumbar intervertebral disc lesions by direct injection of chymopapain. J Bone Joint Surg Br 1967;49B:502–519.

43. Holt EP Jr. The question of lumbar discography. J Bone Joint Surg Am 1968;50:720–726.

44. Simmons JW, Aprill CN, Dwyer AP, Brodsky AE. A reassessment of Holt's data on "The question of lumbar discography." Clin Orthop 1988;237:120–124.

45. Walsh T, Weinstein J, Spratt K, et al. The question of lumbar discography revised: a controlled perspective study of normal volunteers to determine the false-positive rate. J Bone Joint Surg Am 1990;72:1081–1088.

46. Moneta G, Videman T, Kaivanto K, et al. Reported pain during lumbar discography as a function of annular ruptures and disc degeneration. A re-analysis of 833 discograms. Spine 1994;19:1968–1974.

47. Schwarzer AC, Aprill CN, Derby R, et al. The prevalence and clinical features of internal disc disruption in patients with chronic low back pain. Spine 1996;21:776–777.

48. Colhoun E, McCall IW, Williams L, Cassar-Pullicino VN. Provocation discography as a guide to planning operations on the spine. J Bone Joint Surg Br 1988;70:267–271.

49. Gill K, Blumenthal S. Functional results after anterior lumbar fusions at L5–S1 in patients with normal and abnormal MRI scans. Spine 1992;17:940–942.

50. Johnson RG. Does discography injure normal discs? An analysis of repeat discograms. Spine 1989;14:424–426.

51. Flanagan MN, Chung B. Roentgenographic changes in 188 patients 10–20 years after discography and chemonucleolysis. Spine 1986;11:444–448.

52. Saal JA. Dynamic muscular stabilization in the non-operative treatment of lumbar pain syndromes. Orthop Rev 1990;19:691–700.

53. Wagner PC, Grant BD, Bagby GW, et al. Evaluation of spine fusion as treatment in the equine wobbler syndrome. J Vet Surg 1979;8:84–88.

54. Kuslich SD, Ulstrom CL, Griffen SL. The Bagby and Kuslich method of lumbar interbody fusion: history, techniques and two-year follow-up results of United States prospective multicenter trial study. Spine 1997;23:1267–1279.

55. Brodke DS, Dick JC, Kunz DN, et al. Posterior lumbar interbody fusion. A biomechanical comparison, including a new threaded cage. Spine 1997;22:26–31.

56. Tencer AF, Hampton D, Eddy S. Biomechanical properties of threaded inserts for lumbar interbody fusion. Spine 1995;20:2408–2414.

57. Regan JJ, McAfee PC, Mack MJ. Atlas of endoscopic spinal surgery. St. Louis: Quality Medical Publishing, 1995.

58. Brantigan JW. Pseudarthrosis rate after allograft posterior lumbar interbody fusion with pedicle screw and plate fixation. Spine 1994;19:1271–1279.

59. Cloward RB. The treatment of ruptured lumbar intervertebral discs by vertebral body fusion. J Neurosurg 1953;10:154–166.

60. Ray CD. Threaded titanium cages for lumbar interbody fusions. Spine 1997;22:667–680.

61. Brantigan JW, Steffee AD. A carbon fiber implant to aid interbody lumbar fusion. Two-year clinical results in the first 26 patients. Spine 1993;18:2106–2107.

62. Tullberg T, Brandt B, Rydberg J, Fritzell P. Fusion rate after posterior lumbar interbody fusion with carbon fiber implant: one-year follow-up of 51 patients. Eur Spine J 1996;5:178–182.

63. Hinkley BS, Jarenko ME. Effects of 360-degree lumbar fusion in a workers' compensation population. Spine 1997;22:312–323.

PART IV
Low Back Pain and Disability

Chapter 11

Risk Factors in the Development and Management of Low Back Pain in Adults

Steven H. Sanders

The prevalence and cost of acute and chronic low back pain in adults are epidemic throughout the industrialized world. Acute back pain strikes approximately 80% of the adult population at some time in their lives and is the leading cause of absenteeism among workers.[1] Hundreds of millions of adults experience low back pain around the world each year, costing billions of dollars in treatment, lost productivity, and wage replacement. The number of adults experiencing disabling chronic low back pain is rising at exponential rates across countries, with the United States leading the way. Epidemiologic studies indicate anywhere from 5% to 15% of adults experiencing acute low back pain develop a chronic disabling condition. In addition, these chronically disabled low back pain patients appear to consume the vast majority of available health care and compensation dollars.[2,3]

Because many individuals who experience acute and chronic low back pain due to injuries find it difficult to return to gainful employment, medicolegal issues and obstacles have also demonstrated accelerated growth in number and complexity. These medicolegal issues and obstacles have further compounded the ability of health care providers to effectively manage low back pain patients.[4]

The rapidly escalating prevalence of disabling chronic low back pain, accompanied by major increases in cost, has prompted more government-sponsored and independent research projects aimed at better understanding, and possibly predicting, the occurrence of acute and chronic low back pain. As with cardiovascular disease and cancer, one promising area of research has been the identification of significant risk factors that either correlate with or demonstrate, or both, a cause and effect relationship with the occurrence and persistence of low back pain.[5] Through such a process, useful information can be determined, distributed, and applied by health care providers, employers, insurance companies, governmental agencies, and the population at large. The goal is to better detect, treat, and, hopefully, prevent the continued rise of this major health problem.

This chapter is intended to assimilate and interpret this growing research and clinical information base regarding risk factors in acute and chronic low back pain in adults. It reviews and discusses known, probable, and possible risk factors associated with the onset of acute pain and the development of chronic disabling low back pain, including an overview of possible assessment techniques to determine the presence of risk factors. Likewise, recommendations are made, based on existing research and demonstrated clinical practice, on the best methods available to change the risk factors that can be modified.

The focus throughout the chapter is a blend of empirically based information and recommendations for the practicing clinician in rehabilitation medicine to better understand and effectively manage adult low back pain patients.

RISK FACTORS FOR ACUTE AND CHRONIC DISABLING LOW BACK PAIN

This section reviews known and probable or possible risk factors for the occurrence of acute and chronic disabling (i.e., inability to return to work) low back pain. It should be clearly stated that none of the risk factors reviewed has adequate empirical research demonstrating a clear causal effect on low back pain. However, all of the known risk factors have substantial evidence demonstrating that they can predict the occurrence of acute or chronic disabling low back pain, or both. In addition, probable and possible risk factors have enough empirical support to suggest that they may be significant predictors.

Known Risk Factors

Although it is possible to generate a long list of known risk factors, the risk factors with substantial empirical documentation of a predictive relationship with low back pain are summarized in Table 11.1. The table lists risk factors for both acute and chronic disabling low back pain, as well as recommendations for assessing each. The table illustrates 13 risk factors that have been studied and have received substantial research support. Although these risk factors are ordered with regard to their demonstrated predictability of acute or chronic disabling low back pain, or both, not enough data exist to determine any consistent preferential weighting regarding their predictive power. Representative research studies and reviews associated with a given risk factor are referenced in the table, along with references associated with any published assessment instruments recommended.

Back Pain History, Smoking, and Age

Individuals with a history of low back pain or who smoke are at increased risk for acute low back pain (see Table 11.1). These two factors have been repeatedly identified in large-scale studies and are typically assessed within the context of a routine clinical history and interview. Their predictive capabilities for the development of chronic disabling low back pain have not been adequately demonstrated. It is surprising that smoking has not been shown to be predictive of chronic disabling low back pain in research literature. This may be because of a lack of attention to this particular factor in studies focusing on chronic low back pain.

Age is a risk factor that has predictive value for acute and chronic disabling back pain. While the research literature has not been able to delineate discrete age groups, there does appear to be a much higher probability for low back pain within two age groups. For the onset of acute back pain, individuals between ages 25 and

Table 11.1 Known Risk Factors for Acute and Chronic Disabling Low Back Pain

| Risk Factor | Low Back Pain | | How to Assess |
	Acute[a]	Chronic Disabling[b]	
Back pain history[5,6]	Yes	?	Clinical interview
Smoking[5]	Yes	?	Clinical interview
Age[7,8]	Yes	Yes	Clinical interview
Job dissatisfaction[6,7,9–12]	Yes	Yes	Work APGAR[10]
Heavy physical work[5,7–9,11]	Yes	Yes	Social Security Administration and *Dictionary of Occupational Titles* job ratings[13,14]
Severe psychological stress or abuse[15–17]	Yes	Yes	Clinical interview; stress questionnaire[18,19]
MMPI Scale 3 elevation[5,7,8,10,20]	Yes	Yes	MMPI[21]
Depression[5,7,8]	?	Yes	Clinical interview; Beck Depression Inventory[22]
Substance abuse[7]	?	Yes	Clinical interview; drug screens
Low activity/high pain behavior and disability[5,7,23]	?	Yes	Pain behavior lists[24–26]; disability questionnaire[27–29]
Negative beliefs/fear of pain and activity[5,7,30,31]	?	Yes	Belief/fear questionnaire[32,33]
Subjective pain intensity[7,8,34]	?	Yes	Visual analogue scale[35]
Compensation and unemployment[7,36–38]	?	Yes	Clinical interview

MMPI = Minnesota Multiphasic Personality Inventory; ? = undetermined.
[a]Duration of 1–4 weeks and person seeks medical care.[39]
[b]Duration of at least 3 months and failure to return to work.[39–41]

60 years appear to be at significantly increased risk. This is a broad age group, but it specifies some parameters for acute onset. Knowing this age risk factor may be of little value because it is estimated that approximately 80% of individuals in this age range will experience acute back pain. The occurrence of chronic debilitating low back pain appears to increase significantly with individuals older than age 40 years. Again, this is a general parameter, rather than a specific age range.

Job Dissatisfaction and Heavy Physical Work

Job dissatisfaction and heavy physical work have obtained substantial, large-scale research support as risk factors for low back pain. Since the Bigos et al. Boeing study,[10] job dissatisfaction has continued to emerge as an important risk factor for the onset of acute and chronic disabling low back pain. At the clinical level, this is also apparent with patients. This risk factor applies to patients employed outside of the home; however, further study may generalize this finding to individuals not working for pay out of the home. Little research is available assessing general activity satisfaction, whether for pay or not. Formal occupational measures, which are typically too complicated for routine clinical use, exist to measure job satisfaction. The work APGAR measure, originally used in the Bigos et al. study, is useful and recommended. Specifically, this method of measure involves using one question of the seven used by Bigos et al., which states, "I enjoy the tasks involved in my job," followed by a 3-point rating system of almost always, some of the time, or hardly ever. Workers checking hardly ever are at increased risk for the onset of acute low back pain. This technique can also be used for assessing patients at increased risk for chronic disabling back pain.

The role of heavy physical labor has long been appreciated as a risk factor both in the onset of low back pain and development of chronic disabling conditions. Although a variety of workload situations have been studied, exposure to extended vibration, such as truck driving or repeated frequent heavy lifting and twisting, or a combination of these activities, are labor environments and behaviors that are clearly associated with the onset and chronicity of low back pain. As Table 11.1 notes, it is recommended that the rating systems used by the Social Security Administration (SSA) or found in the U.S. Labor Department's *Dictionary of Occupational Titles* be used to classify various jobs. The SSA uses a category rating system, looking at amount and frequency of lifting from sedentary to heavy. Jobs categorized from medium to heavy should be considered heavy physical labor, with the additional review of frequency of twisting, bending, and exposure to prolonged vibration. For the purpose of risk factor identification, it is recommended that patients' physical work conditions be categorized as heavy or not heavy based on SSA ratings.

Severe Psychological Distress or Abuse and Minnesota Multiphasic Personality Inventory Scale 3 Elevation

Severe psychological stress or abuse and Minnesota Multiphasic Personality Inventory (MMPI) Scale 3 elevation move into the psychological and behavioral arena. A rapidly growing body of research demonstrates that individuals who have experienced moderate to extreme emotional distress or abuse (including physical and sexual abuse) are at significantly increased risk for chronic disabling low back pain. When trying to assess this particular risk factor, some difficulty is encountered because there is no gold standard. Sexual, physical, and emotional abuse can be assessed by a straightforward question during the clinical interview. At this point, it is recommended that psychological and emotional stress be assessed with a stressful life events questionnaire. Of the two questionnaires referenced in Table 11.1, the Holmes and Rahe[18] rating scale is the easier to administer and the more extensively used.

The MMPI Scale 3 has also been shown to predict acute and chronic disabling low back pain (see Table 11.1). At least for the onset of acute low back pain, items on Scale 3 associated with lassitude, malaise, and social anxiety are most predictive. Therefore, the ability of Scale 3 to predict appears to be due to its assessment of mood issues.[5] The only way to obtain Scale 3 information is to administer the MMPI. Thus, it may be difficult to routinely assess this particular risk factor within an ongoing clinical setting. It is better to use this risk factor as one identified in a more extensive assessment and evaluation of patients demonstrating other risk factors more easily obtained within the clinical arena.

This completes the basic review of the factors in Table 11.1 predictive of the onset of acute low back pain or both acute and chronic disabling low back pain. The next sections review the remaining risk factors that are primarily associated with the development of chronic disabling low back pain.

Depression

In spite of extensive examination and research, depression has not been found to consistently predict the onset of acute low back pain. However, convincing large-scale studies show that it is a significant risk factor for chronic disabling low back pain. Depression's predictive power has been demonstrated using various measurement techniques across different cultures. In addition to use of the clinical interview, it is recommended that the Beck Depression Inventory be used to assess the extent of depression (see Table 11.1). In general, patients showing moderate to severe levels of depression are at increased risk for chronic disabling low back pain.

Substance Abuse

Of little surprise to individuals working in the pain rehabilitation arena, the evidence supporting substance abuse as a risk factor for chronic disabling low back pain is revealing. This risk includes abuse of prescription drugs, as well as alcohol and street drug usage. Clinical interview and drug screening are recommended when assessing the level of substance abuse (see Table 11.1). It is somewhat perplexing that research literature has not supported substance abuse as a risk factor for the onset of acute low back pain, particularly when smoking has been identified as a risk factor. Although there is no ready explanation for this, it may be a function of the nature of the studies conducted and the subject population. Most research has involved industrial injuries. Individuals with substance abuse problems may disguise the problems at the onset of acute low back pain for fear of job loss or other negative repercussions. Thus, there may be a measurement obstacle in gathering the data regarding substance abuse. Information could be more revealing if data are gathered from work environments in which drug screening is part of the initial evaluation of a worker reporting an acute episode of low back pain. Again, this may be difficult to implement, given current labor laws and protection.

Low Activity, Perceived Disability, and Negative Beliefs and Fears about Pain

Patients exhibiting sedentary or low activity and corresponding high pain behavior, or reporting significant functional disability due to pain, are clearly at increased risk for developing chronic disabling low back pain. This risk factor can be assessed by using one of several pain behavior checklists, the Waddell's sign test, and one of several self-rating disability scales (see Table 11.1). Likewise, negative beliefs and fears about experiencing pain with activity is a consistent risk factor for the development of chronic disabling low back pain. This risk factor usually goes hand-in-hand with the activity, pain behavior, and disability factor, and can best be assessed within the clinical environment using one of the two basic fear avoidance and belief questionnaires (see Table 11.1). Patients scoring in the 75th percentile or higher on assessment questionnaires for either of the two risk factors are considered at significant risk levels.

Subjective Pain Intensity

Research literature shows that the level of subjective pain intensity perceived by the patient can significantly predict the development of chronic disabling low back pain. The clinical standard for assessing subjective pain intensity is the visual analogue scale. However, research has not shown the degree of specificity necessary to allow an actual cut-off point to determine what level of subjective pain the patient must experience for this risk factor to be significant. It is recommended that 75% of maximum level or higher be used as the threshold to consider subjective pain intensity a significant risk factor for developing chronic disabling low back pain.

Compensation and Unemployment

The final risk factor in Table 11.1, compensation and unemployment, has been somewhat controversial over the course of examining low back pain patients.[42] The vast majority of evidence supports the presence of compensation associated with back pain or unemployment predictive of chronic disabling low back pain, or both. Specifically, this risk factor should be assessed by clinical interview, asking the patient if he or she is receiving some kind of financial compensation as a result of his or her low back pain. This compensation may be in the form of work-related wage replacement, health and other insurance benefit coverage, Social Security disability, or private disability insurance. It may also involve a liability settlement for automobile accidents or other injuries encountered in or out of work. Patients demonstrating one or more of these compensation categories are at increased risk, with a cumulative effect typically noted across the categories. Likewise, patients who are at risk of losing, or have lost, their job due to their back pain problem show higher incidences of chronic disability. Embedded in this risk factor is the notion of employability of a given patient. Employability involves the availability of return to work options, as well as transferable skills demonstrated by the patient. In general, patients with few transferable skills and a low chance of being able to return to their prior job are at higher risk.

Probable or Possible Risk Factors

In addition to the factors reviewed in Table 11.1, several other probable to possible factors gain support in research literature. Although these risk factors are not considered primary, evidence is accumulating for their potential inclusion in the known risk factor list. All of these probable or possible risk factors have been studied in the context of their predictive value in the development of chronic disabling low back pain.

Reinforcement and Modeling of Pain Behavior

The environmental and behavioral effects of reinforcement and modeling of overt pain behaviors are well documented.[43] An increasing body of evidence shows that these factors are associated with the development of chronic disabling low back pain.[7,44] However, no quick and straightforward method exists to assess the presence of these variables. It is recommended that questions during the clinical interview about the response of family, friends, and workers to the patient's pain, and if any other influential individuals are experiencing chronic disabling low back pain, be included. Again, the actual level of occurrence for this risk factor to be a predictor is unclear.

Acute Diagnosis and Treatment Approach

There is wide variability and discrepancy in how patients with acute low back pain are diagnosed and managed.[45] Likewise, studies show that this initial diagnostic and management phase with acute low back pain can contribute to the development of chronic disabling low back pain. Several large-scale studies have shown that unless obvious red flag symptoms of major spine pathology exist, diagnosing low back pain as a nonspecific benign problem, with conservative care and a focus on rapid increase in physical function, significantly increases the ability of patients to return to work and general function.[46,47] In contrast, patients given a specific diagnosis of some kind of disk pathology or treated in the typical medical model with multiple diagnostic testing and bed rest, or both, demonstrated a much higher level of chronic disabling low back pain. Again, assessing this particular risk factor is far from standardized, with recommendations to obtain as much information about diagnostic and initial management interventions during the clinical interview as possible. Patients with specific spine pathology diagnoses and mega-workups during their acute pain management could be at increased risk for chronic disabling low back pain.

Activity or Functional Restrictions

A possible additional risk factor within the treatment arena for the development of chronic disabling low back pain is the amount of activity and functional restrictions placed on the patient by health care providers.[48] Although the intent of such a process is typically to protect the patient from further injury, the actual effect may be to indiscriminately prevent the patient from returning to work. True and ongoing functional limits should be recognized and addressed within the care of the patient. However, many times these limits are not scrutinized at the level necessary to place the absolute minimum amount of restriction clinically indicated to promote an increase in function and return to work. The primary method of assessing this possible risk factor is with a functional capacity evaluation, leading to delineation of functional and work restrictions (see Chapter 13 for review of functional performance evaluations). One can assume that this possible risk factor is present in any patient receiving a medium or higher lifting restriction. As with the other previously discussed risk factors, the actual predictability of developing chronic disabling low back pain from this risk factor remains unclear.

CLINICAL APPLICATION OF RISK FACTORS

Having reviewed the known and probable or possible risk factors of low back pain, their integrated clinical application should be discussed further. To repeat, no consistent and convincing data prove a specific cause and effect between any of the risk factors previously discussed and the occurrence of acute or chronic disabling low back pain. Likewise, the evidence does not allow us to weigh the relative contribution across risk factors in predicting low back pain. Thus, the risk factors delineated in Table 11.1 cannot be used in the same fashion as the risk factors for cancer or cardiovascular disease, which have demonstrated cause and effect linkage. Nonetheless, the data are clear regarding the ability of the risk factors outlined to predict the occurrence of acute low back pain or development of chronic disabling low back pain, or both. However, there are no research data delineating how these known risk factors should be used alone or in combination to identify low back pain patients at significant risk. Keeping this in mind, and based on my clinical experience, the following guidelines are recommended when applying the known risk factors delineated in Table 11.1 within clinical practice:

1. Table 11.1 risk factors should not be used as a definitive list of causal variables in low back pain, but, rather, as a preliminary screening checklist to identify patients at higher risk for acute or chronic disabling low back pain.
2. Patients exhibiting five or more acute, or seven or more chronic, disabling low back pain risk factors from Table 11.1 should be considered at high risk.
3. Patients exhibiting at least four of the five known risk factors that predict both acute and chronic disabling low back pain should also be considered at high risk.
4. Patients exhibiting zero or one of the known risk factors should not be considered at significantly increased risk for the occurrence of acute or chronic disabling low back pain.
5. Patients falling between the ranges in numbers 2 through 4 of this list also have some increased risk; however, the actual degree is indeterminable.
6. Patients identified at higher risk should be counseled regarding the presence of identified factors and suggestions given regarding possible changes. Because cause and effect has not been clearly established, recommendations for mandatory change are inappropriate.

The degree of the clinical use of probable or possible risk factors is uncertain. It is recommended that they be assessed and serve to heighten the level of concern, if present. Ongoing research should help clarify their actual role.

These guidelines and recommendations should receive more detailed empirical justification to maximize the use of the current list of risk factors. From clinical experience, these guidelines do allow identification of patients at the most significant risk for acute or chronic disabling low back pain, or both. Given that these patients require the greatest amount of attention and possible intervention, the guidelines serve as a first step to improve overall identification and patient care. More refinement must be accomplished before these, and possibly other, risk factors can reach their full potential of application.

STRATEGIES TO CHANGE AND REDUCE KNOWN RISK FACTORS

Until cause and effect relationships have been determined between the risk factors previously reviewed and low back pain, it is somewhat premature to move too far and fast into developing elaborate strategies to change or influence these factors. If a given factor is not actually causing or contributing to low back pain, then change has little potential benefit in reducing the occurrence of low back pain. Likewise, even if a causal relationship could be established, not all of the risk factors are changeable (e.g., age, history of back pain, history of severe psychological stress or abuse, and initial level of subjective pain intensity). Thus, there are limits in our examination of how we can impact risk factors.

Given these precautions, and in spite of limits, it is still beneficial to discuss some basic ideas regarding risk factor change and, more important, how to better manage patients in the higher risk group. For ease of discussion, the risk factors amenable to change have been grouped by area of similarity, as opposed to their ability to predict acute and chronic disabling low back pain.

Smoking and Substance Abuse

Smoking and substance abuse have been targeted in business and industry as major general health risk behaviors. Likewise, there are a number of private and employee-based programs to help individuals reduce or stop smoking and substance abuse behavior. These do not require review here, but note that such programs should be emphasized for low back pain patients. In general, ongoing education, peer pressure, limited access, and offering discrete and accessible employee assistance programs can result in a reduction in these two risk factors.

Job Dissatisfaction and Heavy Physical Work

Again, I defer to industrial and organizational psychological literature for in-depth discussions about changing job dissatisfaction. In summary, efforts to make the work environment more comfortable, predictable, stimulating, and controllable for the worker typically enhance job satisfaction. In the era of downsizing and out-sourcing, controlling job satisfaction is becoming more and more difficult. Although the degree of physical labor involved in a job is defined by the nature of the job, business and industry are making efforts to reduce the amount of actual physical workload when-ever possible. The use of lifting aids and safety standards can reduce physical demands. Likewise, any effort to reduce the amount of physical fatigue due to pro-longed exposure can enhance and reduce the overall demand. A trend in the wrong direction within business and industry is the implementation of 12-hour shifts. Although this reduces the number of employees, it can significantly increase the risk of initial low back injury, as well as disability.

Severe Psychological Stress, Abuse, and Depression

As with the other risk factors, identification of major stress, abuse, or depression, or some combination of these factors, and allowing the individual an opportunity to learn skills to offset these illnesses, as well as obtain necessary treatment for these problems, are imperative.

Low Activity, High Pain Behavior, Perceived Disability, and Negative Beliefs or Fears about Pain and Activity

Some studies demonstrate that changing perceptions and negative beliefs about activity and pain can reduce the development of chronic disabling low back pain.[32,49–52] Education, activity reinforcement and enhancement, behavioral desen-sitization to activity, and cognitive restructuring interventions to reduce negative beliefs and fears all can change these risk factors.

STRATEGIES TO MANAGE INDIVIDUALS AT HIGH RISK

Specific interventions to change known risk factors may be difficult and, to some extent, premature without the establishment of a clear cause and effect relationship.

There is little doubt, however, that patients at high risk can be managed more effectively, thus reducing the probability of acute low back pain developing into a chronic disabling condition. A number of the studies referenced here substantiate that early detection and intervention with low back pain patients using educational and conservative therapeutic strategies can significantly reduce the risk of chronic disability. Likewise, clinical and research literature has clearly shown that patients experiencing chronic disabling low back pain can be rehabilitated with significant improvement in function and productivity if treated within an interdisciplinary comprehensive pain rehabilitation setting.[53–55] In fact, the American Academy of Physical Medicine and Rehabilitation has adopted practice guidelines to treat chronic nonmalignant pain patients, including low back pain patients, that incorporate all of the elements of interdisciplinary pain rehabilitation in a cost-effective and time-limited model.[40] Thus, it is strongly recommended that patients experiencing acute low back pain at high risk for developing chronic disability be referred for at least an evaluation to a specialty interdisciplinary pain rehabilitation program using the American Academy of Physical Medicine and Rehabilitation–adopted practice guidelines within 30 days of the onset of the acute low back pain. Typically, the cost for such an evaluation should not exceed $800, with the average cost being $500. Most third party payers pay for such an evaluation if they have adequate information about the intent and practical use of any findings (i.e., recommendations to reduce the development of chronic disabling low back pain). This recommendation alone has the potential to dramatically improve the care of high-risk patients and significantly reduce the probability of their acute pain turning into a chronic disabling condition.

The risk factors discussed here, even if not causal, can play an instrumental role. This is true even for individuals with the compensation and unemployment risk factor. Although these patients often exhibit delays, and sometimes not as much functional and clinical improvement, they still can significantly improve.[36,56] Literature has shown that interdisciplinary pain rehabilitation can change many of the known behavioral and emotional or psychological risk factors in chronic disabled low back pain patients with commensurate improvement in function and return to work.[55]

Given the preceding sections on risk factors with low back pain patients, the conclusion of this chapter discusses how to better apply and improve the knowledge base in this important area.

SUMMARY

Identification and use of risk factors with low back pain patients are still in their infancy. Although there are growing research databases on the known risk factors outlined in this chapter, the actual cause and effect on the occurrence of acute, and development of chronic, disabling low back pain require more study. These data enhance the importance of the risk factors and undoubtedly alter the risk configuration. Thus, it is strongly recommended that more systematic cause and effect research be undertaken, particularly on the known risk factors in Table 11.1, which predict both the onset of acute, and the development of chronic, disabling low back pain. As has been demonstrated in the cancer and cardiovascular disease arenas, mainstreaming these risk factors into day-to-day practice requires establishing clinically significant cause and effect relationships with chronic low back pain.

Although this vital cause and effect research is occurring, it is not premature to routinely begin using the risk factor list in Table 11.1 as part of the initial clinical workup for acute low back pain patients. The assessment methods recommended in Table 11.1, for the most part, are brief and user-friendly in the clinical setting, with the exception of the MMPI. Following the guidelines outlined in Clinical Applications of Risk Factors, it is feasible to begin identifying patients at high risk for developing chronic disabling low back pain early in the process. The health care provider should begin looking for these factors in a proactive fashion, rather than waiting to see if a particular patient falls into the 10–20% who do not effectively recover from their low back pain. For patients at high risk for development of chronic disabling conditions, early detection and referral to a specialty program can produce both immediate and long-term improvement.[55,57] If a rehabilitation-based interdisciplinary program using the nationally recognized guidelines already discussed in the section Strategies to Manage Individuals at High Risk are not available,[40] the health care provider should attempt to orchestrate this care whenever possible. Research studies are beginning to demonstrate that something as simple as community-based psychoeducational programs can have a significant positive effect.[58]

These early-detection strategies also should extend to individuals at high risk for the onset of acute low back pain. At least the first six known risk factors outlined in Table 11.1 should be part of routine post-hiring medical examinations for workers. Ideally, the evaluation of the first six risk factors should also extend to the family practice level with routine general medical checkups. Given this information, it is possible to initiate measures to more effectively educate and monitor individuals who are at risk.[59,60]

The critical message is to not ignore the risk factors known to be associated with someone either developing acute low back pain or a chronic disabling condition. Use this information for early detection to promote primary, secondary, and tertiary prevention and intervention whenever possible.

In conclusion, the risk factors discussed in this chapter, and how they are applied and modified, have the potential for making an enormous impact on the occurrence and cost of low back pain in adults. Without incorporating these variables into thinking and clinical practice, advancements in low back pain care will be significantly hampered.

REFERENCES

1. McCaffret E. The impacts of pain: assessing and managing its cost in the workplace. Business and Health Special Report, 1996;14:6–30.
2. Fordyce WE (ed). Back Pain in the Workplace: Management of Disability in Nonspecific Conditions. Seattle: IASP Press, 1995;1–67.
3. Waddell G. Low Back Pain: A 20th Century Health Care Enigma. In TS Jenson, JA Turner, Z Wiesenfeld-Hallin (eds), Progress in Pain Research and Management (Vol 8). Seattle: IASP Press, 1997;101–112.
4. Sanders SH. Why Do Most Patients with Chronic Pain Not Return to Work? In MJM Cohen, JN Campbell (eds), Pain Treatment Centers At A Crossroads: Practical and Conceptual Reappraisal. Seattle: IASP Press, 1996;193–202.
5. Sanders SH. Risk factors for the occurrence of low back pain and chronic disability. APS Bulletin 1995;5:1–5.
6. Papageorgiou AC, Croft PR, Thomas E, et al. Influence of previous back pain on the episode incident of low back pain: results from the South Manchester back pain study. Pain 1996;66:181–185.

7. Turk DC. The Role of Demographic and Psychosocial Factors in Transition from Acute to Chronic Pain. In TS Jenson, JA Turner, Z Wiesenfeld-Hallin (eds), Proceedings of the Eighth World Congress on Pain, Progress, and Pain Research and Management (Vol 8). Seattle: IASP Press, 1997;185–213.

8. Bombardier C, Kerr MS, Shannon HS, et al. A guide to interpreting epidemiological studies on the etiology of back pain. Spine 1994;19:2047–2056.

9. Hassenbring M, Marienfeld G, Kuhlendahl D, et al. Risk factors of chronicity in lumbar disc patients: a prospective investigation of biological, psychologic, and social predictors of therapy outcome. Spine 1994;19:2759–2765.

10. Bigos SJ, Battie MC, Spengler DM, et al. A prospective study of work perceptions and psychosocial factors affecting report of back injury. Spine 1991;16:1–6.

11. Magnusson ML, Pope MH, Wilder DG, et al. Are occupational drivers at an increased risk for developing musculoskeletal disorders? Spine 1996;21:710–717.

12. Burton AK, Tillotson KM, Symonds TL, et al. Occupational risk factors for the first onset and subsequent course of low back trouble. Spine 1996;21:2612–2620.

13. U.S. Department of Labor. Dictionary of Occupational Titles (4th ed). Washington, DC: U.S. Government Printing Office, 1986.

14. Goldman S, O'Neill PI. Social security disability evaluation in axil pain: listed impairments in treating physician's role. Clin J Pain 1990;6:305–310.

15. Croft PR, Papageorgiou AC, Ferry S, et al. Psychological distress in low back pain: evidence from a prospective study in the general population. Spine 1996;20:2731–2737.

16. Linton SJ. The population-based study of the relationship between sexual abuse and back pain: establishing a link. Pain 1997;73:47–53.

17. McMahon MJ, Gatchel JR, Polatin PB, et al. Early childhood abuse in chronic spinal disorder patients. Spine 1997;22:2408–2415.

18. Holmes TH, Rahe RH. The social readjustment rating scale. J Psychosom Res 1967;11:213–218.

19. Sarason IG, Johnson JG, Segal JM. Assessing the impact of life changes: development of the life experiences survey. J Consult Clin Psychol 1978;46:932–946.

20. Gatchel RJ, Polantin PB, Mayer TG. The dominant role of psychosocial risk factors in the development of chronic low back pain disability. Spine 1995;20:2702–2709.

21. Dahlstrom W, Welsh G, Dahlstrom L. MMPI Handbook (Revised Edition). Indianapolis: University of Minnesota Press, 1972.

22. Beck AT, Steer AR. Beck Depression Inventory: A Manual. San Antonio: Harcourt, Brace, Jovanovich, 1987.

23. Ohlumd C, Lindstrom I, Areskoug B, et al. Pain behavior in industrial subacute low back pain. Part 1. Reliability, concurrent and predictive validity of pain behavior assessments. Pain 1994;58:201–209.

24. Turk DC, Wack JT, Kerns RD. Empirical examination of the "pain behavior" construct. J Behav Med 1985;8:119–130.

25. Richards JS, Nepomuceno JS, Riles C. Assessing pain behavior: the UAB Pain Behavioral Scale. Pain 1982;14:193–198.

26. Waddell G, McCulloch JH, Kummel EG, et al. Nonorganic physical signs and low back pain. Spine 1980;5:117–125.

27. Hazzard RG, Haugh LD, Reid S, et al. Early prediction of chronic disability after occupational low back injury. Spine 1996;21:945–951.

28. Smith BH, Penny KI, Purves AM, et al. The chronic pain grade questionnaire: validation and reliability in postal research. Pain 1997;71:141–147.

29. Fairbank CT, Couper J, Davies JB, et al. The Oswestry low back pain disability questionnaire. Physiotherapy 1980;66:271–273.

30. Vlaeyen JWS, Kole-Snijders AMJ, Boeren RGB, et al. Fear of movement/reinjury in chronic low back pain and its relationship to behavioral performance. Pain 1995;62:363–372.

31. Klenerman L, Slade PD, Stanley M, et al. The prediction of chronicity in patients with acute attack of low back pain in a general practice setting. Spine 1995;20:478–484.

32. Waddell G, Newton M, Henderson I, et al. A fear/avoidance belief questionnaire (FABQ) and the role of fear avoidance beliefs in chronic low back pain and disability. Pain 1993;52:157–168.

33. McCracken LM, Zayfert C, Rose RT. The pain anxiety symptom scale: development and validation of the scale to measure fear of pain. Pain 1992;50:67–73.

34. Dworkin RH. Which individuals with acute pain are most likely to develop chronic pain syn-

drome? Pain Forum 1997;6:127–136.

35. Price DD, Bush FM, Long S, et al. A comparison of pain measurement characteristics of mechanical, visual analogue, and simple numerical rating scales. Pain 1994;56:217–226.

36. Rohling ML, Binder LM, Langhinrichsen-Rohling J. A meta analytical review of the association between financial compensation and the experience and treatment of chronic pain. Health Psychol 1995;14:537–547.

37. Rainville J, Sobel JB, Hartigan C, et al. The effect of compensation involvement on the reporting of pain and disability by patients referred for rehabilitation of chronic low back pain. Spine 1997;22:2016–2024.

38. Sanderson PL, Todd BD, Holt GR, et al. Compensation, work status, and disability in low back pain patients. Spine 1995;20:554–556.

39. Spitzer WO, Abenhaim L, Dupuis M, et al. Scientific approach to the assessment and management of activity-related spinal disorders: report of the Quebec Task Force. Spine 1987; 12[Suppl7]:S31–S34.

40. Sanders SH, Rucker KS, Anderson KO, et al. Clinical practice guidelines for chronic nonmalignant pain syndrome patients. J Back Musculoskel Rehab 1995;5:115–120.

41. Agency for Health Care Policy and Research. Clinical Practice Guidelines for Acute Back Pain Management. Rockville, Maryland: U.S. Department of Health and Human Services, 1994.

42. Mendelson G. Compensation and chronic pain. Pain 1992;48:121–123.

43. Romano JM, Turner JA, Jensen MP, et al. Chronic pain patient's spouse behavioral interactions predict patient disability. Pain 1995;63:353–360.

44. Sanders SH. Operant Conditioning with Chronic Pain, Back to Basics. In RJ Gatchel, DC Turk (eds), Psychological Approaches to Pain Management: A Practitioner's Handbook. New York: Gilford Press, 1996;112–130.

45. Cherkin DC, Deyo RA, Wheeler K, et al. Physician views about treating low back pain. Spine 1995;20:1–10.

46. Abenhaim L, Rossignol M, Gobeille D, et al. The prognostic consequences in the making of the initial medical diagnosis of work-related back injuries. Spine 1995;20:791–795.

47. Indahl A, Velund L, Reikeraas O. Good prognosis for low back pain when left untampered: a randomized clinical trial. Spine 1995;20:473–477.

48. Hall H, McIntosh G, Melles T, et al. Effects of discharge recommendations on outcome. Spine 1994;19:2033–2037.

49. Sanders SH, Brena SF. Empirically driven chronic pain patient subgroups: The utility of multidimensional clustering to identify differential treatment effects. Pain 1993;54:51–56.

50. Werneke MW, Harris DE, Lichter RL. Clinical effectiveness of behavioral signs for screening chronic low back pain patients in a work-oriented physical rehabilitation program. Spine 1993;18:2412–2418.

51. Symonds TL, Burton AK, Tillotson KM, et al. Absence resulting from low back trouble can be reduced by psychosocial interventions at the workplace. Spine 1995;20:2738–2745.

52. Rhine WE, Krishna MK, Swanson CE. A prospective study evaluating early rehabilitation and preventing back pain chronicity in mine workers. Spine 1995;20:489–491.

53. Sanders SH, Brena SF. Pain centers: what consumers want to know. APS Bulletin 1995;5:8–11.

54. Lanes TC, Gauron EF, Spratt KF, et al. Long-term followup of patients with chronic back pain treated in a multidisciplinary rehabilitation program. Spine 1995;20:801–806.

55. Turk, DC. Efficacy of Multidisciplinary Pain Centers and the Treatment of Chronic Pain. In MJM Cohen and JM Campbell (eds), Pain Treatment Centers At A Crossroads: A Practical and Conceptual Reappraisal, Progress in Pain Research and Management (Vol 7). Seattle: IASP Press, 1996;257–273.

56. Hadler NM, Karey TS, Garrett J. The influence of identification by workers compensation insurance on recovery from acute back pain. Spine 1995;20:2710–2715.

57. Maruta T, Malinchoc M, Offord KP, et al. Status of patients with chronic pain 13 years after treatment in a pain management center. Pain 1998;74:199–204.

58. LeFort SM, Gray-Donald K, Rowat AM, et al. Randomized control trial of a community-based psychoeducational program for the self-management of chronic pain. Pain 1998;74:297–306.

59. Holmes-Enix D, Lopez SD. How early is early? On-site early return to work programs cut losses and cost. Rehab Manag 1998;11:28–35.

60. Smith MD, McGhan WF. Treating back pain without breaking the bank. Bus Health 1998; 16:50–52.

Chapter 12

Industrial Low Back Pain

Aloysia L. Schwabe, Ernest W. Johnson,
and William S. Pease

Practitioners in various fields frequently encounter patients with work-related complaints of low back pain (LBP). Because LBP is the most common musculoskeletal problem prompting a patient to pursue medical evaluation, physicians should be comfortable and consistent with its management. Physicians treating an individual with back pain who is pursuing a workers' compensation claim should be familiar with the factors affecting the course of an industrial low back injury, as well as the particular workers' compensation system in the state in which he or she is practicing. Many physicians find such claims to be frustrating, both in terms of navigating through a complex system and managing patients with no clear etiology for their continued pain whose disability is refractory to conservative care. Appropriate and comprehensive care should be delivered in a timely fashion to this subset of the general population with the goal of avoiding development of chronic pain and protracted disability. The focus of this chapter is to provide an overview of the etiology, treatment, and rehabilitation of LBP in the industrial setting.

When evaluating a patient presenting with occupational LBP, the physician must decide when and if diagnostic testing is indicated, what type of pain management or therapy prescription is warranted, how often to follow the patient's progress, and when referral to additional specialists or programs is necessary. Additionally, there are questions that should be addressed specifically relating to the occupational nature of the claimed injury (Table 12.1). The physician will be asked to predict how long the injured worker should abstain from particular duties at work or refrain from returning to his or her regular job as a result of his or her back impairment. Recommendations are made for temporary partial or total disability initially. Once patients have been determined to reach maximal medical improvement, vocational rehabilitation may be an option for the patient with permanent partial disability, or a conclusion of total disability may be reached. An algorithm describing the rehabilitation process after a work-related injury is illustrated in Figure 12.1.[1] Note that most patients do not require a formal rehabilitation program. With appropriate medical management, the majority of patients with occupational LBP return to work within the first month after symptom onset.

Table 12.1 Questions Pertinent to Industrial Low Back Pain

Was the injury related to work?
When can the patient return to work?
When has maximal medical improvement occurred?
What is the permanent partial impairment rating?
What is the disability rating?
What is the residual functional capacity?

Clinical Case 1

A 42-year-old construction worker who denies other significant past medical history presents to his primary care physician with a 4-day history of LBP that was acute in onset and has gradually worsened. His current job description involves driving a cement truck and assisting with the pouring of concrete for a new road. His activities include repetitive bending and lifting, as well as some periods of prolonged sitting while driving. He relates the onset of sharp, burning pain in his low back with referral to the left buttock, which began in the evening after an especially long day at work. The discomfort is primarily located just left of the midline lumbar area and over the left buttock without distal extension. He notes exacerbation of his symptoms with lateral rotation of the trunk and bending at the waist. He denies subjective weakness or sensory change, as well as bowel or bladder dysfunction. Valsalva motions do not increase his discomfort. He denies fever or chills. He reports occasional backaches in the past, which resolved quickly with anti-inflammatory medications; however, he asserts that this episode is more severe, and he has not obtained relief with over-the-counter analgesics. He attempted to return to work yesterday after 2 days of bed rest, but noted worsening of his discomfort. His main concern at the present time is whether he has experienced permanent damage to his back, and he does not want to return to work at the risk of making his condition worse. He emphasizes that he enjoys his job and does not want to jeopardize his current standing at work.

On physical examination, he has a normal station and gait. The patient appears to be experiencing discomfort, as evidenced by facial grimacing while climbing onto the examination table, but he does not demonstrate exaggerated pain behavior. Pertinent examination findings include normal sensation and strength, easily elicited and symmetric muscle stretch reflexes, and an absent Babinski sign bilaterally. Straight leg raising (SLR) is limited to 40 degrees on the left due to the patient's complaint of increased LBP; however, leg pain remains absent, and root tension maneuvers did not reproduce or worsen his discomfort. Range of motion of the lumbar spine is limited in flexion or extension and lateral rotation bilaterally with dyssymmetry on lateral bending bilaterally. He has tenderness with vigorous palpation over the left lumbar paraspinal musculature. His diagnosis is LBP without neurologic deficit. In many workers' compensation systems, the diagnosis would be generalized to lumbar strain or sprain.

Given this patient's job description, it is not surprising that he has experienced an episode of activity intolerance secondary to LBP. The worker's job responsibilities and a description of his actions involved in carrying out these duties can help clarify motions that may be causing, or at least contributing to, his current condi-

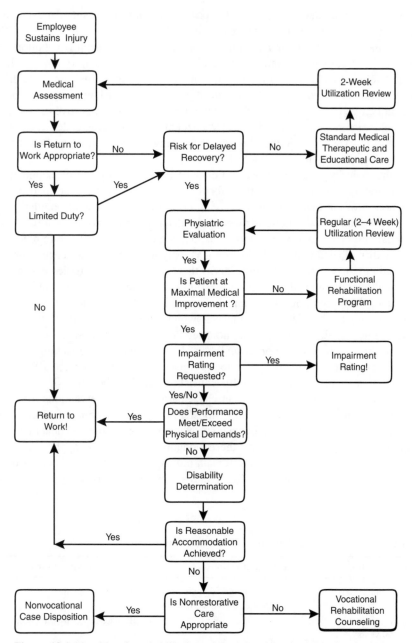

Figure 12.1 Algorithm for rehabilitation of the injured worker. (Reprinted with permission from RD Rondinelli, JP Robinson, SJ Scheer, SM Weinstein. Industrial rehabilitation medicine. Part 4. Strategies for disability management. Arch Phys Med Rehabil 1997;78:S1–S22.)

tion. It has been shown that persons who are heavy laborers, or whose work involves lifting, bending, twisting, repetitive motions, vibrational exposure, and fixed postures, are susceptible to back injury.[2] Whether his back pain is a direct result of an injury sustained on the job is unclear, and a specific causative event frequently cannot be identified. One should also attempt to distinguish between an occupational injury and illness, with the former resulting from a singular event and the latter resulting from cumulative exposures, although this task may prove difficult. Some states allow for an injury to be secondary to repetitive motions or actions. The history and physical examination should aim to identify any red flags suggestive of an underlying condition, which would warrant more immediate diagnostic testing or evaluation.[3] Although most patients have back pain of an unspecified but benign etiology, one should be attentive to findings suggestive of fracture, infection, tumor, or cancer, specifically checking for neurologic deficits (Table 12.2).[4] In this case, no additional diagnostic testing is indicated in the first month after symptom onset in the absence of red flags.

In the majority of cases of occupational LBP, the initial physical examination and laboratory tests and x-rays, if performed, reveal no specific abnormality supporting a clear-cut diagnosis or underlying etiology. In the general population, it has been estimated that a definite diagnosis is determined in only 15% of patients.[5] Potential etiologies for LBP are numerous, but some are more difficult to precisely identify than others (Table 12.3). Pursuing a costly workup in the absence of objective findings may actually do more harm than good. Imaging studies can reveal structural abnormalities that do not necessarily correlate with the patient's symptoms and, therefore, cloud the clinical picture. Patients may take on a sick role while awaiting a scheduled series of tests in which dependency and disability is fostered. Aronoff et al. suggest labeling nonspecific LBP exactly as such, with avoidance of terms such as *sprain* or *strain* when objective findings are lacking.[6] In this case presentation, the patient's condition is consistent with nonspecific LBP.

Conservative management initially consists of limited bed rest, if any, with encouragement toward maintaining activity. Pharmacologic interventions for acute LBP include non-narcotic analgesics, nonsteroidal anti-inflammatory drugs, and muscle relaxants, with the latter being controversial. Topical cold and heat may also help to provide symptom relief, and these modalities can be easily applied at home. The patient should be encouraged to remain mobile and to continue his or her daily routine, if possible. Activity restrictions may be necessary depending on the indi-

Table 12.2 Historic Red Flags for Underlying Condition

Spinal Fracture	Tumor/Infection	Cauda Equina Syndrome
Major trauma—any age	Older than age 50 years or younger than age 20 years	Saddle anesthesia
Minor trauma—older than age 50 years	History of cancer	Bladder/bowel dysfunction
Older than age 70 years	Fever or chills; unexplained weight loss	Neurologic deficits
Prolonged steroid use	Night pain	
Osteoporosis	Supine position increases pain; infection risk—urinary tract infection, intravenous drug abuse, immunosuppression	

Source: Adapted from S Bigos, O Bowyer, G Braen, et al. Acute Low Back Problems in Adults. Clinical Practice Guideline, Quick Reference Guide No. 14. AHCPR Pub. No. 95-0643. Rockville, MD: U.S. Department of Health and Human Services, Public Health Service, Agency for Health Care Policy and Research, December 1994;2.

Table 12.3 Etiologies of Low Back Pain

Musculoligamentous injury (sprain/strain)
Herniated nucleus pulposus with or without radiculopathy
Anatomic changes (fracture, scoliosis, spondylolisthesis)
Degenerative changes of the spine
Facet syndrome (acute versus chronic secondary to arthropathy)
Spinal stenosis
Systemic disease (spondyloarthropathy, infection, local/metastatic cancer)
Myofascial pain/fibromyalgia
Visceral diseases with referral of pain to back

vidual's work description. Further rehabilitation efforts include starting the patient on a home exercise program in an attempt to improve flexibility and strength and to prevent future exacerbations. Patients should be seen frequently in follow-up to monitor their progress. In this case, the patient should have a return appointment in 1–2 weeks. The importance of continuity should be stressed, with the patient understanding that cancellations or no-shows suggest that the clinical course is improving. The treating physician should assess for any changes on physical examination and evaluate the effectiveness of treatment, including interventions for pain management. Additional psychosocial factors should be investigated, because they often impact recovery.

Because this patient already attempted to return to work unsuccessfully with worsening of his symptoms, and he is involved in strenuous activity while on the job, it is reasonable to have him remain off work initially. The patient should be reassured that most cases of LBP are self-limited and that no evidence of neurologic compromise was noted on his examination. If light-duty or modified work schedules are available, these options should be pursued to get the patient back into the work setting as soon as possible. This way, the patient is treated as a valued member of the company for whom accommodations have been made. However, these options are not provided to many workers, and they are expected to return to work without activity restrictions. Supposing that the latter circumstance is present in this scenario, the patient would be forced to remain on temporary total disability until he is fully able to resume his regular work activities in full capacity. There are residual functional capacity guidelines for exertion limitations (i.e., lifting and carrying) available to the physician. During time off from work, a graduated activity and exercise program should be instituted to restore strength, endurance, and confidence. The patient expressed interest in returning to work and job dissatisfaction did not appear to be an issue, although he had concerns about worsening of his symptoms should he return to work prematurely. This is the time to introduce a "use it or lose it" philosophy incorporating negative aspects of prolonged immobility, such as deconditioning. It should be reinforced to the patient that symptom resolution occurs within a few weeks, with the majority of patients recovering within 1 month in most cases of nonspecific LBP. It is also not necessary to ascertain the exact etiology for occupational LBP in the absence of red flags, and it is presumed that most are musculoligamentous in origin.

Clinical Case 2

A 35-year-old assembly-line worker develops LBP with referral to the posterior aspect of the thigh and posterior right leg. His primary care physician has referred him to a physiatrist for further management recommendations, including electrodiagnostic testing. The patient relates feeling a popping sensation in his back 4 weeks ago while lifting a piece of machinery and twisting simultaneously. He immediately noted back pain in the lumbar area, which was followed the next day by referral of pain into the right leg. Initial routine x-rays show no pathology. He denies subjective deficits in strength or sensation. He also reports no change in bowel, bladder, or sexual function. Sitting for prolonged periods exacerbates his symptoms. The patient has been taking narcotics for pain relief and relates poor sleep. There is no prior history of low back injury. He states that he remains off work because even minimal activity exacerbates his pain. This is his first workers' compensation claim.

On physical examination, the patient is noted to ambulate with an antalgic gait. He is able to climb onto the examination table without difficulty, and manual muscle testing reveals no deficits in strength; however, he is unable to perform 10 consecutive toe raises on the right. Sensation is intact. Muscle stretch reflexes are symmetric and easily elicited throughout, with the exception of an equivocal decreased right ankle jerk.

SLR is positive at 50 degrees on the right with root tension maneuvers reproducing his back pain with radiation below the right knee. Range of motion in the low back is limited in both flexion and extension, as well as lateral bending. Diffuse tenderness to palpation is present over multiple lumbar spinal processes and the right lumbar paraspinal musculature.

In this scenario, referral to a specialist for electrodiagnostic testing is warranted as the patient's radicular pain has persisted over the course of a month without clear-cut deficits apparent on physical examination corresponding to a specific neurologic level. His history and examination findings suggest possible involvement of the S1 nerve root, and this diagnosis is supported by findings on electrodiagnostic testing, including an abnormal right H-reflex. Electrodiagnostic testing allows for diagnosis and prognosis for neurologic recovery, whereas imaging may yield only diagnostic information. At this point, deferring diagnostic imaging, such as magnetic resonance imaging (MRI) or computed tomography, is reasonable while a comprehensive treatment plan is initiated. Imaging tests may reveal evidence of anatomic nerve root compromise correlating with the clinical and electrodiagnostic findings; however, these studies are usually reserved for invasive treatments. In this situation, the patient should be followed every 1–2 weeks to monitor for neurologic compromise with evidence of progressive weakness, sensory change, loss of reflexes, or bowel or bladder difficulties, or both. In the absence of new deficits, his radiculopathy should be managed conservatively without surgical intervention. Referral to a surgeon to discuss management options is appropriate in the setting of progressive neurologic deficits or cauda equina syndrome. Surgery is not indicated for persistent pain complaints alone.

In addition to performing electrodiagnostic testing, the physiatrist formulates a treatment and rehabilitation plan for this patient. He has been placed on temporary total disability by his primary care physician. Now, 6 weeks after his injury, he is continuing to receive narcotics for pain relief. Transitioning the patient to non-narcotic analgesics is ideal to prevent future dependence. A course of oral steroids may decrease nerve root inflammation and thereby reduce the amount of pain medication needed; however, this intervention may have decreased effectiveness as symptom duration increases. The patient could benefit from a physical therapy program emphasizing proper body mechanics and posture, as well as an exercise program progressing from early to advanced lumbar stabilization exercises.

The physician should attempt to identify any individual risk factors that could affect the course of recovery. These factors include job dissatisfaction and stressful relationships existing within the workplace with peers and superiors. Marital discord, sedentary lifestyle, low education level, history of substance abuse, and depression are among many psychosocial factors associated with chronic LBP.[7] When these characteristics are identified, psychological evaluation and counseling as part of the treatment plan are indicated. Potential financial disincentives to recovery should also be explored, as well as pending litigation, especially when improvement over a reasonable time course is lacking.

Options for getting patients back into the workplace in various capacities include gradual return to work or light duty that can be incorporated into a work conditioning program. Larger companies have case managers who are usually in contact with the managing physician and should be available by phone for questions. Smaller employers may not have a standard protocol for dealing with injured workers, and coordination of care may be more challenging in this circumstance. The physiatrist may also recommend that a job site evaluation and analysis be performed. There may be ways to modify the patient's workplace or tasks to improve body mechanics and eliminate problem spots that place the patient at risk for injury. Given the presence of a neurologic deficit, specific concerns, such as strength and balance requirements for climbing ladders and scaffolding, should be addressed. Many employers have personnel trained in ergonomics who are specialized in job site analysis. A portion of these accommodations in the work setting may fall within the Americans with Disabilities Act.

Clinical Case 3

A 38-year-old male warehouse stocker with a history of prior back injury returns to his physiatrist after an acute exacerbation of his LBP symptoms. Approximately 3 years ago, he underwent L4–L5 diskectomy secondary to a herniated nucleus pulposus causing progressive weakness in his left lower limb. After the surgery, he had improvement in foot dorsiflexor strength to 4/5 on the left and relief of his radicular pain; however, he continued to have LBP. After an extensive rehabilitation course, including a work conditioning program, he returned to work 3 months after his surgery. Since that time, he has occasional flare-ups with worsening of his back pain from baseline. One week ago, he attempted to support a crate that was slipping off of a shelf in the warehouse when he experienced excruciating pain acutely. He denies weakness in his lower limbs, changes in sensation, or bowel or bladder dysfunction.

On physical examination, the patient ambulates with an antalgic gait. He has difficulty heel walking on the left, and manual muscle testing reveals slightly weaker ankle dorsiflexion on the left, but these findings are similar to those of previous examinations. There is no new weakness or change in muscle stretch reflexes on examination as well. The patient does have increased pain with an SLR maneuver on the left while supine at 45 degrees, but SLR has been limited to 50–60 degrees in the past.

For this patient, his exacerbation of pain should be managed similarly to an acute episode of LBP. He sought medical attention soon after his symptoms began, which portends a more favorable outcome compared to those who have a delayed presentation. In light of his prolonged disability in the past, this patient should be followed at least every 2 weeks to monitor pain management and functional status. After his symptoms have improved, he would benefit from a regular exercise program. Job analysis and job redesign may help prevent future recurrences as well.

Clinical Case 4

A 46-year-old nurse presents on referral from her primary care physician after slipping and falling approximately 2 months ago at the nursing home where she is employed. She complains of constant, aching pain in her lumbosacral region with shooting pains into her proximal lower limbs. She notes that her legs are weak, and states that she must use a cane to ambulate. She also reports circumferential numbness in a stocking distribution below the knees in both lower limbs, which has been worsening over the past year. There is no loss of bowel or bladder function. She has a history of diabetes diagnosed 5 years ago, for which she takes an oral hypoglycemic agent. She presented to her primary care physician approximately 1 week after the accident when her pain did not improve with bed rest and over-the-counter analgesics. Her physician ordered plain films, which were unremarkable, and started her on a nonsteroidal medication, as well as a muscle relaxant. When her pain did not improve, she saw a chiropractor, but thought that this intervention actually worsened her pain. She then returned to her primary care physician who obtained a lumbosacral MRI, which was interpreted as multilevel degenerative changes.

Further inquiry into her job history reveals that this is the second work-related back claim that she has filed. She was off work for 4 months 2 years ago after "pulling her back out" while assisting with a patient transfer. She has changed jobs frequently in the past and is currently dissatisfied with her present job. She has a graduate equivalency diploma and would like to return to school to find better employment. She denies a history of substance abuse. She has a history of depression, but stopped taking antidepressants 3 years ago. She relates poor sleep since the fall due to constant pain.

On physical examination, she demonstrates exaggerated pain behavior. She lurches to her left side while ambulating with her cane. She moans throughout range of motion testing, which is markedly limited in all directions. There is tenderness diffusely with palpation over the spinous processes and paraspinal musculature in the lumbosacral region. She is able to walk on her heels and toes but she leans heavily on her cane to maintain her balance. While seated, she has give-way weakness (no detectable effort by the patient) on manual muscle testing. Sensation to light touch and proprioception is decreased in both lower limbs. Reflexes are symmetric and intact throughout, except for decreased ankle jerks bilaterally, and toes are downgoing bilaterally. SLR in the seated position does not provoke pain, but when supine, the patient complains of shooting pains into her legs with less than 30 degrees of motion on SLR bilaterally.

In this setting in which examination findings are inconsistent, as demonstrated by decreased effort on manual muscle test with preserved ability to toe-to-heel walk and a negative sitting SLR compared to a positive supine SLR, it is even more difficult to ascertain the true etiology of a patient's back pain. Her decreased sensation in her lower limbs and decreased ankle jerks are suggestive of diabetic neuropathy, which is confirmed with electrodiagnostic testing. Otherwise, there is no suggestion of neurologic compromise, with her prior MRI correlating with these findings. The patient should be reassured that her examination findings and diagnostic workup do not suggest skeletal or neurologic injury, and it should be reinforced that her pain will subside with time. Again, maintaining activity should also be stressed. Because 8 weeks have already elapsed since the time of injury, this patient's injury is classified as subacute. She deserves close follow-up, ideally weekly, as attempts are made to treat her pain conservatively. A comprehensive interdisciplinary rehabilitation program is indicated if limited or no progress has been made within the month after her initial visit because she is at risk for developing chronic pain complaints. By including various professionals in one setting, multiple goals, including conditioning, education, psychological well-being, and pain management, can be addressed.

Exaggerated pain complaints and examination inconsistencies, such as those illustrated in this case presentation, are fairly common in the industrial population because individuals often believe that they must show that they are injured or ill to substantiate a workers' compensation claim. However, outright malingering is actually rare. As mentioned previously, identifying psychosocial factors that could contribute to disability and impede rehabilitation is especially important when treating patients with work-related LBP. In this scenario, it is critical. The concern is that the longer this patient remains off work, the more difficult it will be to get her back to work. She has already admitted that she is dissatisfied with her job. Given her history of depression, her job dissatisfaction, and exaggerated pain behavior, psychological consultation as part of her rehabilitation plan is indicated. Of note, a disability syndrome has been described to characterize those patients who appear resistant to rehabilitation efforts. Proposed explanations for ongoing disability and delayed recovery include fear of reinjury, low self-esteem, estrangement from the workplace, reversal of roles within the family, and the perception that their chances for success in competitive employment are low.[8]

After an appropriate and adequate course of conservative therapy and rehabilitation efforts have been undertaken and sufficient time has elapsed for recovery to occur, the physician should determine if the patient has reached maximal medical improvement. In this situation, although the patient has reached maximal medical improvement, she is not able to function in her prior capacity. An impairment rating and disability determination are then made based on objective findings rather than persistent pain complaints. Her depression plays a role in this assessment because her examination findings and functional residual capacity may reflect what she will do versus what she can do. A referral to a vocational counselor and ongoing psychiatric or psychological counseling for the preceding problems listed is recommended.

Clinical Case 5

A 43-year-old male truck driver who was involved in a work-related motor vehicle accident is referred for an independent medical examination after being off work for the past 9 months secondary to persistent low back strain. He states that he has seen multiple specialists who have tried everything for his pain without success. He reports that he continues to require medication with propoxyphene napsylate and acetaminophen (Darvocet) throughout the day to make his pain bearable. His activity level has declined, and he spends the majority of his time on the sofa or in bed; however, he has difficulty sleeping. Standing and ambulating aggravate his pain. He was noted to enter the examination room with an antalgic and labored gait. He notes generalized weakness throughout his body. He describes pain circumferentially shooting into legs proximally. He also complains of vague sensory changes with patchy areas of numbness in his legs bilaterally. There is no change in bowel or bladder function.

He becomes emotional while describing the circumstances of his injury and then expresses anger toward the individual who is at fault. He resents his employer who fired him due to damage to the truck, although the patient was not responsible for the accident. In addition to taking multiple Darvocet tablets throughout the day, he admits to frequently self-medicating with alcohol. He also smokes one pack of cigarettes per day. His relationship with his wife has become strained because she is now the sole financial support for the household. The patient has a high school diploma with 2 years of technical schooling.

Workup to date has included plain films and an MRI, which were unremarkable. Treatment has consisted of multiple analgesics, with the patient denying any response to nonsteroidal anti-inflammatory drugs. He states he was switched to Darvocet from oxycodone and acetaminophen (Percocet) approximately 6 months ago. A course of oral steroids within the first month of his injury did not help. Physical therapy with ultrasound and massage only provided temporary relief immediately after sessions. He refuses to exercise because he asserts that any activity exacerbates his discomfort. A transcutaneous electrical nerve stimulation unit has also been tried unsuccessfully.

His examination reveals exaggerated pain behavior with frequent moaning and wincing. Range of motion of his lumbosacral spine is severely limited, with the patient complaining of increased discomfort with only slight movement. Forward trunk flexion is limited to 40 degrees, and extension is limited to 20 degrees. Palpation over his spinous processes and paraspinal musculature reveals diffuse tenderness, but not involuntary guarding. Manual muscle testing reveals ratchety or give-way weakness in the lower limbs bilaterally. He staggers when attempting to toe or heel walk bilaterally. Sensation testing reveals sensory loss in a nonphysiologic distribution. Reflexes are difficult to elicit in the lower limbs with downgoing toes bilaterally. SLR is limited to 30 degrees bilaterally, with the patient noting severe back pain provoked by the maneuver. With distraction, a negative sitting SLR is demonstrated bilaterally. Electrodiagnostic testing, including H-reflexes, reveal no abnormalities.

At this point, this patient is considered to have chronic LBP, as his symptoms have persisted for longer than 3 months. It is safe to conclude that his symptomatology is consistent with chronic pain syndrome, with his entire focus revolving around his intolerable pain. These patients remain the most challenging to treat within the industrial system. It is not uncommon to see workers' compensation case files that extend over a several-year period in patients with the chronic pain syndrome (Figure 12.2) Patterns of behavior are difficult to alter, with patients resistant to rehabilitation efforts as if they do not want to recover. Frequently, secondary gain is what motivates them. Only a minority of patients with chronic pain syndrome return to work, despite costly and intensive rehabilitation programs. This has become even more of a problem to society as chronic pain and long-term disability

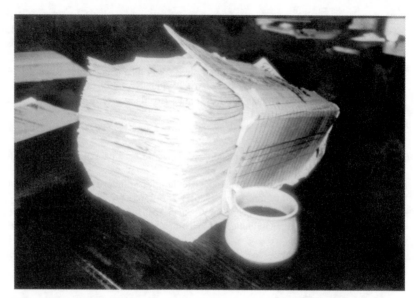

Figure 12.2 Bureau of workers' compensation case file for claim extending over a 3-year period.

are becoming more socially acceptable.[9] It would be helpful to be able to predict during the acute stage which patients, after an occupational back injury, would progress to chronic pain syndrome; however, this remains difficult.

SUMMARY

Industrial LBP in the United States has been extensively researched due to the profound and widespread social and economic effects resulting from this prevalent condition. Direct and indirect costs related to medical care, lost wages, decreased productivity, and litigation are enormous and escalating. Industrial LBP is a complex entity, and, often, multiple factors impact its presentation, medical and rehabilitation course, and outcome. Although workers' compensation programs were intended to be no-fault systems, litigation is still commonplace. This litigation stems from the inherent complexity of the various systems involved and the burden of proof required to determine that the disability is work related. The challenge is to deliver comprehensive medical care and rehabilitation in an era of cost containment.

REFERENCES

1. Rondinelli RD, Robinson JP, Scheer SJ, Weinstein SM. Industrial rehabilitation medicine. Part 4. Strategies for disability management. Arch Phys Med Rehabil 1997;78:S21–S28.
2. Andersson GB. Epidemiologic aspects on low-back pain in industry. Spine 1981;6:53–60.

3. Bigos S, Bowyer O, Braen G, et al. Acute Low Back Problems in Adults. Clinical Practice Guideline No. 14. AHCPR Pub. No. 95-0642. Rockville, MD: U.S. Department of Health and Human Services, Public Health Service, Agency for Health Care Policy and Research, December 1994;15–20.

4. Bigos S, Bowyer O, Braen G, et al. Acute Low Back Problems in Adults. Clinical Practice Guideline, Quick Reference Guide No. 14. AHCPR Pub. No. 95-0643. Rockville, MD: U.S. Department of Health and Human Services, Public Health Service, Agency for Health Care Policy and Research, December 1994;2.

5. Deyo RA, Rainville J, Kent DL. What can the history and physical examination tell us about low back pain? JAMA 1992;268:760–765.

6. Aronoff GM, DuPuy DN. Evaluation and management of back pain: preventing disability. J Back Musculo Rehab 1997;9:109–124.

7. Bigos SJ, Spengler DM, Martin NA, et al. Back injuries in industry: a retrospective study. Part III. Employee-related factors. Spine 1986;11:252–256.

8. Robinson JP, Rondinelli RD, Scheer SJ, Weinstein SM. Industrial rehabilitation medicine. Part 1. Why is industrial rehabilitation medicine unique? Arch Phys Med Rehabil 1997;78:S3–S9.

9. Waddell, G. Keynote address for primary care forum. Low back pain: a twentieth century health care enigma. Spine 1996;21:2825–2828.

Chapter 13

Functional Performance Evaluation in Patients with Low Back Pain: Methods, Procedures, and Issues

Karen S. Rucker and Michael D. West

Thousands of persons' lives are disrupted every day because of functional limitations caused by back pain. According to a poll of Americans, one-fourth of adults report having pain strong enough to interfere with their daily activities every month.[1] Not only can pain be debilitating, it can be costly, causing more than $55 billion a year in lost work days.[2]

The sensation of pain is subjective and, therefore, not directly measurable. Thus, the inability to identify specific organic pathology in many patients with persistent pain, continued reports of pain after the correction of pathologic conditions, and continued complaints of pain after the expected period of resolution of an injury have led to a lack of consensus about basic definitions and inconsistencies in measurement and assessment techniques.[3,4]

There is no way to prove or disprove the presence of pain in a particular person.[5] Pain is inferred by verbal and nonverbal expressions or actions, referred to as *pain behaviors*. Fordyce lists these behaviors as verbal complaints of pain and discomfort; nonlanguage sounds, such as moans and sighs; body posturing and gesturing, including limping and rubbing the painful body part or area; and displays of functional limitations or disability, such as reclining for excessive periods of time.[6] Other pain behaviors have been noted, such as the frequent reliance on health care by seeking medical consultation, excessive use of nonessential medications, multiple surgeries, therapy, and work disability.[5,7] These pain behaviors are influenced not by the pathologic process identified, but, often, by the effects of naturally occurring learning processes and social reinforcement.[8]

Because patients in pain demonstrate large individual differences in response to injury, many believe these pain behaviors should be the focus of assessment and treatment, rather than subjective pain reports, which are often used.[3] Pain behaviors, it is suggested, may offer a more useful assessment of responses referring to pain.

Portions of this manuscript are excerpted from KS Rucker, MD West. Functional Performance Evaluation in Patients with Chronic Pain. In GM Aronoff (ed), Evaluation and Treatment of Chronic Pain (3rd ed). Baltimore: Williams & Wilkins, 1999;603–615.

Other commonly used measures of functional limitations from pain are measures of the patient's capabilities as perceived by the patient, family members, and physicians.[4] These functional capacities typically include ability to perform basic self-care functions (e.g., dressing, bathing) or to engage in strenuous activities, such as sports, housekeeping, or manual labor. A worldwide literature search that identified more than 600 function-related evaluations from 20 different countries was funded by the Social Security Administration and conducted by the primary author in 1996.[9] It is significant to note that the majority of functional assessment instruments relied on self reports of symptoms, which frequently do not agree with more objective measures, such as patient observations or results of physical examinations.

Across the country, functional performance evaluations (FPEs) have become big business with rehabilitation programs and physical therapy groups. FPEs are used for a number of purposes, including to predict the ability to return to a former job, for pre-employment testing for potential jobs, and for determination of functional limitations for compensation purposes. FPEs are intended to measure a person's performance of specific tasks, and, from this viewed performance, predict the ability to perform those specific tasks and related tasks, usually in a work environment. There is no nationally accepted standardized functional capacity evaluation or procedure; there is great variation in the tasks measured, the length of time over which performance is evaluated, the qualifications of the evaluator, and the use of the data produced. A large number of tests are published evaluating a wide and diverse range of abilities; however, measuring and predicting ability to perform specific tasks are limited and impacted by many factors that are difficult to control. Pope identified many of these factors, including patient discomfort or pain, medications, gender, body weight, motivation, fatigue, fitness, and fear of injury.[10]

The focus of this chapter is on FPEs, which are used to assess and predict the performance of a person with chronic back pain and chronic pain syndrome, as opposed to acute and subacute low back pain. Despite the increasing medical and economic impact of chronic back pain, many aspects of pain assessment and treatment remain unclear.[3] What follows are some general guidelines of what should be expected from FPEs.

UNDERSTANDING THE TERMINOLOGY

Since the introduction of functional performance testing, various terms have been used interchangeably to identify the same test, including *functional capacity assessments*, *functional abilities assessments*, and *functional capacity evaluation*. Because of this confusion in terminology, these individual tests do not always reflect the same areas being assessed.[8] This confusion is often a result of inappropriately applied labels.[11] Therefore, it is important that the distinction among these terms be made when ordering, performing, and interpreting assessments.

A *screening evaluation* can be an assessment to identify general status and assist the physician in referring persons to the appropriate treatment or rehabilitation program. It is based on interviews or tests that are designed according to skills. An *assessment* is an investigation of the abilities, or strengths, and limitations, or weaknesses, of a particular body function and comparison to expected levels (i.e., the norm). An *evaluation*, therefore, is simply a measurement appraisal process designed to find values or amounts that describe performance levels.[11]

The distinction between capacity and ability also should be made. *Capacity* is the limits of the anatomic, physiologic, and psychological systems for the individual. These capacities are dependent on gender, age, body type, etc. *Ability*, on the other hand, reflects human capacities as modified by individual behavioral attitudes, in addition to external factors, such as injury, pain, and environmental and social stressors.[11]

Understanding the difference between physical, functional, and work-related attributes is important to the complete comprehension of functional performance testing. For these purposes, *physical attributes* include static and dynamic muscular strength, flexibility, mobility, alertness, steadiness, gait, balance, posture, coordination, and muscular and cardiovascular endurance. *Functional measures* comprise sitting, standing, walking, kneeling, squatting, lifting, carrying, pushing, pulling, and manual dexterity. *Work-related factors* are those job demands that are specific to the job or occupation in question (i.e., lifting 50 pounds frequently).[11]

TYPES OF FUNCTIONAL PERFORMANCE EVALUATIONS

FPEs are a means of testing such parameters as lifting and carrying capability, positional tolerance, general endurance level, and ability to lift to certain heights. Work capacity testing tends to be more job specific, and requires more assessment in actual job-task simulation to be truly appropriate. The primary distinctions are cost and time spent in testing.[12] A typical functional performance test is performed over a 2-day period for a total of 4–6 hours, whereas work capacity can require a full week.

Several types of evaluations have been described in the area of human performance testing[11]:

1. *Physical capacity evaluation* measures the maximum levels of physical performance of the individual (i.e., maximum weight that can be lifted, number of stairs climbed, and number of times reaching overhead). These measurements, in turn, assess fundamental parameters, such as strength, flexibility, and endurance.
2. *Functional abilities assessment* assesses the acceptable level of performance at a certain point in time and usually produces data regarding parameters, such as lifting, carrying, walking, and standing. The patient is not pushed to a maximum performance level.
3. *Work-related assessments* test the individual's ability to meet or exceed the physical demands of the work, with specific reference to the job and the tasks involved (e.g., duration, load, repetition). Among these demands are standing, walking, sitting, lifting, carrying, pushing, pulling, climbing, balancing, stooping, kneeling, crouching, crawling, reaching, handling, fingering, feeling, talking, hearing, and seeing. These factors constitute the basic elements of this type of assessment. A number of different types of work-related assessments are used for different purposes. These are summarized in Table 13.1.

FUNCTIONAL PERFORMANCE EVALUATION ROLES

The FPE process involves various people, the physician, the functional performance evaluator, and the patient.[11] Each person plays a vital role in the outcome of the FPE and the subsequent treatment and rehabilitation protocol identified.

Table 13.1 Components of Commonly Used Work-Related Evaluations

Work tolerance screening	Performance of simulated activities reflecting critical job requirements
	Requires performance in same sequence and frequency as job
	Typically a 4-day assessment
	Requires detailed job description
	Difficult to duplicate extrinsic factors, such as heat, glare, stress
Fitness for duty	Assesses ability to perform critical job requirements
	For worker off only short time
	Useful for workers in hazardous jobs
Work hardening	Progressively increases worker's physical ability to accomplish job requirements or maximize ability
	Rehabilitation of entire body, as well as specific injury
	Includes instruction in posture and body mechanics
	Daily progression in hours (i.e., from 3–4 hours to 6–8 hours)
	Length of time usually 3 weeks
	Can use in conjunction with light duty or part-time work
Work conditioning	1–2 hours per day, 3–5 days per week
	General conditioning exercises
	Some specific return to work activities
	May precede work hardening
On-site job analysis	To determine if job description accurately reflects job responsibilities
	Assessment of equipment and supplies
	Measurement of number and heights of lifts, bends, and reaches
	Assess other factors, such as uneven ground, work area congestion, awkward equipment

Physician

The physician is the first to examine the patient to formulate a medical diagnosis and an appropriate medical treatment plan. This treatment plan can include the use of exercises, physical therapy, medications, surgery, or referrals for specialty consultations, education, or counseling.[13] The physician is asked to determine the ability of the patient to perform functional tasks and return to work or other daily activities. Because this often cannot be determined under the confines of a physician office visit, the physician will refer the patient to a functional performance evaluator to measure his or her functional performance and limitations.

After assessing the measurements obtained through the FPE, the physician looks for any discrepancies that may exist between those findings and the present medical diagnosis.[13] This includes consideration of present and future physiologic and biomechanical concerns of the patient.

Functional Performance Evaluator

The functional performance evaluator determines the ergonomically safe level of function of the patient through objective testing and using physician-determined parameters and guidelines when provided.[14] Objective information regarding functional performance enables the physician and rehabilitation team to design an appropriate rehabilitation protocol. The functional performance evaluator is responsible for preparing written and oral reports on the physical abilities and limitations of the evaluee, which are then used in the interpretation of (1) true physical impairment, (2) functional abilities and deficits, (3) symptom magnification, (4) physical abilities versus physical demands of a potential job, (5) need for further treatment, and (6) options for continued rehabilitation.[13]

It is essential that the functional performance evaluator have a thorough understanding of the neuromusculoskeletal system. This includes muscle, nerve, soft tissue, and bone physiology, along with normal and dysfunctional characteristics of each. The physical therapist and orthopedically trained occupational therapist most often have this professional preparation.[13] Occupational and physical therapists specializing in the prevention and management of musculoskeletal disorders possess the perspective and expertise to evaluate and make recommendations to the physician regarding the patient's current functional capabilities and, where applicable, return-to-work potential.[15,16]

Patient

The primary role of the patient (evaluee) in the FPE process is to voluntarily and actively participate in his or her own rehabilitation.[13] To do this, the patient should understand why the FPE is being performed, including perceived benefits and outcomes. The patient is to be informed of all treatments recommended and delivered to him or her before initiation of the treatment.[17] With this knowledge, the patient is able to make an informed decision concerning compliance with the rehabilitation plan. The patient has the right to refuse any treatment; however, if compensation benefits are an issue, they may be terminated or suspended as determined by law.

FACTORS AFFECTING FUNCTIONAL PERFORMANCE EVALUATIONS

FPEs are primarily conducted as the result of an individual's report that he or she is disabled or impaired and unable to return to work. The patients for whom this issue is most common are those who report that their chronic pain is restricting them from returning to their previous employment or to any employment at all.[3] Chronic pain and chronic pain syndrome complicate the assessment of functional performance immensely due to the variability of how pain impacts individuals, the inability to measure pain, the many psychosocial factors that accompany pain, fear of increasing pain, fear of injury or reinjury, the impact of single efforts versus repetitive efforts on pain, and the impact of effort exerted over time on pain. Because of the chronicity of their condition, these patients present for an FPE with considerable environmental and psychosocial and behavioral factors that can influence their conduct during the evaluation.[3]

Environmental Factors

Because the rehabilitation process involves such a wide array of parties, including physicians, the functional performance examiner, third-party payors, employers, attorneys, case managers, and family members, this multitude of outside influences can play a significant role in the success of the rehabilitation effort. These same parties can also affect the outcome of the FPE.

Physicians

Physicians often look to the results of an FPE to assist them in making a decision regarding a patient's treatment, rehabilitation, and, ultimately, his or her functional capacity. Thus, the expressed or implied expectations of use of the results of the FPE may directly influence the examiner's selection of tests, as well as the presentation and interpretation of the results.[3] Furthermore, advice or restrictions (or both) placed on the patient by the physician may affect the amount of effort expended during the FPE and his or her willingness to attempt certain functional tasks. The physician should communicate to the evaluator the purpose of the assessment and any specific questions to which they are seeking answers.

Third-Party Payors

Another significant influence is the role of the insurance company and other third-party payors. This group is responsible for payment of the medical care, including the FPE, while also pushing for cost containment and case closure.[3] In addition, the rehabilitation consultant, who is often hired by the insurance company, is commonly responsible for managing the evaluation process in chronic pain cases and determining the person's level of return to work. With this goal in mind, rehabilitation consultants may have already formed impressions of the patient's functional abilities or limitations well before the FPE referral, and will seek to obtain information needed to test their own hypotheses.[3]

Employers

Employers can have a significant impact on the outcome of FPEs. Depending on the relationship between employee and employer, and the employee's belief about the future health of the company (i.e., pending layoffs, restructuring), these factors can significantly influence the patient's performance on the FPE.[3] This relationship can impact the employee's desire to return to work or lack of desire. It is helpful for the physician and evaluator to be aware of the employer and employee relationship.

Attorneys

When the employee and employer relationship is questioned due to mistrust of the employer, observations of previous cases at the company, or when there is a question of fault related to the injury, complex litigation and other legal issues represent an important factor that may affect the outcome of FPEs.[3] Attorneys often coach their clients on how to behave and what to say during the FPE process. This, in turn, can affect the patient's performance indirectly and directly. Again, it is important for the evaluator to be aware of these issues that can influence performance and interpretation of the assessment.

Test-Specific Factors

Clinical research tends to show that self-report assessments of status frequently do not agree with more objective measures, such as observations of the patient or results of physical examinations.[18] Many persons either underreport or exaggerate their symptoms for a number of reasons. For example, underreporting may occur because patients believe they are actually getting better when, in actuality, they are simply accepting or adjusting to their new, diminished status. Or, they may under-report symptoms in acquiescence to the examiner, as a defense mechanism, or because they have unrealistic beliefs about their conditions. Exaggeration of symptoms may result from attempts to gain recognition of their pain, a desire to receive assistance or rehabilitative services that might otherwise be unavailable, a belief they are more limited than they are, or fear of exacerbating pain.

The evaluator's determination of his or her role in the FPE process is often guided by the environmental factors discussed previously. For example, referral sources, including insurance companies and attorneys, can exert considerable influence on the examiner regarding preconceived opinions of the patient's capabilities or legitimacy of his or her symptoms.[3] In addition, if the examiner has had previous contact with the patient and is aware of his or her functional abilities, the physician may deviate from the testing protocol to confirm his or her own impression. Thus, the attitudes and behaviors of the evaluator can have a significant impact on the evaluation process, including test selection, test administration, interpretation of the data, and reporting of the results.[3]

The amount of experience the functional performance evaluator has with a specific type of assessment affects the conduct of the test (i.e., standardization or lack of, use of normative data) and the interpretation of the results. After considerable use, some examiners begin to personalize and adapt the testing to their own preferences and expertise, often causing the results to be invalidated, and eliminating the opportunity to collect standardized data.[3]

Most important, the evaluator's own beliefs about pain and how it is expressed determine how observed behaviors are interpreted. Likewise, if the examiner believes that a patient is providing his or her best effort, then pain complaints during the testing may be taken more seriously; however, if the patient is viewed as exaggerating the pain or even frank malingering, the examiner's attitudes, and how the FPE is conducted, also change.[3] Testing procedures can be significantly influenced by potential examiner bias. This can involve a rephrasing of instructions by the examiner based on his or her familiarity with the patient. Likewise, patients look to the evaluator to decide when they should stop the testing, with questions such as "My back is hurting, do you want me to keep going?" If the examiner is being cautious, possibly for medicolegal reasons, then he or she may indicate to the patient that it is okay to stop the task. Conversely, if the examiner is suspicious of the patient's effort, he or she may push the patient to do more. As the functional capacity evaluator, it is important to recognize that subtle but very influential cues by the examiner, including simple changes in voice tone or facial expressions, can significantly alter the verbal message being given to patients.[3] Evaluators should use consistent task-specific endpoints and general endpoints to avoid deviating from the test protocol (Table 13.2).

Rating the intensity of pain is a common component in the evaluation of individuals reporting pain.[3] The relevance of these reports, however, becomes less significant when dealing with chronic pain patients because other factors enter into the

Table 13.2 Task-Specific Endpoints and General Endpoints

Task-specific endpoints
Shortness of breath
Dizziness
Pause between repetitions >7 seconds
Decreasing weight
General endpoints
Psychophysical—voluntary test termination
Aerobic—achievement of 85% of age-determined maximum heart rate
Safety—anthropometric safe limit or 55–60% of body weight
Completion of maximum repetitions

Source: Adapted from TG Mayer, RJ Gretchel. Functional restoration for spinal disorders: the sports medicine approach. Philadelphia: Lea & Febiger, 1988.

picture, including emotional distress and depression, which may influence the level of pain perceived.[19] Because many chronic pain patients tend to focus heavily on their pain, continual questions about pain during testing may negatively influence patients' performance by directing their attention to the pain.[3] Standardized cheerleading responses should be used, such as "Let's keep trying," "Do the best you can," and "Can you continue?" For consistency, the evaluator should use each statement once per task in the same order.

Psychosocial and Behavioral Factors

It should be recognized that unique characteristics specific to the individual patient can influence the results of the FPE. Many of these characteristics involve behavioral or psychosocial factors, or both, including self-efficacy expectations and fear-induced avoidance of activity, interpretation of meaning of pain (i.e., supposed to live with it versus creating more injury), and litigation.

A *self-efficacy expectation* is explained as a personal conviction that one can successfully perform certain behaviors in a given situation.[20] Therefore, if a patient has a negative perception of his or her physical capabilities, this leads to an inability to perform the activities because of these perceptions of incapacity, creating a vicious and endless circle.[21] Furthermore, for many chronic pain patients, the fear of pain is strong enough to make them avoid situations or behaviors that they believe will cause them further harm. In turn, these already formed expectations of what activities will cause harm guide their choice of what activities will be attempted and with how much effort, and what activities will be avoided.[3] Avoidance learning, therefore, reduces the opportunity to disprove these expectations, creating a vicious circle. Thus, the motor impairment seen in many chronic pain patients is due, in part, to the patient's avoidance of certain types of motor activity because of expectations of pain.[3]

These and other psychosocial factors are thought to have a substantial impact on patients' performance on functional capacity tests. This presents a challenge to the evaluator who, often, as a physical or occupational therapist, is not trained in, or even comfortable with, evaluating psychosocial factors. Nevertheless, Rudy and colleagues suggest that these factors should be addressed because not doing so limits the therapist's ability to thoroughly understand the scope of the problems contributing to the patient's disability, as well as the ability to achieve maximal outcomes.[3] However, it is noted that, to address psychosocial factors appropriately, psychometrically sound instruments should be used. This is not to suggest the use of comprehensive and costly psychological assessments, but rather, the examiner should use brief, cost-effective psychosocial screening instruments and be trained as to how to interpret data obtained from the instrument.[3] Then, if significant psychosocial factors are found during the screening, referral to a psychologist may be warranted.

Sincerity of Effort

It is difficult to predict a patient's performance at work or on a functional evaluation. It is even more complicated when a patient reacts inappropriately or magnifies his or her symptoms. In a pain study at Virginia Commonwealth University's Medical College of Virginia in Richmond, funded by the Social Security Administration,[22] a broad sample of patients (18%) were believed by the physicians to have an exaggerated response or magnified symptomatology. The same physicians were then asked to predict what type of effort the patient would give if a functional capacity evaluation was performed. The physicians predicted that of these patients, 40% would give a maximum effort, 33% would give a moderate effort, 10% would give minimum effort, and 2.6% would give no effort at all.

Sincerity of effort is critical to the FPE process.[23] The main goal of functional performance testing is to identify what a patient can and cannot do from a functional perspective. The testing is based on the assumption that the evaluee will cooperate and will do his or her best when performing the various tasks involved in the test. If this cooperation does not exist, the abilities of the evaluee will be inaccurate, and the conclusions drawn from the evaluation will be erroneous.[23]

When discussing the issue of sincerity of effort, a differentiation must be made between malingering and magnification or exaggeration of symptoms. Chronic pain patients may magnify or exaggerate their symptoms for many reasons other than feigning an illness or disability.[18] For example, patients may magnify symptoms in an effort to gain recognition of their pain, which otherwise may not produce objective findings. They may assert a need to magnify their symptoms to be believed and to get the attention that they think is appropriate for their discomfort. In addition, magnification of symptoms may also represent pain behaviors,[22] that is, patients may have a fear of pain in the area being tested and, consequently, avoid tasks that they perceive will bring on that pain.

Malingering, on the other hand, is defined as *the conscious and deliberate feigning of an illness or disability.*[22] It involves the fabrication of symptoms and complaints to achieve a specific goal. Many pain specialists, as well as representatives from the Commission on the Evaluation of Pain, believe that malingering is readily detected using appropriate medical and psychological tests.

It is important to recognize that there are many behaviors that can be associated with malingering and magnification or exaggeration of symptoms, including grimacing, groaning, and use of a cane. Many clinicians tend to label these behaviors as *chronic pain behaviors*, which is misleading because patients with chronic or acute pain can and do use the same behaviors, consciously and subconsciously, to express the experience of pain, and sometimes intentionally to call attention to themselves or to manipulate people and situations for secondary gain.[24] Nevertheless, these behaviors can be judged as appropriate or magnified, acute or chronic, only when a complete understanding of the pathologic process in a given patient is known.

Often, confirming sincerity of effort is not as simple as making behavioral observations. For various reasons, including secondary gain or fear of pain, some patients will not put forth maximum effort when participating in functional performance testing. To address this propensity to expend less than maximum effort, the degree of effort expended should be evaluated using grip tests, isometric strength tests, and so forth. These methods are based on the assumption that people who are performing to their maximum capability will give a consistent performance, whereas patients who perform submaximally will not.[25] Specific tests using the Jamar dynamometer have proved effective in determining sincerity of effort and are discussed in the section Measurement of Effort.

CHARACTERISTICS OF AN EFFECTIVE FUNCTIONAL PERFORMANCE EVALUATION

What makes an effective FPE? Insufficient reliability and validity of existing FPEs make their application somewhat questionable and confusing to physician and evaluator alike. Because of this lack of standardization, however, it is up to the physician and evaluator to determine which evaluation will provide the information needed to make the best decision for the patient. In doing so, various factors have been identified that ideally should be addressed in the selection and use of any functional test, including safety, reliability, validity, practicality, and use.[26]

Safety

Any testing performed on the patient should be safe and not be expected to lead to reinjury or new injury. This can be assured by complete understanding of the patient's injury, including pathology, the ergonomics of the injury, and the patient's understanding and use of correct body mechanics and ergonomics. In addition, FPEs should be administered only by trained personnel and under the supervision of the attending physician.

Reliability

Test scores should be reliable across evaluators, patients, and the time of day the test is administered.[26] Various qualified professionals should be able to administer the FPE. The two most important methods of establishing reliability are inter-rater reliability and test-retest reliability (intrarater reliability).[25] *Inter-rater reliability* refers to the ability of a test to produce similar scores when administered by different, similarly trained administrators.[27] Consistency must be maintained to ensure that significant differences in scores are not a result of the use of different examiners. *Test-retest (or intrarater) reliability* ensures that consistency of measurements is maintained by the same examiner over time.[27] This consistency is achieved by determining an appropriate interval of time that is long enough to minimize a learning effect from the first test for the subject and examiner, but short enough that the patient's medical condition will not change significantly between tests.[25]

Validity

A measurement is considered valid if it measures the attribute it claims to measure.[27] The interpretation of a test score should be able to predict or reflect the patient's performance in a target work setting, and the test must focus on primary physical job demands.[26] Different types of validity represent different ways to support the attributes measured. Of these, the most important is criterion-related validity. This method compares scores from the test in question with other independent measures of the same attribute.[25] There are two types of criterion-related validity. *Predictive validity* measures the ability to predict future occurrences (i.e., to predict return to work and at what level). *Concurrent validity* identifies patients who are currently performing in a certain way in an independent setting. An example of concurrent validity would be if FPE scores distinguish between patients who are currently unable to perform heavy manual labor and patients who are currently performing heavy manual labor successfully, then the FPE would demonstrate good concurrent validity.[25]

Practicality

FPEs should be practical and cost effective. We cannot rely on expensive equipment and lengthy periods of administration by highly trained professionals, or we are going to price ourselves out of the market. Matheson and colleagues define cost as *the direct expense of the test procedure, plus the amount of time required of the patient, plus the delay in providing the information derived from the procedure to the referral source.*[26] Furthermore, the equipment used should be widely available and inexpensive.

Use

Because the need for and use of FPE results involve various parties, including physicians, payors, referral sources, and employers, the usefulness of the FPE should meet the needs of all the parties. Therefore, the FPE should help the treating physician to determine the patient's ability to return to work, when the patient has reached his functional plateau, and at what functional level the patient is likely to return to work.[26]

In addition to the aforementioned factors, the domains of the variables used in FPEs should be covered as comprehensively as possible. One method of determining comprehensiveness is to review how many of the U.S. Department of Labor's 20 physical demands of work are addressed.[28] It is not enough, however, to simply use various domains. Rather, each domain should be evaluated thoroughly and produce an objective, specific, and quantifiable score, not just a pass or fail score.[25]

In addition to meeting the aforementioned requirements of an effective FPE, the testing should also be spread out over time. The evaluation should take place over at least a 4-day period to assess the cumulative effect of increased activity to the worker's pain. This allows the examiner to identify activities that may aggravate the injury and whether the pain level decreases after completing the aggravating activity or remains consistent. It should be expected that the worker's pain will increase gradually, due to the nature of testing throughout the day; however, it is whether this pain continues into the next morning that is most important.[29] If the worker reports severe or incapacitating pain over the next several days after testing, this suggests a poor response to activity, perhaps poor technique used, or fibromyalgia. Conversely, if the worker reports having no muscle soreness at all on the second or third day of testing, the question should be raised as to whether the patient gave a maximal effort.

EVALUATION

The goal of the FPE is to measure an individual's current physical abilities. To meet this goal, the objectives of an FPE are (1) to determine if an individual is able to safely meet the physical demands of a general category of job; (2) to quantify the physical impairment and functional performance of the injured worker; and (3) to assist in determining guidelines for the development of a vocational rehabilitation plan.[13]

Choosing the Appropriate Test

When assessments are ordered, the therapist should know the goals of the evaluation so that an appropriate test can be designed. The therapist should be creative, adapting the evaluation to the realistic ability of the worker and the practical resolution of the case.[29] The therapist should have the clinical knowledge to design programs that minimize unnecessary strain on the injured area.

Many evaluations are requested on individuals who have been out of work 6 months or longer, and who will likely not return to their previous employment.[29] Performing the wrong test at the wrong time can lead to underestimating a worker's potential employment opportunities or injuring the worker, thus prolonging time out of work. The order of testing should be flexible to obtain maximal performance. For example, if a patient has a knee disorder, floor-to-waist lifting should be postponed until the end of the evaluation to avoid potential increase in pain due to aggravation of the injury.[29] This option may not be indicated in the report, but should be made available to and discussed with the physician.

The safest plan for all injured workers whose jobs require strenuous activity is to have a *fitness-for-duty evaluation* before return to work. If the worker does not pass this evaluation, a *work hardening program* should be initiated to improve the areas in which the worker was unable to perform. When the worker is able to perform critical job requirements, a *work tolerance screening* should be performed before returning to the physician. If the worker has been deemed unable to return to previous employment, a *vocational evaluation* may be done to identify more appropriate job types. The work hardening program can then focus on alternatives for employment, and, again, discharge of the patient when critical job requirements can be performed.[29] If a worker complains of reinjury or a new injury, the physical therapist should be able to recognize the problem and refer the patient in a timely manner to the physician for evaluation and further treatment, thereby preventing delays in treatment or increased injury.

Test Components

History and Complaint

Although there exists great variation in the realm of functional performance testing, as has been demonstrated in this chapter, several essential components are shown to be effective methods of assessing a patient's functional limitations. Information regarding the specific injury is obtained from medical records and patient interviews. Initial questions should include how the injury occurred and what residual deficits were sustained as a result of the incident. The therapist should then become familiar with the treatment course thus far, pertaining to this particular injury, including the level of relief, if any, provided by this treatment. Assessment of cardiovascular risk factors should also be performed at this stage.

After these questions are answered, the therapist should attempt to identify how the patient views his or her injury, and subsequent limitations or deficits as a result of that injury. Important to obtain during the medical history is the patient's history of previous injuries. History of previous injuries could signal additional problems, which may require observation.[16] Because pain can interfere with function, the therapist should include an assessment of the patient's experience of pain, and the degree to which he or she perceives that pain interferes with function.[15] The use of pain diaries is the most common method of assessing activity.[30] Usually, pain diaries consist of forms that are completed by the patient on a daily basis, which track the levels of pain and activity. Pain drawings have also been helpful in assessing a person's pain.

Physical Examination

The purpose of the physical examination is to quantify true physical impairment, rate symptom magnification, determine the injured worker's perception of his or her own disability, and list the specific quantifiable patient problems. The performance of this examination provides the functional evaluator an opportunity to identify and evaluate the potential risks or contraindications for performing the functional portion of the FPE. Therefore, the purposes of the neuromusculoskeletal examination are to determine if the patient is medically stable and does not have any contraindications for testing, to quantify physical impairment for potential permanent impairment rating, for any post-testing comparisons, or for any comparisons to functional limitations, if necessary. During the physical examination, the focus is on the patient's functional capabilities. Specific goniometric measurements are not as critical in and of themselves as they are in relation to the job's physical demands and the worker's ability to perform those job demands.[16]

The physical examination should include observation and documentation of the overall appearance of the injury. After this observation and documentation, evaluation of active range of motion should be made by instructing the patient to perform active range of motion movement patterns and noting any gross deficits. Often, further evaluation is recommended via a goniometer, and the evaluation of passive range of motion is also performed. Discrepancies in active and passive motion should signal a need for further exploration.[16]

Lifting

The assessment of lifting is a vital component of any FPE. Before initiation of the lifting portion of the evaluation, the therapist should be familiar with what the maximum lifting capabilities of the worker are going to be in the actual work setting. This familiarity should also include the frequency of this lifting, the size of the material being lifted, and the manner in which the material will be lifted (i.e., waist to floor, floor to overhead). Before lifting tasks begin, the therapist should review with the patient proper body mechanics needed in performing the tasks. This review should be made verbally and demonstratively.[16]

During the performance of the lifting tasks, the patient should be instructed to stop if there is any discomfort. On completion of the evaluation, the therapist should re-evaluate the worker's physical status with regard to pain, and discuss with the patient his or her current pain level, possibly using the pain drawing sheet again.[16]

Functional Working Postures

A general FPE should include a variety of tests in each of the functional working postures, including sustained postures and repetitive motions, as well as the handling of materials. Some evaluations only estimate the worker's tolerance for sitting, standing, and walking instead of observing and measuring these actions during the use of other tests. The report should reflect how the data were collected. For example, while observing for signs of symptom magnification, the worker's tolerance for sitting or standing can also be documented. Likewise, by having the worker perform various activities in different locations, his or her tolerance for walking can be observed and measured.[29]

Measurement of Effort

There has not been significant research regarding measurement of effort, with the exception of research on the use of a hand dynamometer to measure grip strength, which has been shown to be a reliable indicator of effort. It has been demonstrated that when the five positions of the hand dynamometer are graphed, maximal effort produces a bell curve across the five positions, with the greatest grip force occurring between two and four. Conversely, true weakness produces the same-shaped curve, but with reduced force at each position.[31] Therefore, an abnormal curve seems to demonstrate evidence of submaximal effort.[23]

Another test used to identify submaximal effort was developed by Hildreth et al.[32] The rapid exchange test requires patients to perform the five-position hand grip test with the dynamometer set at the position at which the greatest force occurred. The subjects are then instructed to switch hands rapidly on the dynamometer, maximally gripping each time.

Some researchers have recommended the use of electromyograms (EMGs) to measure sincerity of effort.[23] The theory is that because EMGs are able to measure overall neural drive, then sincere maximal hand grip tests could be distinguished from faked maximal tests by the detection of differences in amplitude and frequency data of the EMG.

Based on the research performed on these tests, a positive rapid exchange test and a flat curve for the five-position grip test, all with low-amplitude EMG data in someone with low back pain, would provide good (some clinicians would say conclusive) evidence of malingering.[23] However, according to Hoffmaster et al.,[33] clinicians who suspect malingering should not simply use one test for confirmation. Instead, the evaluator should have the patient participate in the five-position grip test and the rapid exchange grip test. If further confirmation is warranted, EMG measurements can, according to some clinicians, provide additional data that even a skilled malingerer should find difficult to circumvent.[23]

Report

Many physicians, employers, third-party payors, and so forth look to the evaluation report to make decisions regarding the injured worker's ability to safely return to work. Findings also enable the worker to make clear work restrictions, rather than vague ones, such as no repetitive motion or light work only.[16] Tests performed should be clearly defined or described within the report. The report should provide a clear picture of what the worker did (e.g., number of lifts, distance carried or walked). Most of the tests performed should be able to be duplicated from the information provided in the report. The actual work performance should be given in a format that is understandable, and the report should not consist solely of the examiner's opinion. Furthermore, the report should detail inconsistencies noted by the therapist during the worker's performance on the tests, and should provide specific examples of these inconsistencies. If any tests were administered but not completed, this information should also be included in the report.

The effect of each activity on the estimated pain level should be documented in the report. This documentation should include clinical observations on the ease of movement and inability to maintain proper form and balance. From this report, the physician should be able to easily identify activities that are particularly aggravating to the worker's pain, as well as activities that can be performed easily. This information is helpful in determining potential employment options.

All data or scores should be explained or interpreted. Norms and their sources should be provided or indicated for all items. If norms are not available for a particular test, the report should provide a reasonable and justifiable interpretation. If a job description is used, specific reference should be made regarding the demands of the specific job, or to jobs in that work category.[11]

The summary section of the report should address the original questions or reasons that led to the referral. Narratives should be individualized and specific to the evaluee. If the report includes recommendations, these should be problem and goal oriented and provide details for implementation.[11] Recommendations should include specific information regarding appropriate timing of return to work and at what capacity (full- or part-time).

SUMMARY

In low back and chronic pain patients, physical examinations and x-ray and laboratory findings have not correlated well with pain complaint, disability, or functional abilities. Lack of correlation combined with the wide variability in how physicians assess impairments that cause disability makes the FPE a critical factor in determining function, disability, and return to work. However, to date, no valid, scientific data from controlled studies exist to determine the accuracy of these testing programs. The Commission on the Evaluation of Pain and the Institute of Medicine have placed significant emphasis on the need for FPEs.

In 1992, after a review of available functional muscle testing protocols, Malcolm Pope wrote that science has not kept up with the marketing of this industry.[10] No uniformly acceptable series of activities and no standardization of the evaluations are out there. As can be seen from the scope of this chapter, the focus of assessments can vary from analysis of a single job and specific job task, to a more comprehensive assessment designed to be applicable across multiple job settings. No valid, scientific data from controlled studies can be used to determine the accuracy of these tests. Women, the elderly, minorities, and persons with disabilities have been particularly underrepresented in the few studies that have been performed. Yet, despite the limitations, FPEs are used clinically and provide a snapshot of a person's capabilities.[8]

From the review of the functional testing instruments discussed, it appears that the direction of functional assessment instrument development is to incorporate not only somatic complaints and symptoms, but also the impact of symptoms on the fulfillment of social roles and expectations, including home management, self-care, engagement in social and leisure activities, financial self-support, well-being, and employment.

As physicians continue to be asked tough questions by insurance companies, employers, and even the patient, such as, "When can the patient return to work?" "What are the restrictions?" and "Can he or she get disability?" the vital need for standardized, valid, and reliable FPEs will continue to be evident.

REFERENCES

1. Mellman Lazarus Lake Inc. Presentation of Findings, Mayday Fund 1993. Washington, DC: Mellman Lazarus Lake Inc, 1993.
2. Naisbitt's Trend Letter. New York: Morrow, 1993.
3. Rudy TE, Lieber SJ, Boston JR. Functional capacity assessment: influence of behavioral and environmental factors. Journal of Back and Musculoskeletal Rehabilitation 1996;6:277–288.
4. Rucker KS. Standardization of chronic pain assessment: a multiperspective approach. Clin J Pain 1996;12;94–110.
5. Osterweis M, Kleinman A, Mechanic D, eds. Pain and Disability—Clinical, Behavioral, and Public Policy Perspective. Committee on Pain, Disability and Chronic Illness Behavior. Washington, DC: National Academy Press, 1987.
6. Fordyce WE. Behavioral Methods for Chronic Pain and Illness. St. Louis: Mosby, 1976.
7. Vasudevan SV, Monsein M. Evaluation of Function and Disability in the Patient with Chronic Pain. In PP Raj (ed), Practical Management of Pain (2nd ed). St. Louis: Mosby Year Book, 1992.
8. Vasudevan SV. Role of functional capacity assessment in disability evaluation. J Back Musculo Rehab 1996;6:237–248.
9. Rucker KS, Wehman P, Kregel J. Analysis of Functional Instruments for Functional Assessment Instruments for Disability Rehabilitation Employment Programs. Report Submitted on Completion of SSA Contract #600-95-21914, 1996.
10. Pope MH. Clinical Efficacy and Outcome in the Diagnosis and Treatment of Low Back Pain. New York: Raven Press, 1982.
11. Abdel-Moty E, Compton R, Steele-Rosomoff R, et al. Process analysis of functional capacity assessment. J Back Musculo Rehab 1996;6:223–236.
12. Keane GP, White AH. Back rehabilitation programs: sorting through the options. J Back Musculo Rehab 1991;1:29–36.
13. Trinkle KL, Hart DL, Bunger SD. Roles and responsibilities of team members in the functional capacity evaluation and rehabilitation of the injured worker. J Back Musculo Rehab 1993;3:61–67.
14. Hart DL, Isernhagen SJ, Matheson LN. Guidelines for functional capacity evaluation of people with medical conditions. J Orthop Sports Phys Ther 1993;18:682–686.
15. Schultz-Johnson K. Assessment of upper extremity–injured persons' return to work potential. J Hand Surg [Am] 1987;5:950–957.
16. Williams K. Functional capacity evaluation of the upper extremity. Work 1991;1:48–64.
17. Coy JA. Autonomy based informed consent; ethical implications for patient noncompliance. Phys Ther 1989;69:826–833.

18. Bech P. Rating Scales for Psychopathology, Health Status and Quality of Life: A Compendium of Documentation in Accordance with the DSM-111-R and WHO Systems. Berlin: Springer-Verlag, 1993.
19. Waddell G, Frymoyer JW. Acute and Chronic Pain. In MH Pope, GB Andersson, JW Frymoyer, DB Chaffin (eds), Occupational Low Back Pain: Assessment, Treatment, and Prevention. St. Louis: Mosby Year Book, 1991.
20. Bandura A. Self-efficacy: toward a unifying theory of behavioral change. Psychol Rev 1977;84:191–215.
21. Schmidt AJ. Cognitive factors in the performance level of chronic low back patients. J Psychosom Res 1985;29:183–189.
22. Rucker KS. Pain Assessment Instruments Development Project. Final report upon completion of SSA Contract #600-90-0263, 1996.
23. Simonsen JC. Validation of sincerity of effort. Journal of Back and Musculoskeletal Rehabilitation 1996;6:289–295.
24. Decker MJ. A response to redefining chronic pain programs for the injured worker population. Journal of Back and Musculoskeletal Rehabilitation 1993;3:88–90.
25. Lechner D, Roth D, Straaton K. Functional capacity evaluation in work disability. Work 1991;1:37–47.
26. Matheson LN, Mooney V, Grant JE, et al. Standardized evaluation of work capacity. J Back Musculo Rehab 1996;6:249–264.
27. Feinstein AL, Josephy BR, Wells CK. Scientific and clinical problems in indexes of functional disability. Ann Intern Med 1986;105:413–420.
28. U.S. Dept of Labor, Employment and Training Administration. Dictionary of Occupational Titles (4th ed, rev). Washington, DC: U.S. Government Printing Office, 1991.
29. Carruth MK. Commentary: ???FCE-WTS-WH-WCE-FFD-WC??? Journal of Back and Musculoskeletal Rehabilitation 1993;3:86–94.
30. Follick MJ, Ahern DK, Laser-Wolston N. Evaluation of a daily activity diary for chronic pain patients. Pain 1984;19:373–382.
31. Stokes HM. The seriously uninjured hand—weakness of grip. J Occup Med 1983;25:683–694.
32. Hildreth DH, Breidenbach WC, Lister GD, Hodges AD. Detection of submaximal effort by use of the rapid exchange grip. J Hand Surg [Am] 1989;14A:742–745.
33. Hoffmaster E, Lech R, Niebuhr BR. Consistency of sincere and feigned grip exertions with repeated testing. J Occup Med 1993;35:788–794.

Chapter 14

Assessment and Treatment of Chronic Low Back Pain: The Multidisciplinary Approach

Hubert L. Rosomoff and Renee Steele Rosomoff

In 1994, the Agency for Health Care Policy and Research of the U.S. Department of Health and Human Services identified acute low back problems in adults as a major health care delivery issue. The panel of 23 multidisciplinary experts defined back problems as *activity intolerance due to back-related symptoms* and acute as *limitations of less than 3 months' duration*. The clinical practice publication, *Acute Low Back Problems in Adults: Assessment and Treatment*, was to serve as a guideline for all practitioners who deal with low back pain, both at the primary level and at the specialist level.[1] An attempt was made to produce an algorithm that would guide the practitioner in a step-wise fashion to the diagnosis and treatment for individuals in this defined group. However, this monograph addressed acute low back problems only, as the panel did not wish to grapple with the complexity of chronic low back pain, wherein psychosocial factors, behavioral aberrations, and vocational issues assume an increasingly larger proportion of the problem that need to be resolved, specifically in the rehabilitation effort.

How much of a problem is low back pain? Most people report low back problems at some time in their lives, and it is estimated that four out of five individuals have major back pain during their lifetimes. National statistics indicate a general yearly prevalence in the U.S. population of 15–20% and, among working-aged people, 50% admit to back symptoms each year. In fact, back symptoms are the most common cause of disability for persons younger than age 45 years. At any given time, approximately 1% of the U.S. population is chronically disabled because of back problems and another 1% is temporarily disabled. Annually, approximately 175 million workdays are lost per year, with an additional $20 billion of lost productivity. Low back problems are expensive. The total cost to society is difficult to calculate, but it is estimated that annual societal costs of back pain in the United States range from $20 to $50 billion. This estimation does not include nonmonetary costs of low back problems, which can also be substantial. The inability to function normally at work and during other daily activities impacts patients and their families. This loss of productivity is not only potentially catastrophic to the individual, but it also clearly impacts the Gross Domestic Product.

CHRONIC PAIN ASSESSMENT

The observation by Mixter and Barr in 1934,[2] which proposed that the herniated disk would produce what we now call a *root syndrome*, was an attractive hypothesis. The validity of this observation appeared to be substantiated by surgical removal of the herniation with resultant resolution of the symptomatology. The question of whether a herniated disk does, in fact, produce pain was addressed by Rosomoff in a signal publication in 1985.[3] This paper was a reasoned set of observations combined with clinical and experimental evidence that supported the contention that herniated disks with nerve root compression do not always produce pain, and that alternative nonsurgical methods provide successful treatment, even for manifest disk herniations or lumbar stenosis.

Some descriptions of patient histories sound like the classic herniated disk, but that could just as easily be representative of lumbar myofascial pain syndromes, in which pain distribution is identical, and there is a paucity of neurologic change.[4] The soft tissue examination demonstrates outstandingly painful, tender, or trigger points in the muscular system with limited motion in the back, hips, and legs, mimicking the herniated disk syndrome.

It is the premise of this article that disordered soft tissue structures are responsible for initiating biochemical alterations associated with hyperalgesia and chronic pain. These structures are extraspinal in the surrounding paraspinal muscles, buttocks, hips, and legs. These peripheral sites and syndromes are treatable by alternative medical approaches, and treatment restores function and alleviates pain without the need for correcting the intraspinal pathologic entities that have been traditionally designated as the cause of pain and neurologic deficit.

In 1970, Rosomoff[5] proposed and carried out an operation called *Dorsal Arch Resection*, which was based on the theory that bony or soft tissue intrusion into the spinal canal acts like the arm of a pincer to compress the nerve. This condition can be corrected by total removal of the posterior half of the spinal canal, leaving the nerve roots and dural sac without any chance of compression from the remaining structures. This approach was applied to failed back syndrome patients who met all of the requirements for surgical intervention of that era, such as intractable pain, neurologic deficit, and impaired function. The operation appeared to be successful, until the following scenario unfolded. Rosomoff placed his postoperative patients in an intense and vigorous rehabilitation program. This program was designed to identify and treat the previously mentioned myofascial syndromes as the follow-up treatment to surgical removal. His therapists found that the patients had great difficulty in carrying out an intense rehabilitation program immediately postoperatively because rehabilitation requires learned physical and mental behavior, which are difficult to acquire in the early, painful postoperative state. The therapists suggested that the patients be put into a rehabilitation program to learn its elements for 2 weeks preoperatively until the program is then interrupted for surgery and carried out to conclusion. This procedure seemed eminently wise and feasible. As such, all patients who were referred for surgery were told that they should enter a 2-week rehabilitation program preoperatively and then surgery would be carried out. This plan was initiated, and the surgical and rehabilitation outcome was rewarding. As time went on, and, particularly, as the patients were examined for a baseline the night before surgery, it became apparent that the indications for surgical intervention were disappearing, simply as a result of the rehabilitation program, and that surgery was no longer indicated. When this observation became clear, a moratorium on surgery was called and all patients were told that they should undergo the rehabilitation program as they did previously, for 2 weeks, and if they did not improve, they would undergo surgery. During the 6-month moratorium, no patient needed to undergo surgery because they all improved significantly. This finding brought the whole concept on which surgical intervention had been based into question.

Biochemically, cell membranes of the injured soft tissues break down to arachidonic acid, which is then biosynthesized into prostaglandins, thromboxane, monohydroxy fatty acids, and leukotrienes.[6-8] These individually and collectively are involved in the reactions to injury, producing hyperalgesia, vascular instability, and an inflammatory reaction, with loss of function.[9] The symptoms produced depend on the relative proportions of these substances at the site of injury. For example, prostaglandins produce vasodilatation, and the area feels warm. Thromboxane produces vasoconstriction, and the part feels cold. The leukotrienes produce inflammation leading to the development of focal tender or trigger points. These substances, when interacted with polypeptides, such as bradykinin and histamine, or in the presence of excessive mechanical stimulation, create a nociceptive impulse transmitted to the central nervous system.[10] These chemical reactions are inhibited by steroids, aspirin, and related products, effects that then provide a rationale for pharmacologic treatment.[11] Even more interesting, however, is the reversal of these same phenomena by focal physical forms of therapy, such as application of ice, which, parenthetically, has been well established as a method for limiting or averting tissue reaction to injury.[12] Vigorous activation of the musculoskeletal system also limits the reaction to injury because enkephalins are released at two to three times the baseline levels. This response serves as an endogenous pain control system.[13] It follows, then, that therapeutic application of these basic principles should lead the physician to prescribe the use of ice and vigorous exercise as alternatives to the traditional trials of bed rest, analgesics, and muscle relaxants.

There further ensues a number of secondary effects, such as sustained muscle contraction, referred pain, and autonomic reflex change. These phenomena, in fact, are major components of the chronic state. The muscle contraction is not reflex, as was once thought. It is, in fact, a chemical phenomenon, wherein the traumatized muscle releases calcium ions, which combine with adenosinetriphosphatase to create an uncontrolled contraction, leading to pain, tenderness, vasoconstriction, and decreased blood supply, resulting in an energy-deficit contracture. It is this inflammatory reaction and accompanying decreased muscle length that produce the restricted range of joint movement and tendon and fascial shortening. The result is functional disability and chronicity. Of further clinical interest is that immobilization, a traditional mode of treatment, and emotional tension are prime contributors to the production of disability, hence the conclusion that acute treatment programs should avoid immobilization and chronicity may be prevented by incorporating alternative relaxation and behavioral modification techniques to eliminate tension and stress when these elements are recognized.

Physicians frequently do not seek or do not report in detail abnormal movements of the back; soft tissue abnormalities; restricted ranges of motion in the back, hips, or legs; or the presence of muscle tenderness and/or trigger points as might be seen with myofascial syndromes. To this end, it is mandatory that a soft tissue examination be done and all musculoskeletal and myofascial abnormalities be identified. This is particularly important because myofascial syndromes may masquerade as lumbar disk syndromes. When done thoroughly, a comprehensive physical examination can reveal multiple areas of tenderness, trigger points, and restricted ranges of motion in the back, hips, and legs. These can perpetuate mechanical dysfunction, continued strain, muscle fatigue, and pain. The difference, with respect to restricted ranges of motion and muscle tightness in the chronic state, is the ease of reversibility during the acute phase and the extreme difficulty of stretching contracted painful muscles in the chronic state. Even when this is recognized, many physical medicine facilities instruct their therapists to stop when stretching reaches the point of discomfort; when, in fact, stretching is only productive when the well-trained therapist pushes beyond the pain to achieve gradual and progressive release and lengthening of the pathologic structures.

A common syndrome is the quadratus lumborum. The pain usually begins with a quick, stooping movement when the torso is twisted, as in gardening and scrubbing. Pain is perceived at the iliac crest or greater trochanteric area, sometimes in the lower abdomen and groin. There also may be pain over the sacroiliac joint area and deep in the midbuttock. Symptoms are manifest with walking, twisting, stooping, turning in bed, and rising from a chair. Coughing or sneezing aggravates the pain, so that this phenomenon is not a necessary sign of free fragment disk herniation. Pain is felt in climbing steps, and there may be severe pain at night which awakens the patient. The examination finds guarded movements when walking, lying, or rising. There is a pelvic tilt when standing. There is limited flexion and extension in the spine with paraspinal tenderness. There sometimes is a leg-length discrepancy, and the radiologic studies may show a small hemipelvis.

Associated with the quadratus lumborum syndrome is the iliopsoas syndrome, which also may produce ipsilateral paraspinal pain or anterior thigh pain, or both. Gait is carried out with external rotation and flexion at the hip. Posture is stooped, with a flattened lordotic curve, and extension is limited due to contracture of the iliopsoas muscle. There may be tenderness deep in the femoral triangle, as well as deep in the pelvis.

Perhaps the most confounding syndromes are those of the gluteal muscles, which produce leg extension pain in the sciatic distribution. The gluteus maximus produces pain in the buttock, coccyx, medial sacrum, and lateral iliac crest; the gluteus medius produces pain more deeply in the midbuttock and posterior thigh area; and the gluteus minimus produces pain in the lower buttock, posterior thigh, and calf or lateral thigh and leg radiating towards the ankle. It is easy to see how these syndromes can be confused with so-called classic descriptions of radiculopathy.

Another heralded syndrome is that of the piriformis, which produces low back and sacroiliac-type pain with discomfort deep in the buttock, hip, posterior thigh, and, again, sciatica. There is tenderness over the sciatic notch and weak abduction and external rotation at the hip. The diagnosis is best made by feeling the tight piriformis muscle by way of a rectal examination, but this diagnosis can be often inferred from the clinical history, and treatment is similar to that of the gluteal syndromes. It is the gluteal and piriformis syndromes that produce restrictive ranges of motion about the hips, which contribute to weightbearing pain. It is a common experience to find that this abnormality, which is seen in nearly all of the chronic low back disorders, is uncommonly sought and uncommonly diagnosed. Many years of reviewing recorded examinations for low back disorders attests to this observation, which emphasizes the need for understanding this mechanism for low back pain and, beyond that, its treatment. Unless these mechanical impairments of posture, gait, movement, and weight displacement are addressed therapeutically, the patient will remain in pain. Moreover, this treatment should be combined with a functionally restorative program to prevent recurrent pain and disability.

Reduced physical functional capacities and performance may lead an individual to become depressed and anxious, particularly when he or she has a nonadaptive personality style. Fear may become a formidable barrier if the perception is that a permanent injury has occurred that, by activation, may produce further loss of function. To this can be added the problems of dependencies, such as narcotics, barbiturates, and muscle relaxants, supplemented by alcohol. Patients also become dependent on back braces, stimulators, and other such equipment, further reinforcing their perception that they are seriously disabled. Marital problems, role reversal, and disruption of the family unit may also occur. Low self-esteem, guilt, loss of motivation, and, often, suicidal ideation are seen in these patients. Loss of identification is not limited to the shift in the patient's position in the family circle; it is compounded by a loss of vocational identification for those previously employed. Patients become more focused on their pain; they think they are helpless, hopeless, and disability oriented. Social withdrawal takes place, involving isolation, with accompanying dependence on television for stimulation and distraction. Prolonged immobilization compounds the pain-depression cycle. Physical, behavioral, and socioeconomic factors compound one another, and the family circle commonly reinforces the ensuing disability by subjugating their own needs while assuming the patient's responsibilities. They, too, become frightened, angry, and protective. The progression of events has now evolved into major behavioral reactions. Repeated unsuccessful attempts to relieve the patient of his or her pain and mental burdens through a series of unrewarding treatments, including bed rest, traction, ineffective physical therapy, drugs, x-rays, myelograms, and unsuccessful surgery, result in a fearful, untrusting, uncooperative patient. This iatrogenic failure frustrates the physician, who then advises the patient to seek psychiatric help because he or she has not responded to prolonged medical or surgical treatment, further implying that it's all in the patient's head. If the patient is receiving workers' compensation, an employer may be compounding the issue by an uncaring attitude, unsympathetic pose, or threat to fire the worker and/or refusal to modify the job to accommodate the injury. Moreover, a well-intentioned lawyer may discourage the patient concerning rehabilitation efforts and a weary insurance adjuster, who has authorized many forms of treatment approaches in hopes of bringing the claim to closure, also begins to blame the patient for the unsuccessful treatment. The overall result is a patient who now has chronic pain and is impaired physically; is weak and inactive; is drug- and alcohol-dependent, hostile, untrusting, and frightened; believes he or she is helpless and hopeless; is unable to live independently; has marital and sexual problems; is anxious, depressed, and angry; has no job and no motivation; and is disabled and disability oriented. Where does one start to treat such a person, this "low back loser?"

TREATMENT OVERVIEW

The management of the back-injured individual is far from simple. An early referral to an experienced medical provider may prevent the simple lumbar sprain from becoming a catastrophe. Moreover, this early referral may avoid the behavioral consequences that are prone to develop if chronicity becomes established.

The low back loser is a victim of the system, and the cost for early multidisciplinary treatment is less than the cost that the victim exacts if the loser profile develops. The treatment system, therefore, should be capable of identifying these problems early, and then deal with them in a comprehensive way. These problems can be categorized as sensory, perceptual, psychologic, psychosocial, and environmental.

The immediate natural reaction of humans to injury and pain is rest or immobilization. Persistent immobility increases pain; causes disuse, atrophy, and weakness; slows healing; and demineralizes bone, resulting in functional disabililty.[14] Conversely, activity increases endorphin levels, which becomes an endogenous source of pain control, decreasing pain and facilitating healing.[13] Furthermore, working through pain produces the phenomenon of stress-induced analgesia.[15]

Stress-induced analgesia is a keystone to successful treatment. If stress (i.e., pain) is applied continuously without interruption, pain transmission will cease. In simplistic terms, it is like an overload to an electrical system, which blows the fuse or circuit breaker. The patient is pain-free for a period, which is a golden opportunity to apply usually pain-provoking therapy, like muscle stretching, before the circuit resets. Coupled with exercise-induced endorphin release, treatment can be advanced, but the patient and the treating professional should overcome the natural fear of pain, which is frequently equated with injury.

Most therapists are taught to limit or halt treatment when the patient complains of pain, which, by this concept, is when treatment should begin. To functionally progress, it is necessary to activate muscles intensively 8–10 hours per day. Not only is there a decrease in pain, but there is also an effect on depression. A sense of well-being is induced, mobility is increased, and analgesic intake is decreased. Importantly, drug withdrawal is eased, and detoxification can be achieved quickly with a minimum of side effects. With this conceptual background, let us discuss the role of the pain specialist and pain center.

The data of the usual clinical course show that 74% of the initial group of patients with nonspecific pain have good pain control and can return to their previous productive lives (Figure 14.1). Twenty-five percent, however, experience persistent symptoms beyond the first 4 weeks. These individuals should be re-evaluated referable to history and physical findings. Plain x-rays may now be indicated to be certain that an occult lesion has not been overlooked and a sedimentation rate is appropriate to rule out inflammation or infection. Conservative measures, particularly involving physical therapy, should be pursued in a more intense fashion. Occupational therapy may be added to review those occupational factors that may be influencing the outcome. Particularly, this refers to proper body mechanics and work-site factors that come under the aegis of ergonomics.

During the next 3 weeks, 9% of patients spontaneously recover, leaving 16% with chronic pain and disability. If this process does not resolve within the next 3 weeks, then consultation with a specialist is indicated. This should be with a musculoskeletal expert or pain medicine specialist to identify specifically myofascial syndromes that may have been overlooked or never treated, or other psychosocial barriers to recovery. It is important that the pain medicine consultant understand the rehabilitation model because the invasive techniques that commonly are applied by some members of this group are usually not indicated.

In the period from 7 weeks to 3 months, another 4% of patients return to work, leaving 12% who remain symptomatic. Although originally proposed that a multidisciplinary team re-evaluate the patient at 3 months to include the psychosocial

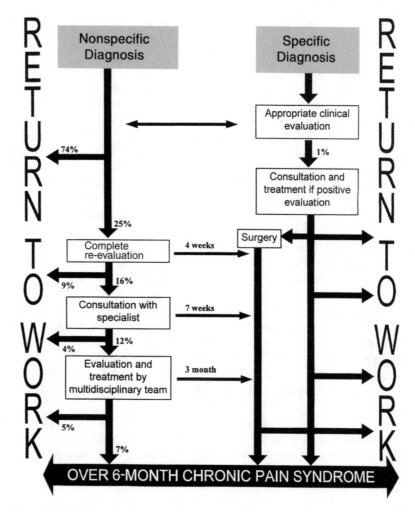

Figure 14.1 Critical path for the management of low back pain.

aspects of pain and ergonomic assessment, it is clear now that the 7-week mark is probably the better time to start this process because it becomes more cost effective if done earlier. The process at 3 months results in another 5% of patients who return to work, leaving 7% of the original population with chronic pain syndromes. It should be pointed out that none of the task forces that has studied this problem have been willing to deal with the chronic pain patient, but this is a most costly group of patients who cannot be ignored. They should be evaluated by a multidisciplinary pain center that is comprehensive in its approach.

PAIN TREATMENT FACILITIES: SELECTION CRITERIA

Patients with chronic pain present a clinical challenge because of the vast amount of time and the diagnostic and therapeutic resources they consume. The impact of even one such patient in a typical family practice can be substantial. Despite high costs, multidisciplinary pain clinics and centers can be cost-effective by reducing long-term use of medical services and returning patients early to employment or previous lifestyle. Physicians should consider referral when serious reduction of functional status is due to chronic pain, or when pain is becoming a major focus for the patient and family. The problem of chronic pain is a powerful practical example of the importance of an illness or injury compounded by the complexity of the patient's beliefs, experience, family, workplace, community, and health care system. Seen from this perspective, it is predictable that these multifaceted problems are more amenable to a multidisciplinary treatment approach than to a series of single therapeutic interventions. Furthermore, primary care physicians are often in a position to treat conditions like lower back pain before they become chronic. Thus, they may be in a uniquely powerful position to prevent the development of the chronic state by aggressively promoting early diagnosis, treatment activity, and return to work, while addressing any impediments to recovery, such as patient misperceptions about the nature of the condition, an overprotective family, or problems in the workplace. Pain treatment facilities were developed specifically to treat pain that is intractable and chronic.

There are between 1,500 and 2,000 pain treatment facilities in the United States.[16] These facilities generally differ in their staff makeup, size, philosophy, and treatment approach to the chronic pain patient. Usually, the philosophy and treatment approach are dependent on the training or specialty, or both, of the medical or program director. This variability in approach has blurred the distinction between the different types of pain treatment facilities in the minds of physicians and the public.[17]

Treatment goals of multidisciplinary pain facilities have been stated as follows: reduction or elimination of pain; reduction or elimination of medication intake; correction of physical abnormalities, like posture, gait, and range of motion; reduction of psychiatric or psychological impairment, or both; education of chronic pain patients in the roles that emotions, behavior, and attitudes play; improvement of activities of daily living; improvement of level of function in social, familial, and household roles; improvement or restoration, or both, of strength and functional status; restoration of vocational and avocational role functions; and education on the ways of maintaining rehabilitation gains and avoidance of reinjury. Initially, the efficacy of multidisciplinary pain facilities in treating chronic pain was questioned. Evidence from well-designed outcome studies, however, indicates that multidisciplinary pain facilities do return chronic pain patients to work. The increased rates of return to work are due to treatment, and the benefits of treatment are not temporary. Criteria for referral to a pain treatment facility are outlined in Table 14.1.[18,19]

Physicians should differentiate clearly between acute pain and chronic pain.[20] Chronic pain is a continuous noxious input, like that of acute pain, but modulated and compounded by the prolonged or recurrent nature of the chronic state and complicated by a multitude of economic and psychosocial factors. Pain behavior has been defined as any and all outputs of the patient that a reasonable observer would characterize as suggesting pain, including, but not limited to, posture, facial expressions, verbalizing, lying down, taking medications, seeking medical assistance, and receiving compensation.[21] A list of identified pain behaviors is presented in the following tabulation:

Table 14.1 Indications for Multidisciplinary or Other Pain Center Referrals

Major inclusion criterion
   Chronic pain or chronic benign pain lasting longer than 3–6 months in duration
Minor inclusion criteria
   Severe pain behavior
   Presence of nonorganic physical findings
   Impaired functional status or perceived functional impairment, or both
   Disability perception
   Discrepancy in perceptions between physician and patient on ability to function
   Drug abuse, dependence, or addiction
   Significant psychopathology associated with chronic pain
   Failed back surgery syndrome
   Patient refused or denied surgery
   Myofascial pain syndrome and fibromyalgia
         Diagnosis of somatoform pain disorder (psychogenic pain)
         Unsuccessful conservative management
         No response to one isolated mode of treatment (e.g., physical therapy alone)
Exclusion criteria
   Inability to understand and carry out instructions
   Aggressive or violent behavior, or both
   Imminently suicidal
   Unwillingness to participate in a pain center program, as this can lead to noncompliance,
      uncooperativeness, and unsuccessful behavior modification process
   Unrealistic expectations of what can be accomplished (seeking an immediate cure)
   Unstable medical conditions (e.g., uncontrollable high blood pressure or congestive heart
      failure)

Sits stiffly	Moves slowly
Limps	Walks bent forward
Stands bent forward	Shifts frequently in position
Has distorted gait	Grimaces
Holds painful part	Rubs painful part
Moans	Groans
Writhes	Uses cane
Takes medication for pain	Moves in guarded fashion
Rests frequently	Uses prosthetic devices
Uses heat or ice	Avoids physical activity

The presence of significant pain behavior should be a reason for pain treatment facility referral.

A high percentage of chronic pain patients display decreased functional status or impairment, or both. When the functional impairment is perceived to be a severe problem, the patients may believe that they cannot live normal lives ever, or as long as they have pain. Their level of functioning is inversely proportional to their perceived pain. Severely decreased functional status is an indication for pain treatment facility referral.

Patients with chronic pain perceive their pain as a disability limiting their functional status.[22] The perception of pain as a disability is such a national problem that the Social Security Administration Commission on the Evaluation of Pain recommended the development of a listing of impairment due primarily to pain.[23] This last point demonstrates the importance of the concept of perceiving pain as a disability. Disability perception is another indication for pain treatment facility referral.

Drug abuse, dependence, and addiction are reported in the range of 3.2–18.9%.[24] Although these diagnoses are reported in a significant percentage of chronic pain patients, little evidence proves that addictive behaviors are common. At issue is whether patients with physician-perceived drug problems are best treated at pain treatment facilities or drug and alcohol treatment facilities. Detoxification in pain treatment facilities where simultaneous pain treatment is available appears to be the better route. Physicians' perception of drug problems, therefore, is an indication for pain treatment facility referral.

Patients with chronic pain being treated at pain centers have been reported to experience a wide range of psychiatric conditions. These include depression, drug dependence abuse and/or addiction, anxiety, irritability and/or anger, suicidal ideation, and memory and/or concentration problems. These data are supported by epidemiologic community studies, which indicate a strong relationship between chronic pain and depression.

The issue of depression is important, not only as a potential target symptom for treatment, but also because it is possible that coping strategies may differ in depressed chronic pain patients. Patients with chronic pain may over-rely on passive avoidance coping activities in response to life's stresses, including pain. These coping activities may be a function of depressed mood.[25] It is likely that faulty coping activities are best addressed in a pain center setting, where patients can be taught to improve their coping abilities. Therefore, severe depression is an indication for pain treatment facility referral, but a facility with on-site psychiatric treatment should be chosen.

Failed back syndrome has been described as *persistent or recurrent back pain, sciatica,* or *other impairments that exist after back surgery or noninterventional treatment.*[26] Failed back syndrome can occur in as many as 40% of postoperative patients, and this syndrome represents the reason for a large number of pain center admissions. It is also claimed that these patients are characterized by drug misuse, reactive psychiatric problems, and unappreciated psychiatric and psychosocial problems that existed before surgery. Reoperations on this group of patients usually meet with limited success. The second operation may be only successful for 40–50% of patients, whereas the third and fourth operations are successful for 20–30%, and 10–20% of patients, respectively.

It has been demonstrated that some of these patients have disturbed back or hip muscles and loss of muscular support. These abnormalities may lead to increased biomechanical strain that results in disability. Improvement with pain facility treatment for patients who have had a number of surgical procedures can be as successful as for patients without surgeries.[27] Patients with one or more unsuccessful neck or back surgeries are candidates for pain treatment facility referral, especially if behavior abnormalities or drug problems, or both, are present.

Some patients who are thought to have surgically remediable conditions sometimes refuse or are denied surgery for medical reasons. These patients can be placed into a physically supervised exercise and conditioning program. At 1-year follow-up, 84% of all such patients are improved.[28] Thus, a patient who refuses surgery or is a candidate for surgery but has risky concomitant medical problems should be considered for possible pain facility referral. It should also be noted that myofascial pain syndromes can be associated with acute radiculopathy and can persist after successful surgery.[29]

Fibromyalgia is a nonarticular disease characterized by musculoskeletal aches and pains, tender points at specific sites, fatigue, morning stiffness, and sleep disturbance. Ninety percent of patients with fibromyalgia have low back pain, and 24% of these patients are disabled because of their pain. In addition, many patients with fibromyalgia display psychological problems that could be related to the consequence of their disease process. The presence of low back pain or cervical pain, disability, and psychological problems also makes these patients candidates for pain treatment facility referral.

Somatoform pain disorder (conversion) has the essential feature of a preoccupation with pain in the absence of adequate physical findings to account for the pain or its intensity. The preoccupation with pain then serves as the major criterion. Patients with chronic pain and this diagnosis should be considered for pain treatment facility referral, especially if other forms of chronic pain treatments have been unsuccessful.

A particular body of literature alleges that many patients experiencing chronic low back pain cannot be assigned a diagnosis conforming to a specifically defined disease. The lack of objective physical findings in such patients has led to the designation of chronic intractable benign pain.[30] This type of pain is thought to be a central phenomenon, which is made worse by sensory input. Poor adaptation makes pain the focus of the patient's life. Patients so classified are often evaluated for behavioral abnormalities and often become candidates for the diagnosis of psychogenic pain. Presumably, no physical findings indicative of an organic dysfunctional or pathologic process are present. Such a presumption is not supported by facts.

In a study that addressed this issue, 90 patients with back pain were isolated from a group of 283 mixed chronic pain patients who conformed to the diagnosis of chronic intractable benign pain.[31] None had neurologic deficit; all radiologic studies were unremarkable. Almost all (97.6%) had tender or trigger points and multiple other non-neurologic abnormalities. Seven categories of abnormalities were identified: tender or trigger points, decreased range of motion, nondermatomal sensory abnormalities, contracted muscles, abnormal gait, miscellaneous physical signs, and decreased range of motion at the hips. Patients had an average of three of the seven categoric findings, led by myofascial syndromes and other soft-tissue changes. Almost one-half (45.6%) had nondermatomal sensory changes; this condition is physiologic dysfunction, not malingering or hysteria.[32]

The investigators made the following conclusions:

1. Chronic intractable benign pain patients without objective findings can be shown regularly to have musculoskeletal disorders.
2. Myofascial syndromes are the source of nociception in these patients.
3. Criteria for the specific diagnosis of myofascial pain syndrome are demonstrable in 97.6% of the patients.
4. Multiple physical findings (average = 3.1) are usual.
5. The demonstration of such physical findings invalidates the chronic intractable benign pain concept.

[PLINARY TEAM

of Miami Comprehensive Pain and Rehabilitation Center has more than 80 full-time personnel in six divisions: (1) neurologic surgery serving primarily as consultants; (2) physical medicine and rehabilitation directing the application of all physical medicine modalities and treatments; (3) nurses trained in rehabilitation and behavior modification who monitor patient progress and serve as case managers; (4) a behavioral division, which has psychiatrists and psychologists who are assigned as counselors to each patient and who administer biofeedback, behavioral modification, or other applicable techniques; (5) vocational rehabilitation specialists who evaluate and direct job placement; and (6) an ergonomic division that simulates the job and adapts the patient or work site, or both, while computing daily achievement goals.

To enter the system, the patient should undergo evaluation over a 3-day period. A problem-solving group attempts to identify the medical, behavioral, vocational, financial, social, and other significant problems of the patient. The approach is comprehensive and holistic and patient selection criteria are broad. The patient should have the ability to understand and carry out instructions, should be compliant and cooperative, and should not have aggressive or disruptive behavior. Patients with schizophrenia, manic-depression, or other major psychiatric disorders are not precluded as long as these conditions are well controlled. Lastly, the patient, the family, and significant others, such as the lawyer, the employer, and the insurer, should be accepting of the program. Workers' compensation, liability cases, multiple surgeries, long histories of invalidism, or drug abuse are not exclusionary conditions.

The average program lasts 4 weeks on an inpatient or outpatient basis, or a combination thereof. Inpatient status is preferred for difficult, complicated cases, but it is not always possible, as dictated by reimbursement status. It should be understood clearly that, in a tertiary referral center, few "simple," early primary care–type patients are seen. We receive the most complex, "court of last resort," salvage cases.

Physical Medicine and Rehabilitation

Physical medicine has the goal of restoring body function to normal, or its closest equivalent. Because myofascial contracture is a common denominator in the low back disorders that we see, the first phase of management is muscle stretching and restoration of full range of motion in the joints of the hips, back, and lower extremities. This therapy includes gait retraining, because of acquired maladaptive patterns; postural adjustment; proper use of effective modalities; elimination of adjunct equipment, when possible; strength and endurance conditioning, with instruction of body mechanics; prevention of reinjury; vocational or avocational requirements; sexual counseling; and, lastly, a home maintenance program.

Modalities, when evaluated as unimodal therapy, may not show clear-cut evidence of effectiveness.[33] They appear to be useful, however, in combination, which makes statistical evaluation more difficult. Nonetheless, scientific rationale exists for some. Ice application with lowering of temperature is known to decrease nerve conduction to the point of anesthesia, and the inflammatory reaction is contained with a reduction of chronic changes.[34,35] To be effective, the body part should be packed in ice for periods in excess of 30 minutes. Heat seems to soften muscle preparatory to stretching. An adjunct vapo-coolant helps to block the stretch reflex and makes lengthening easier.

Traction is useful for certain specific indications. Conceptually, we apply traction to stretch muscle groups, not to distract the spine or to release nerve entrapment. We do not believe that distraction can be effected with the weights that we use, and the principle of entrapment is not tenable. Therefore, traditional pelvic or leg traction is not used. Gravity traction is applied for iliopsoas contractures in the patient with a spinal flexion deformity or inability to extend the back, or both.

Autotraction is an important technique that allows three-dimensional placement of the spine by rotating, flexing, or extending the unit as the patient imposes his or her own body force by pushing and pulling.[36] The self-applied force of autotraction does not exceed that which could be potentially injurious, but it releases tight paraspinal muscles. Autotraction does not decompress the nerve root, as was the concept of its originators.[37,38]

Trigger point desensitization is indicated. Liberal use of ice is the preferred method of treatment, but like the other modalities (i.e., ultrasound, electrical stimulation, and neuroprobe) it is only an adjunct to stretching. Heat and massage also are used, but, again, as adjunct treatment to enhance muscle lengthening and supple movement.

Transcutaneous electrical neural stimulation (TENS) is used infrequently and only with patients who are TENS responders and who can be assisted with a difficult detoxification for which the TENS gives short-term relief as the drugs are withdrawn. TENS is not given to the patient beyond this period; it has no role in long-term therapy. Conceptually, it is to be emphasized that we are aiming for resolution of the painful disorder by physical restitution, not by an attempt at distraction or at coping by learning to live with pain.

Passive, then active ranging of motion is essential, especially around the hips and, in particular, the hip rotators. Hamstring lengthening is another mandate, because hamstring tightness affects back movement. Full ranges of back motion are the ultimate goal, so flexion and extension exercises are instituted without prejudice for the proponents of either type. Both flexion and extension exercises are necessary.

A full compendium of exercises is employed, as described in any standard physical therapy textbook, to establish full ranges of motion throughout the lower body with supple muscles and fluid movement. As this is being achieved, muscle strengthening and cardiovascular conditioning are added to the regimen with monitoring of those patients who have associated medical problems.

Dance therapy is an interesting adjunct because patients with pain often perform to music when, seemingly, they cannot move their bodies on command. When a specific muscle group is weak, functional electrical neuromuscular stimulation and muscle re-education are implemented.[39] This technique can produce rapid and dramatic increases in muscle recruitment patterns and muscle strength, and foot drop braces can be discarded.

Occupational and recreational therapy concentrates on body mechanics. Sitting, standing, walking, lifting, and driving tolerances are established and brought to normal levels of function. Pacing of activity is taught. Assistive equipment is used infrequently and only on specific indication. Energy-saving techniques are taught. Posture and gait are corrected because most patients are found to have poor posture and maladaptive gaits.

Activities of daily living are reviewed for home and work, looking for the proper use of body mechanics, with correction as needed. Driving evaluation is conducted and proper transfers are taught. Diversionary activities are reviewed and eye, hand, and leg coordination and tolerances are established. Education and vocational goals are set and job simulation is begun.

Job simulation and work conditioning are other concepts that we introduced to pain center management in the early 1990s. This is the ultimate goal of achievement for the working-aged group, but it does not exclude students or the elderly, who receive instruction for their needs. With respect to these problems, the occupational and physical therapists team with vocational counselors and ergonomists to develop the treatment plan.

Vocational Rehabilitation

Vocational rehabilitation counselors analyze factors of employment, such as age, education level, work history, supervisory and peer relationships, job requirements, job skills, transferable skills, date and circumstances of injury, return to work since injury, and, most importantly, motivation and compliance. This type of program cannot be successful without the patient's full attention or effort. If the patient does not give both, he or she is not accepted. The vocational goal is full functional activity and return to previous employment. Retraining is recommended rarely. Even the heaviest physical activity capacities have been achievable in most patients.

Behavioral Management

Behavioral management is a key issue. Nearly 20% of Americans experience one or more emotional disorders, so the low back injury patient may be harboring such a problem. Our study of pain population patients found 62.5% to have anxiety disorders and 56.2% to have current depression.[40] These conditions were commingled with other less prevalent disorders. Only 5.3% of 283 patients were found to have no psychiatric diagnosis.

This study questions the criteria for the diagnosis of psychogenic pain. Pure psychogenic pain is probably rare when defined as a psychological factor directly leading to pain. However, all pain, as perceived by the patient, is real, regardless of cause. Most bodily pain is a combination of factors (e.g., physical stimuli and mental events). Mental and emotional states may be from a situation arising out of circumstances of the moment, from a background of past personal experiences with pain, or from personality characteristics.

Behavioral analysis considers compliance, achievement level before injury, activity level after injury, functional capacities, anxiety, depression, personality disorders, marital status, role reversal, and family history. Psychological services offer biofeedback and relaxation training. Group and family therapy deal with social interactions, return to environment, employment, and disability versus wellness, with an emphasis on function, not pain.

Individual counseling is given when needed, including sexual counseling. Every patient has an assigned counselor who monitors daily progress and reinforces the goal of physical restoration. Relaxation training includes coping approaches, muscle re-education, meditation and distraction, guided imagery, autosuggestion (especially to be used with physical activity), and tape supplements, which enhance live therapy. Stress management is incorporated into the behavioral sessions.

Weekly family groups explore the goals of the patient with the spouse or other family members. How to respond to pain without fear is discussed. Communication is an important subject. The roles of the various family members are defined, including distribution and responsibility. Experiences and frustrations are shared. These sessions facilitate the return to home, hopefully to an environment that now fosters wellness, not disability.

Biofeedback may be a pain control method, but we use it as a muscle tension and relaxation technique. Surface electromyographic biofeedback is used to regulate muscle tension, especially when an activity may, by past experience, have been pain provoking. Reduction of muscle tension correlates well with reduction of pain.[41]

Our psychological assessment instrument is the Millon Behavioral Health Inventory Assessment. This instrument tests psychogenic attitudes, such as chronic tension, recent stress, premorbid pessimism, future despair, social alienation, and somatic anxiety. This instrument is not a predictor of outcome, nor should it, or any other instrument, such as the Minnesota Multiphasic Personality Inventory, be used for that purpose. We are trying to find out what the patient is like so that the treating staff can interact with the individual in a manner that he or she is willing to accept. The patient has to be the partner in a rehabilitative process; otherwise, the effort will not succeed.

The behavioral staff regulates detoxification from drugs. As stated earlier, this process is carried out rapidly while pursuing intense activation. Endorphin release helps ameliorate withdrawal, and symptoms are generally minimal.

Ergonomics

In the early 1990s, industrial engineering and ergonomics were introduced into the Pain Center.[42] Ergonomics studies the worker in his or her environment, trying to match the physical capabilities to the industrial task. This process may require designing and redesigning of the workplace and the tools that are used. The goal is to condition the worker with regard to strength, posture, and flexibility, while eliminating fatigability.

The engineers see the human body as a machine, working with levers and acting as a mechanical crane. Proper lifting dictates carrying the weight close to the body; the more bulky the weight, the more difficult it is to carry, and the less efficient the handling of manual materials. The objectives are human comfort, optimum efficiency of the man-machine system, safety and prevention, health, and work satisfaction. Work satisfaction is an important issue.

Measuring outcome is a big problem. To account for psychophysical variants, a measure of back strength in back pain patients was developed, called *Acceptable Maximum Effort*.[43] This method is highly reliable and useful in determining treatment outcome. Reliability coefficients for all strength measurements are greater than 0.90.

The level of voluntary muscular effort beyond which the patient's level of pain becomes unacceptable is the principle. Patients are tested before, during, and after treatment. Back and leg strength may more than double in a 4-week treatment period, which is also true for composite strength. Human performance evaluations track overall strength, pace, reactions, hand steadiness, flexibility, level of cooperation, level of effort, ranges of motion, gait, posture, and pain level. The bottom line is to make the achievement level match or exceed the task demand.

The ergonomists also analyze the patient's anthropometric measurements, from which ideal layouts for chairs, desks, home furniture, work site equipment, and condition can be developed and printed out by computer. The pain program is a 6-day per week program for 4 weeks, with 8–10 hours of activity per day. Therapeutic time schedules allow the individual to have alternating, but consecutive, periods of major exertional and nonexertional activity.

By the time of discharge, patients may have achieved the best physical condition in their lifetimes. Usually, by 1 week, patients are ambulatory and independent in activities of daily living with decreasing levels of pain. They are approaching full ranges of motion with increasing strength in 2–3 weeks. Relief of pain is not the end point, but functional restoration is. At the end of 4 weeks, sometimes 6 weeks, the patients have achieved full functional levels of activity. If a neurologic deficit has been present, motor strength may recover in 2–3 weeks, sensation in 2–3 months, and reflexes in 3 months. Complete pain relief is attained in one-third of patients; in the remainder, the pain may dissipate over time or become controllable for functional comfort.

PAIN CENTER EFFECTIVENESS

Are multidisciplinary pain centers effective? The answer is yes, by virtue of pain reduction, elimination of opioid medication, increase in functional activity, return to work, decreased use of the health care system, closure of disability claims, and proved cost-effectiveness.[44]

Furthermore, only 21% of patients who were disabled or unemployed before back surgery returned to full-time employment postoperatively; 14 of 38 patients who were working before surgery retired prematurely (before age 60 years). Thus, the net gain in employment after surgery was approximately 7% (7 of 102 patients). Only 36% of industrially injured patients receiving surgery for back pain return to work after surgery and, at 5-year follow-up, only 25% of patients with spinal cord stimulator implants return to work.

By comparison, treatment at multidisciplinary pain clinics, based on a meta-analysis of 3,080 patients, found savings in medical expenditures equal to $9,548,000 and savings in indemnity expenditures equal to $175,225,000, with a total savings of $184,772,050.

In 1981, our center reported that 86% of all patients treated returned to full activity, with 70% fully employed and another 16% who were physically capable of full employment, but could not be placed at work because of prejudice against their medical history of low back disorder. Among the 86% who were fully active, there was no clear-cut difference between compensation and noncompensation class cases.[45] In a study conducted in 1994, the return rate to full function and work was again 86%, although the patients had some residual discomfort that eventually remitted or was controlled at a low level of intensity.[46] The 14% who did not return to full function were highly complex patients with major behavioral problems. Cassisi et al. conducted an independent study of injured workers referred to our pain center for treatment.[47] Follow-up was obtained in 61% or 143 patients. The sample was divided among five groups: participants in the University of Miami Comprehensive Pain and Rehabilitation Center program (n = 39), patients not approved by insurance (n = 30), patients who declined participation (n = 46), participants in other programs (n = 14), and dropouts (n = 14). Of the 39 patients who completed the Comprehensive Pain and Rehabilitation Center program, only 13% were working at the time of entry into the program, whereas 69% were working at a mean follow-up of 2 years. Not included in this analysis are the patients who were fit to return to work by their own self-report but could not find employment. If these patients were added to the number who returned to work, the total would have approximated 86%. In a separate group of 30 patients whose admission was denied by the third-party payor, the employment rate increased from 21% to only 41%. The Cassisi study is notable in that this represents an independent assessment by a disinterested third party not linked with our center.

Current data from the University of Miami Comprehensive Pain and Rehabilitation Center are displayed in Figure 14.2. A 92% improvement in functional status, a 66% reduction in pain, and a 62% return to employment or a work-ready state, together with a 93% patient satisfaction rate with treatment, are strong testimony to the effectiveness of multidisciplinary pain center treatment.

As favorable as these data are, questions still require resolution, and some patients have problems that cannot be eliminated with the available time limits. Room for improvement always exists. We submit, however, that the multidisciplinary, comprehensive approach to the management of low back disorders is the mode of management for these complex patients.

To summarize, we have emphasized prominence, underdiagnosis, and undertreatment of myofascial components of refractory low back pain syndromes; erroneous past tendency to focus on absent objective findings as support for psychogenic formulation; importance of comprehensive evaluation and treatment

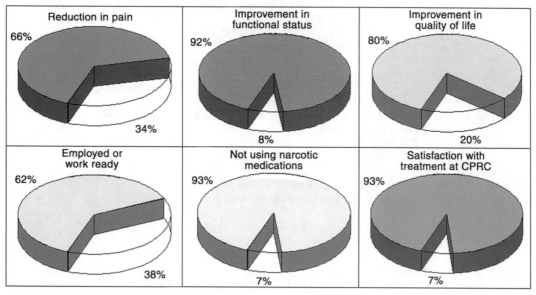

COMPREHENSIVE PAIN AND REHABILITATION CENTER
PROGRAM EVALUATION SYSTEM
November 1989 through June 1998
OUTCOME RESULTS AT DISCHARGE (N=1731)

Figure 14.2 Comprehensive pain and rehabilitation center (CPRC) program evaluation system.

defined as *including careful physical examination and treatment planning, as well as attending psychosocial vocational and ergonomic factors*; and data supporting substantial functional restoration and decreased future medical usage deriving from intensive, comprehensive, rehabilitation approaches, such as we have described.

REFERENCES

1. Bigos S, Bowyer O, Braen G, et al. Acute Low Back Problems in Adults: Clinical Practice Guideline No. 14. AHCPR Publication No. 95-0642. Rockville, Maryland: Agency for Health Care Policy and Research, Public Health Service, U.S. Department of Health and Human Services, December, 1994.
2. Mixter WJ, Barr JS. Rupture of the intervertebral disc with involvement of the spinal canal. N Engl J Med 1934;211:210–215.
3. Rosomoff HL. Do herniated disks produce pain? Clin J Pain 1985;1:91–93.
4. Travell JG, Simons DG. Myofascial Pain and Dysfunction: The Trigger Point Manual. Baltimore: Williams & Wilkins, 1983.
5. Rosomoff HL. Neural arch resection for lumbar spinal stenosis. Clin Orthop 1981;154:83–89.
6. Granstrom E. Biochemistry of the Prostaglandins, Thromboxanes, and Leukotrienes. In JJ Bonica, U Lindblom, A Iggo (eds), Advances in Pain Research and Therapy (Vol 5). New York: Raven Press, 1983;605–615.
7. Juan H. Prostaglandins as modulators of pain. Gen Pharmacol 1978;9:403–409.
8. Moncada S, Ferreira SH, Vane JR. Pain and Inflammatory Mediators. In JR Vane, SH Ferreira (eds), Inflammation Handbook of Experimental Pharmacology. Berlin: Springer, 1978;558–616.
9. Higgs GA, Moncada S. Interactions of Arachidonate Products with Other Pain Mediators. In JJ Bonica, U Lindblom, A Iggo (eds), Advances in Pain Research and Therapy. New York: Raven Press, 1983;617–626.
10. Ferreira SH. Prostaglandins: Peripheral and Central Analgesia. In JJ Bonica, U Lindblom, A Iggo (eds), Advances in Pain Research and Therapy. New York: Raven Press, 1983;597–603.
11. Higgs GA, Flower RJ, Vane JR. A new approach to anti-inflammatory drugs. Biochem Pharmacol 1977;28:1959–1961.
12. Rosomoff HL, Clasen RA, Harstock R, et al. Brain reaction to experimental injury after hypothermia. Arch Neurol 1965;13:337–345.
13. Carr DB, Bullen BA, Skrinar GS, et al. Physical conditioning facilities the exercise-induced secretion of beta-endorphin and beta-hypoprotein in women. N Engl J Med 1981;305:560–563.
14. Cailliet R. Soft Tissue Pain and Disability. Philadelphia: FA Davis, 1980;1–313.
15. Lewis JW, Cannon JT, Liebeskind J. Opioid and non-opioid mechanisms of stress analgesia. Science 1980;208:623–625.
16. Steele-Rosomoff R. The pain patient. Spine 1991;5:417–427.
17. Fishbain DA, Rosomoff HL, Steele-Rosomoff R, Cutler BR. Types of pain treatment facilities and referral selection criteria. Arch Fam Med 1995;4:58–66.
18. Fishbain DA, Rosomoff HL, Goldberg M, et al. The prediction of return to work after pain center treatment: a review. Clin J Pain 1993;9:3–15.
19. Cutler BR, Fishbain DA, Rosomoff HL, et al. Does non-surgical pain center treatment of chronic pain return patients to work? A review and meta-analysis of the literature. Spine 1994;19:643–652.
20. Fishbain DA, Rosomoff HL. What is chronic pain? Clin J Pain 1990;6:164–166.
21. Turk DC, Matyas TA. Pain related behaviors: communication of pain. APS Journal 1992;1:109–111.
22. Riley JF, Adhera DIT, Follick MJ. Chronic low back pain and functional improvement: assessing beliefs about their relationship. Arch Phys Med Rehabil 1988;69:579–584.
23. Turk DC, Rudy TE, Stieg RL. The disability determination dilemma: towards a multi-axial solution. Pain 1988;34:217–229.
24. Fishbain DA, Steele-Rosomoff R, Rosomoff HL. Drug abuse, dependence, and addiction in chronic pain patients. Clin J Pain 1992;8:77–85.

25. Weickgerant AL, Slater MA, Patterson TL, et al. Coping activities in chronic low back pain: relationship with depression. Pain 1993;53:95–103.
26. Long DM, Filtzer DL, Bendebba M, et al. Clinical features of the failed back. J Neurosurg 1988;69:61–71.
27. Rosomoff HL. Non-Operative Treatment of the Failed Back Syndrome Presenting with Chronic Pain. In DM Long (ed), Current Therapy in Neurological Surgery. Toronto, Ontario: BC Decker, 1985;200–202.
28. McCoy CE, Selby D, Henderson R, et al. Patients avoiding surgery: pathology and one-year lift status follow-up. Spine 1991;[Suppl]:S198–S200.
29. Rosomoff HL, Fishbain DA, Goldberg M, et al. Are myofascial pain syndromes (MPS) physical findings associated with residual radiculopathy? Pain 1990;[Suppl 5]:S396.
30. Crue BL, Pinsky JJ. An approach to chronic pain of non-malignant origin. Postgrad Med J 1984;60:858–864.
31. Rosomoff HL, Fishbain D, Goldberg M, et al. Physical findings in patients with chronic intractable benign pain of the back and/or neck. Pain 1989;37:279–287.
32. Wall P. The Role of the Substantia Gelatinosa as a Gate Control. In JJ Bonica (ed), Pain. New York: Raven Press, 1980;205–231.
33. Deyo RA. Conservative therapy for low back pain: distinguishing useful from useless therapy. JAMA 1983;250:1057–1062.
34. Rosomoff HL. The effects of hypothermia on the physiology of the nervous system. Surgery 1956;40:328–336.
35. Rosomoff HL, Clasen RA, Hartstock R, et al. Brain reaction to experimental injury after hypothermia. Arch Neurol 1965;13:337–345.
36. Larsson U, Choler U, Lidstrom A, et al. Autotraction for treatment of lumbago-sciatica: a multicentre controlled investigation. Acta Orthop Scand 1980;51:791–798.
37. Lind GAM. Auto-Traction: Treatment of Low Back Pain and Sciatica. Sweden: Sturetryckeriet, Diss. Linköping University, Linköping, 1974.
38. Natchev E. A manual on autotraction treatment for low back pain. Folksam Scientific Council Publ, 1984;B:171.
39. Abdel-Moty E, Khalil TM, Rosomoff RS, et al. Computerized Electromyography in Quantifying the Effectiveness of Functional Electrical Neuromuscular Stimulation. In SS Asfour (ed), Ergonomics/Human Factors IV. New York: Elsevier, 1987;1057–1065.
40. Fishbain DA, Goldberg M, Meagher R, et al. Male and female chronic pain patients categorized by DSM-III psychiatric diagnostic criteria. Pain 1986;26:181–197.
41. Khalil T. Asfour SS, Waly SM, et al. Isometric Exercise and Biofeedback in Strength Training. In SS Asfour (ed), Trends in Ergonomics/Human Factors IV. New York: Elsevier, 1987;1095–1101.
42. Khalil TM, Asfour SS, Moty EA, et al. New Horizons for Ergonomics Research in Low Back Pain. In RE Eberts, CG Eberts (eds), Trends in Ergonomics/Human Factors II. New York: Elsevier, 1985;591–598.
43. Khalil TM, Goldberg ML, Asfour SS, et al. Acceptable maximum effort (AME): a psychosocial measure of strength in back pain patients. Spine 1987;12:372–376.
44. Turk DC. Efficacy of Multidisciplinary Pain Centers in the Treatment of Chronic Pain. In MJM Cohen, JN Campbell (eds), Pain Treatment Centers at a Crossroads: A Practical and Conceptual Reappraisal. Progress in Pain Research and Management (Vol 7). Seattle: IASP Press, 1996;257–273.
45. Rosomoff HL, Green CJ, Silbret M, et al. Pain and Low Back Rehabilitation Program at the University of Miami School of Medicine. In LKY Ng (ed), New Approaches to Treatment of Chronic Pain: A Review of Multidisciplinary Pain Clinics and Pain Centers. National Institute on Drug Abuse Research Monograph Series 36. Washington DC: U.S. Government Printing Office, 1981;92–111.
46. Cutler R, Fishbain D, Rosomoff HL, et al. Does nonsurgical pain center treatment of chronic pain return patients to work? A review and meta-analysis of the literature. Spine 1994;19: 643–652.
47. Cassisi JE, Sypert GW, Salamon A, et al. Independent evaluation of a multidisciplinary rehabilitation program for chronic low back pain. Neurosurgery 1989;25:877–883.

RECOMMENDED READINGS

Boden SD, Davis DO, Dina TS, et al. Abnormal magnetic-resonance scans of the lumbar spine in asymptomatic subjects. J Bone Joint Surg Am 1990;72:403–408.

Doita M, Kanatani T, Harada T, et al. Immunohistologic study of the ruptured intervertebral disc of the lumbar spine. Spine 1996;21:235–241.

Ehni G. Significance of the small lumbar canal: cauda equina compression syndromes due to spondylosis. J Neurosurg 1969;31:490–494.

Elsberg CA. Experiences in spinal surgery: observations upon 60 laminectomies for spinal disease. Surg Gynecol Obstet 1913;16:117.

Epstein JA, Epstein BS, Lavine L. Nerve root compression associated with narrowing of the lumbar spinal canal. J Neurol Neurosurg Psychiatry 1962;25:165.

Gargano FP, Jacobson RE, Rosomoff HL. Transverse axial tomography of the spine. Neuroradiology 1974;6:254–258.

Gronblad M, Virri J, Tolonen J, et al. A controlled immunohistochemical study of inflammatory cells in disc herniation tissue. Spine 1994;19:2744–2751.

Kanerva A, Kommonen B, Gronblad M, et al. Inflammatory cells in experimental intervertebral disc injury. Spine 1997;22:2711–2715.

MacNab I. Negative disc exploration: an analysis of the causes of the nerve root involvement in sixty-eight patients. J Bone Joint Surg Am 1971;53:891.

MacNab I. The Mechanisms of Spondylogenic Pain. In C Hirsch, Y Zotterman (eds), Clinical Pain. New York: Pergamon Press, 1972;89–95.

Mehler WR. Some Observations on Secondary Ascending Afferent Systems in the Central Nervous System. In RS Knight, RP Dumke (eds), Pain: Henry Ford Hospital International Symposium. Boston: Little, Brown, 1966;11–32.

Rosomoff HL. Do herniated discs produce pain? Clin J Pain 1985;1:91–93.

Rosomoff HL. Evaluation of Surgical and Conservative Therapy of Lumbar Disc Lesions. In B Nashold, Z Hrubec (eds), Lumbar Disc Disease: A Twenty-Year Clinical Follow-Up Study. St. Louis: Mosby, 1971;1–139.

Rosomoff HL. Neural arch resection for lumbar spinal stenosis. Clin Orthop 1980;154:83.

Rosomoff HL, Johnston JDG, Gallo AE, et al. Cystometry as an adjunct in the evaluation of lumbar disc syndromes. J Neurosurg 1970;33:67.

Rosomoff HL, Johnston JDG, Gallo AE, et al. Cystometry in the evaluation of nerve root compression in the lumbar spine. Surg Gynecol Obstet 1963;117:263.

Rosomoff HL, Rosomoff RS. A Rehabilitation Physical Medicine Perspective. In MJM Cohen, JN Campbell (eds), Pain Treatment Centers at a Crossroads: A Practical and Conceptual Reappraisal, Progress in Pain Research and Management (Vol 7). Seattle: IASP Press, 1996;47–58.

Saal JS, Franson RC, Dobrow R, et al. High levels of inflammatory phospholipase A2 activity in lumbar disc herniations. Spine 1990;15:674–678.

Smyth MJ, Wright V. Sciatica and the intervertebral disc: an experimental study. J Bone Joint Surg 1958;40:1401–1418.

Spitzer WO, LeBlanc FE, Dupuis M, et al. Scientific approach to the assessment and management of activity-related spinal disorders: a monograph for clinicians. Report of the Quebec Task Force on Spinal Disorders. Spine 1987;12:51–59.

Takahashi H, Suguro T, Okazima Y, et al. Inflammatory cytokines in the herniated disc of the lumbar spine. Spine 1996;21:218–224.

Vane JR. Pain of Inflammation: An Introduction. In JJ Bonica, U Lindblom, A Iggo (eds), Advances in Pain Research and Therapy (Vol 5). New York: Raven Press, 1983;597–603.

Verbeist H. A radicular syndrome from developmental narrowing of the lumbar vertebral canal. J Bone Joint Surg 1954;36B:230.

Wall PD. Physiological Mechanisms Involved in the Production and Relief of Pain. In JJ Bonica, P Procacci, CA Pagni (eds), Recent Advances on Pain: Pathophysiology and Clinical Aspects. Springfield, Illinois: Charles C. Thomas, 1974;36–63.

Weinstein PR, Ehni G, Wilson CG. Lumbar Spondylosis: Diagnosis, Management and Surgical Treatment. Chicago: Year Book, 1977;115–132.

Chapter 15

Medicolegal Issues in Acute and Chronic Low Back Pain Management

Steven H. Sanders and R. Norman Harden

This chapter discusses important medicolegal issues and obstacles that impact the management of acute and chronic low back pain. This chapter is a partial extension of Chapter 11 in that medicolegal issues and obstacles (at least in the United States) can take on risk factor qualities that significantly influence the course of low back pain for a given patient. These legal issues may influence the clinical management of low back pain or enhance the probability that acute low back pain will develop into a chronic disabling condition, or both. Unlike Chapter 11, this chapter does not have rich scientific support. Rather, the areas discussed are based on clinical experience and common practice since the 1980s.

Specifically, this chapter focuses on discussing the legal issues and factors that tend to complicate and reduce the chances of successful resolution of an acute back pain injury, thus increasing the chances for a chronic and many times disabling condition. Although the topics discussed are far from definitive, they are representative of most of the major variables encountered in clinical practice that can significantly influence outcome. It should be noted that the term *legal* is being used loosely to include not only state and federal laws, but also all of the various factors and issues embedded in managing the low back pain patient over and above day-to-day clinical care.

FEDERAL AND STATE LAWS

At the federal level, some important basic laws are directed primarily at American workers to protect their rights and support basic medical care that clearly can influence the low back pain patient's recovery. Although all of these laws (Occupational Safety and Health Administration regulations, the Americans with Disabilities Act [ADA], and the Social Security Disability Act [SSDA]) are intended to help, not all of them do. The Occupational Safety and Health Administration guidelines have shown a slow but steady increase in comprehensiveness and threshold criteria for acceptance. On one hand, this increase theoretically improves workers' safety. On the other hand, it can inadvertently reduce the chances of an injured worker returning to his or her former job. For example, a worker who is exposed to hazardous material may be required to wear certain protective gear and administer protocols for cleanup that can become difficult or uncomfortable subsequent to a low back injury. Thus, the worker is unable to resume such a position, despite the fact that with some modification in how the job is done, safety would not be compromised.

The ADA is intended to reduce discrimination against workers who have identified disabilities. To some extent, this law has not been thoroughly tested in the courts; therefore, its real potential use is still not completely clear. It may have produced a potential false sense of security for workers returning to work after a low back injury. This is particularly true if the workers are looking for another kind of work within a company that is not aware of their prior back problems. Although one hopes that former low back pain patients would not experience hiring discrimination, the reality is that this discrimination happens daily. The ADA may give employers potential capability to reduce the willingness to change and incorporate modified work situations for returning workers. To some extent, this is due to the ADA inadvertently defining the terms of employment. The ADA states that you cannot discriminate against a person due to a disability as long as that disability does not interfere with the person's ability to do a job. Thus, if the low back pain patient cannot do the job as defined by the employer, then the ADA is harder to use in the employee's defense. It can set the occasion for the employer to be much less willing to adapt and work with the low back pain patient to modify the job situation to accommodate the return to work.

At the state level, the laws determining the hiring and firing of employees can have significant impact on the low back pain patient's ability to resume some kind of work. "At will" states provide employers with much more latitude regarding discharging individuals with and without cause. An injured low back pain worker in an "at will" state is much more likely to lose his or her job once his or her sick-leave benefits and any disability benefits run out. Unemployment is a risk factor for chronic disabling low back pain. Likewise, state statutes and regulations for the insurance industry, including workers' compensation and private health insurance, can impact the low back pain worker's ability to return to work. It is not uncommon for premium rates to increase with return of injured workers and/or lack of insurability in changing jobs or companies at the discretion of the insurance carrier. This particular issue cuts across state and federal laws with legislation in process to reduce some of this discrepancy in the form of "insurance portability" legislation to help remove this stress and potential obstacle. For the most part, this legislation is new and has not been tested. Thus, its actual potency is unknown.

LIABILITY AND LITIGATION

A number of factors and issues influence the low back pain patient injured on the job or elsewhere where there is an assumed liability on the part of someone or some company for the injury. This section provides an overview of those factors, as well as liability and process issues with which the physical medicine and rehabilitation provider may be confronted. Although the special case of workers' compensation is addressed in the section Workers' Compensation, there is some overlap with the process and potential malpractice issues reviewed here. In addition, this section offers some recommendations for dealing with the myriad of potential medicolegal problems inherent in low back pain patients.

Personal Injury Cases

Individuals involved in nonwork site injury or motor vehicle accidents often have an almost instant recognition of the need to document damages. Whenever there is an injury with potential liability from someone other than the patient, a lawsuit can become a major factor influencing the acute management and the probability of developing chronic low back pain. In this country, billions of dollars are spent, and sometimes wasted, toward this end. The potential for financial gain and "retribution" for such an injury on the patient's part can be potent and sustain low back pain complaints and presentation. The potential for financial gain should not be assumed to be the most important factor or present in all low back pain patients. In the case of personal injury, however, it should be processed and appreciated.

The nature of documenting damages or minimizing liability, or both, on the part of the patient (plaintiff) and the individual or company being sued (defendant) can be a setup to perpetuate chronicity, particularly because in most cases it is primarily dictated by third party insurers. They have no real interest in the clinical status of the injured party, but rather maximizing or minimizing settlement, depending on what side they are on. The process is a setup for multiple and megadiagnostic workups and treatments, escalating frustration and distress, stalling and delaying case resolution, and sometimes creating elaborate strategies to discredit the injured. Most of these tactics tend to impair recovery and promote chronicity. Likewise, they can significantly complicate and fragment treatment efforts. Recall that one possible risk factor is the nature of managing the acute injury, and personal injury cases can promote the wrong management approaches.

Before talking about the best approach and recommendations in dealing with personal injury cases, let us look at the actual steps involved in such litigation. Assuming the injured person obtains an attorney (the insurance companies always will), the first step is typically to attempt a settlement that does not involve filing a lawsuit. Most insurance carriers prefer to do this if they see some exposure to liability because it is typically more cost-effective. Usually, this involves the attorneys reviewing the medical reports, establishing who is at fault, and discussing possible settlement terms. In the meantime, the patient is being seen for initial evaluation, diagnostic workup, and establishment of a treatment plan. This is implemented and passage of time ensues to see if recovery and increase in function and reduction in low back pain occurs. The time frame on this initial step is anywhere from 2 to 12 months, depending on the internal protocols for the insurance carriers. If recovery does not occur within this time frame and a settlement is not reachable through the carriers in concert with the patient, then a lawsuit is typically filed by the patient. With the lawsuit, the need for documentation, either for or against damages and chronicity, significantly escalates. The physician and other health care providers may be asked to submit additional evidence or the patient may be asked to see one or more additional practitioners for independent medical evaluation, or both. This is typically done during the "discovery" phase of any litigation, meaning discovering all the facts and nature of the particular case which are necessary for the attorneys to go to trial.

Once the litigation process starts, it is difficult for the patient to effectively improve without significantly jeopardizing the integrity of the case. Thus, it is at least a momentary but very potent factor to sustain pain behaviors. During this time, the health care providers may be asked to participate in a deposition, where they actually testify before the two attorneys and a stenographer to be used later during trial or to gather more information to prepare the case, or both. Likewise, either side may use an expert witness, which typically constitutes another health care provider who is asked to review the case, examine the patient, and present his or her impressions and opinions as evidence. The treating physician may be asked to serve in this capacity. The discovery phase can last anywhere from 3 months to, more typically, 6 to 24 months, with both sides "jockeying for position" and attempting to build their cases where possible. At some point, the two parties may agree to a settlement, either before or during trial. If settlement is not reached, the trial proceeds to a verdict in civil court as determined by a jury.

Having briefly outlined the generic process, let us now look at its potential effects, along with recommendations on proper patient management. By definition, the time frame and need to demonstrate damages can be potent factors to perpetuate chronicity for the low back pain patient. Likewise, the increased potential for poor continuity and improper intensity of care can enhance chronicity. Thus, the personal injury liability and litigation process can be hazardous to the low back pain patient's health. There are, however, certain fundamentals that can help the patient get through this process without leading to chronic disabling low back pain.

First, it is essential that the focus remain on providing good clinical care to resolve the level of pain and significantly improve the patient's physical functioning. How the patient is managed clinically depends on when he or she is actually seen. This may not be at the onset, but rather later in the process as a specialty service. If that is the case, decisions must be made regarding any additional diagnostic tests and treatment based on the clinical presentation and existing adequacy of prior diagnostic workups. Judgment can be swayed by either the plaintiff or defense positions. Maintain your medical integrity. If the patient is seen shortly after the injury, it is recommended that the practice guidelines for management of acute low back pain advocated by the Agency for Health Care Policy and Research (AHCPR)[1] be followed.

A second fundamental recommendation is to help the patient maintain focus on clinical improvement and not case settlement. Although the variables discussed thus far can influence chronicity, we are clearly not seeing some magical cure and instant relief of chronic low back pain and dysfunction with case settlement.[2] These patients may show some reduction in overall emotional distress; however, most of them continue to be functionally disabled and still experience some level of now chronic low back pain. This is an important point to make with the patient. Although the lawyers, judges, insurance companies, and so forth can go home after the case is completed and forget about it, the patient may be left with a significant disabling chronic pain problem. Likewise, there may be no funds left to acquire the necessary rehabilitation to improve the patient's condition. Thus, the time to obtain and focus on improvement is not after case resolution, but before. Although this can be a frustrating and difficult process for both the health care provider and the patient, if each can remember why he or she is involved (to help the patient improve physically and restore function), this can offset some of the negative effects of the litigation process. Finally, as was noted in Chapter 11, early referral to a specialty interdisciplinary pain rehabilitation program can significantly improve the patient's chances for meaningful improvement, despite ongoing litigation issues.

Attorney's Agenda

It is important to appreciate the motivation and intent of the plaintiff and defendant attorneys in personal injury litigation. These motives can significantly influence the development of a chronic disabling condition. This is not to say that it is the intent of the legal process and the attorneys involved to produce chronic disabling back pain; however, inadvertently, this is a real possibility. Understanding the fundamental reason for this involves appreciating the primary goals and objectives within the legal system. These objectives include maximizing protection of the client's legal rights while maximizing the financial outcome of the case. For the plaintiff (patient) attorney, the objective involves obtaining the highest dollar settlement or benefits, or both, possible. In contingency cases, this is reinforcing for the patient's attorney. For the defendant attorney, it involves minimizing damages and dollar amounts, thus saving money. For both attorneys, the longer and more complicated litigation becomes, the higher the fees. These goals can come into direct conflict with the low back pain patient's ability to significantly improve function. The more loss of function over time and higher pain and discomfort demonstrated, the higher the potential damage settlement to the plaintiff (patient) and the more the financial rewards for his or her attorney. This translates into messages of maintaining a chronic disabled condition and maximizing medical care and expenses, which figures into determining damages. The patient cannot improve while maintaining such a state. This sets the condition for developing chronic disabling low back pain.

On the defendant's side, the attorney may delay the process even further by extending the discovery period to "wear the patient down." Assuming the patient has not been able to sustain any ongoing employment because of the injury or does not have any disability coverage, the loss of income over time can be a potent factor in reducing the patient's willingness to proceed with the suit for months to years. Thus, for the defendant attorney, the longer and more complicated the case, the more fees and potential for lower damages if the patient becomes more willing to eventually settle to stop the process. Again, the intent is not to "hurt" the patient, but the effect can set up two diametrically opposed goals with regard to clinical improvement.

For the health care provider, the most appropriate position to take is to continue to encourage the patient to take care of himself or herself physically and emotionally, leading to improvement in long-term function. This message should also be communicated, whenever possible, to the attorneys. The concept of winning the case and not losing the client should be emphasized.

Managed Health Care

There have been increasing liability and contractual trends within managed health care that can significantly influence the clinical outcome for low back pain patients. With the general position that managed health care has focused on cost reduction, it is not surprising that the overall effect has been to foster minimal and fragmented care. To some extent, this effect could be positive if it resulted in offering more conservative and cost-effective treatment for acute low back pain. However, there has been a tendency to limit cost for those patients showing more chronic pain profiles, resulting in inadequate and insufficient treatment with increased potential for development of chronic disability. Theoretically, the physician makes the determination regarding the treatment plan. In actuality, most managed health care contracts have maintained strong control over definitions of "medical necessity." Thus, in an effort to reduce cost, denial for interdisciplinary pain rehabilitation has become commonplace.[3] Likewise, the cost savings appeal of less expensive pharmacologic or one-time procedural "fixes" for the developing chronic disabling low back pain patient have been promoted without the benefit of positive outcomes for these modalities. The result of all of these factors is to significantly increase the chances of the patient developing chronic disability with low back pain.

There are some changes occurring in the managed health care marketplace to offset this trend. These changes are occurring primarily at the state level and involve increasing the patients' rights to appeal and actually hold the managed health care company liable for decisions regarding care. In addition, a movement is occurring at the federal level to challenge the Employee Retirement Income Security Act (ERISA), which has exempted many of the managed care companies from responsibility and liability in influencing the nature of medical care for patients whom they are supposed to cover. Thus, all is not lost in this area, with momentum building to protect patients' rights both at the state and federal level. One recent movement is the Patient Access to Responsible Care Act (PARCA), which is being considered in the U.S. Congress.

As far as recommendations for health care providers who deal with managed health care companies, the following points should be remembered. First, to state the obvious, read your contracts. Particularly, read those sections that define medical necessity and outline who makes that determination, as well as delineation of both the provider and patient appeal process. These sections should define who is liable and responsible for what, with the managed health care company taking responsibility along with the provider when appropriate. The provider should not leave the terms of the contract up to the managed health care company. It may be necessary to enlist the help of an attorney in this matter, given the changing nature of the market and laws. Be sure there is a defined appeals process that has some legitimacy. The core issue involves a denial of care that the provider believes is necessary and the managed health care company says is not necessary. This denial of care puts the provider in a difficult clinical and, many times, legal position. Again, the primary motives from the managed health care company are typically to save money, not effectively treat the patient. Such mentality is penny wise and pound foolish if it interferes with the care necessary to prevent chronic disabling low back pain. It is, nevertheless, the nature of the marketplace.

Providers should not expect a great deal of cooperation from the managed health care company to go along with their recommendation once it has been ruled "not medically necessary." In cases in which the low back pain patient falls into the high-risk category for developing chronic disabling pain, the provider should document this categorization and send an appeal letter to the managed health care company objecting to their position. Likewise, the patient should be encouraged to file an appeal to overturn this position. Although the provider runs the risk of being dropped from the managed health care company's provider list, increasing litigation challenges such an action if based solely on making an appeal. It is important for the health care provider to make a clinical position statement, document this statement, and encourage the patient to do the same through the appeal process. This is good practice, and also protects against unnecessary malpractice issues. It is important to be a patient advocate with regard to what is medically necessary. Usage of any and all recognized practice guidelines can help make a rational, empirically based case.[1,4] Do not sit idly by with patients who are at high risk for developing chronic disabling low back pain. When a provider does this, everyone loses.

In general, the legal rights of the low back pain patient and regulations for managed health care companies are in the process of significant change and hopefully improvement. A host of state and federal laws are being reviewed to protect patients from discriminatory cost savings at the expense of care and access areas. Although the outcome of this legislative movement is not yet certain, some good could emerge from it.[5]

Medical Malpractice

The subtle and sometimes blatant influences of medical malpractice risks are not unique to managing low back pain patients. However, in light of the probable or possible risk factors addressed in Chapter 11, malpractice issues do influence the management, and, therefore, the likelihood of low back pain developing into a chronic disabling condition. In spite of our best efforts and wanting to think otherwise, the underlying threat of a malpractice suit can insidiously affect practice decisions. This usually takes the form of excessive workups for acute low back pain to rule out serious spine pathology or other physical etiology. Because such a workup is a probable risk factor, it can lead to perpetuating the problem. Likewise, fear of medical malpractice suits can result in placing too many return to normal activity restrictions and delaying reactivation for too long.

Although malpractice risks cannot be ignored, the health care provider can do certain things to minimize the risk while inadvertently perpetuating an acute low back pain problem. It is recommended that, whenever possible, the overall guidelines proposed by the Agency for Health Care Policy and Research[1] be used in managing the acute back pain patient. These guidelines promote a judicious diagnostic workup and conservative care for a proper period of time. They are less likely to promote the development of a chronic disabling condition. Likewise, because they represent federally sponsored national guidelines, they can be used as sound justification and corroboration of practice. Embedded in these guidelines are recommendations to offer conservative treatment over time and promote reactivation as much as possible. This philosophy also helps to guide practice against excessive activity restrictions. The guidelines also promote moving to more comprehensive evaluation and assessment within an interdisciplinary pain rehabilitation model if the patient is not recovering within a reasonably short period of time.

The issue of excessive activity restriction lacks nationally recognized guidelines for direction in clinical practice to offset malpractice risk. For the moment, the best recommendation is to use objective functional capacity evaluation information, as available, to determine true restrictions. Restrictions should not be applied based solely on subjective "medical opinion," if possible. The more restrictions that are not justified, the less likely the patient will be able to return to work. As discussed in Chapter 11, unemployment is a risk factor, increasing the chances of chronic disabling low back pain. Thus, using as reliable and valid an assessment of restrictions and functional limitations as possible reduces the chances of inadvertently overrestricting a patient for fear of more injury in returning to work and a subsequent malpractice suit. Although functional capacity evaluations are far from an exact and completely objective science, this information can be useful in making suggestions about functional restrictions in a clinically appropriate fashion, without becoming too defensive regarding the potential for a malpractice suit.

With respect to minimizing malpractice concerns with the chronic disabled low back pain patient, referral to an interdisciplinary pain rehabilitation program that follows guidelines endorsed by the American Academy of Physical Medicine and Rehabilitation is highly recommended.[4] If referral is not possible, then use of these empirically based guidelines, as closely as possible, is highly recommended. Again, although use of these guidelines does not provide a guarantee against malpractice, it can reduce the risk and deal with any issues that arise.

Having highlighted some important liability and litigation issues, let us now look in more detail at the special circumstances within workers' compensation, Social Security Disability (SSD), and private disability, which can further influence the occurrence of acute and, more importantly, the development of chronic disabling low back pain.

WORKERS' COMPENSATION, SOCIAL SECURITY DISABILITY, AND PRIVATE DISABILITY

Because of the potential depth and frequency of encounter, the special influences and situations within the workers' compensation, SSD, and private disability systems need individual attention. As has been the case throughout this chapter, the focus is not on specific nuts and bolts of the systems, but rather on highlighting and discussing major factors that can influence the occurrence of acute or development of chronic disabling low back pain.

Workers' Compensation

As already noted, 80–90% of individuals sustaining a work-related low back injury successfully return to their prior jobs. Individuals who do not return to work, however, can face a myriad of issues within workers' compensation systems across states that may influence the development of chronic disabling low back pain. Although cause and effect have not been demonstrated at the empirical level within clinical practice, the effect of workers' compensation on low back pain patients is seen on a daily basis. Although each state has its own workers' compensation law and system with a multitude of variations across states, some fundamental principles and factors can be found.

In general, all of the factors discussed within the personal injury liability arena also apply to low back pain patients receiving workers' compensation. There may be more statutory structure within a state's rules and regulations about second opinions and documentation; however, the factors involved in case building and defending (limiting liability) are present within a workers' compensation low back pain case. In addition, unlike personal injury cases, the low back pain patient injured on the job is eligible to receive wage replacement. This can be a significant reinforcer of pain behavior under certain circumstances, particularly if the individual loses his or her job in the process.

As Table 11.1 in Chapter 11 notes, receiving compensation is a risk factor for the development of chronic disabling low back pain. This should not be viewed as simply "paying people to be sick."[6] In some cases, it can be part of trapping the patient within a system that does not allow any exit without a great deal of struggle, especially in those cases where there is an unfriendly return to work environment from the employers in the community. This is made even worse in the states in which there are no time limits on workers' compensation coverage. Although more states are passing legislation to limit such coverage, this has not occurred across all states.

Another significant influence on workers' compensation is the degree of control by the underwriting insurance company in association with the employer over treatment for the injured worker. In some states, insurance carriers and employers are able to strongly influence whether patients receive quality, effective care for their low back pain problems. So, there is even less choice than seen in the typical managed health care arena. This may lead not only to a lack of continuity of care but also to significant escalation in distress, anger, and, at times, depression on the part of the patient. These are all known risk factors for the development of chronic disabling low back pain. Thus, the workers' compensation system can exacerbate or induce a number of the factors known to be associated with chronic disability. In addition, the 10–20% of injured workers who do not improve within 3–6 months gradually move from an anticipated manageable financial expenditure to a potentially major financial liability for the insurance carrier and employer—In other words, from someone injured on the job who needs help to recover and return efficiently to work to an angry, depressed patient with potential for ever increasing and long-term financial liability.

Although the health care provider is helpless to make any immediate change in a state's workers' compensation system, the same recommendations in the liability and litigation section are appropriate here. That is, stay focused on what is important for meaningful physical and emotional improvement, resist the pressure from the carrier and employer to dictate treatment, use practice guidelines wherever possible, get the patient involved in interdisciplinary pain rehabilitation as soon as possible, and be careful not to excessively restrict the patient regarding work-related behaviors.

Social Security Disability

Although the workers' compensation system is predominantly state dictated, SSD falls under federal jurisdiction. Theoretically, it should be uniform across states. Although this is true on paper, the interpretation of the law can vary dramatically from state to state. By definition, the low back pain patient must be chronically unable to do "any gainful work" to qualify for SSD. Thus, several influential factors are embedded within the SSD system that can affect the patient before receiving this benefit. For patients who see SSD as their best hope for financial and medical assistance, the system requires them to be chronically and totally disabled. This means disabled from doing any type of consistent work for pay for at least 12 months.

The probability of actually getting an award the first time is extremely low for most low back pain patients. Thus, to pursue the system further, the patient must then appeal the ruling, which can take at least another 6 months or longer. As with the liability and litigation factors, this mandates continuation of total disability during all this time to qualify. Although the system was not intended to work this way, low back pain patients who are willing to make a second or third appeal over a 2–3 year time frame typically stand an excellent chance of finally getting SSD. This may become a self-fulfilling prophecy. The patient has to be chronically disabled to get the award, and the process of getting the award forces him or her to be chronically disabled. Even if there is a reasonable chance for a significant increase in function and productivity, pursuit of SSD makes this chance virtually impossible.

Once a patient receives SSD for chronic low back pain, it is extremely unlikely that the patient will ever get off disability. The system does not allow a true opportunity for gradual re-entry into the work setting without major financial consequences. Additionally, employers are strongly reluctant to hire someone who is, or recently has been, on SSD, the ADA notwithstanding. In short, SSD is a potential breeding ground for chronic disabling low back pain in its current form. This is not to say that the system is fundamentally bad or does not help a great many individuals who truly need it. Rather, the steps and chronicity involved in getting an award, coupled with the extreme difficulty escaping the system once an individual is in it, can be potent factors influencing the establishment and perpetuation of chronic disability.

As with workers' compensation, the health care provider is not in a position to change SSD. However, it is recommended that, at the very least, everything should be done to help the patient avoid pursuing this course of action just as a "safety net." Specifically, it is important to do everything possible to enhance function and return to productive behavior. Although determination of SSD is a legal, not medical, decision, the health care provider can educate the patient regarding the extreme level of functional limitations required to enter the system, and that the patient will likely become dependent on SSD once there. By the same token, if it is clear that the patient is totally disabled with little, if any, chance for returning to some kind of work, it is appropriate to support this position. There can still be some benefit in reducing the fallout from chronic disabling low back pain by reducing the distress and financial or emotional uncertainty factors for a truly disabled patient. This can translate into reduction of the need for ongoing health care once in SSD.

Private Disability

Many low back pain patients are covered under private disability insurance, either through their work or individual policies. The potential and actual influence of private disability coverage is not as clear as seen within workers' compensation and SSD. Most private disability policies have a different definition of disability that focuses more on a person's ability to do the work they were primarily engaged in at the time of their illness or injury. Thus, the requirement of chronic disabling low back pain is not present for many of these private policies. Likewise, the time when the policy is initiated is typically much shorter, ranging anywhere from 3 to 6 months. These policies can also have a transitional process for return to work to reduce the financial burden on the patient. Thus, private disability policies may not be so compelling with regard to chronic disabling low back pain.

An area in which private disability may be more potent in setting the stage for chronic disabling low back pain is the rate of wage replacement. Typically, these policies are written to continue paying at two-thirds of the worker's current salary. Likewise, this wage replacement can be tax exempt. In addition, most policies have a premium waiver clause so the premiums are paid as long as the person maintains his or her disability status.

A second potential area to enhance the probability for developing chronic disabling low back pain is the vagueness in defining disability. Each policy typically has its own requirement for defining disability, with much less rigor and structure in gathering information to determine this than is seen with SSD. In many cases, it simply requires that the treating physician sign a form stating that the patient is unable to perform his or her work. No additional documentation or corroboration may be required. Such a subjective approach makes it much easier to "document" and maintain a state of chronic disabling low back pain. Once on private disability, the review process can be much less stringent than it is in workers' compensation or SSD. Thus, if the patient is so inclined and given the level of wage replacement, remaining in the private disability category can be quite appealing, particularly if the policy gives latitude to continue to engage in some kind of work for pay to further supplement income.

Although the health care provider also cannot change the private disability process, he or she is in a position to significantly influence the database determining disability. Likewise, he or she can assist the patient in maximizing function and return to productive behavior whenever possible. As far as determining the level of disability, it is recommended that the rehabilitation physician request as much information as possible about the nature of the patient's job, including specific physical and stamina demands. Simply checking a question on an insurance form, such as "Is this patient disabled to do their current job?—yes or no," is not good practice without clear delineation of the actual demands of the job and as much objective information as possible regarding the patient's ability. More private disability carriers are becoming much more proactive and aggressive when trying to truly rehabilitate the chronic disabled low back pain patient. The health care provider should reinforce these efforts whenever possible.

MORE PRACTICAL CLINICAL GUIDELINES

The pain rehabilitation clinician must serve many masters. The traditional sacrosanct patient and physician relationship is a charming historic note. Now payors and attorneys must be included in the decision-making team, and all players have rights and responsibilities. The majority of chronic low back pain patients should retain counsel to assist with the complexities of the compensation system in disability and personal injury. Forensic law is increasingly complex, and the necessity of attorney involvement is likely to increase, rather than decrease, over time.

In the era of managed health care and more fiscal accountability, the payor is assuming an increasingly active role in deciding who gets what type of health care. The "bottom line" philosophy is often counterproductive for chronic low back pain patients, and payors should be educated to not be penny wise and pound foolish. It is the clinician's responsibility to not only educate the payor of the value of interdisciplinary care, but also to help demonstrate promises and benefits of this care. Likewise, physicians have proven over time that they are unable to control costs. Thus, they should be sensitive to the need for externally managed health care and accept responsibility for negotiating cost-effective care. Physicians must also resist the temptation to unnecessarily pursue the highest possible technology, or treatments that hold the best remuneration.

Diagnosis

Chronic low back pain is a biologic, psychological, and sociologic phenomenon. It is the responsibility of the clinician to accurately identify the lesion or the problem in each of these areas. In terms of the biomedical diagnosis, it is important that the best possible taxonomy for diagnosis be used. The International Association for the Study of Pain Task Force on Taxonomy has developed such a criteria, called *Classification of Chronic Pain.*[7] Other best sources of diagnostic criteria are the *Classification and Diagnostic Criteria for Headache Disorders, Cranial Neuralgias and Facial Pain* (of the headache classification committee of the International Headache Society)[8] and the *Primer on the Rheumatic Diseases* published by the Arthritis Foundation.[9] The diagnostic categories as proposed by the *International Classification of Diseases, Ninth Edition* are suboptimal. Although they often must be included for billing purposes, these categories should be supplemented by the more rigorous criteria as mentioned.

The psychological diagnoses should be based on the most current version of the *Diagnostic and Statistical Manual* of the American Psychiatric Association.[10] The sociologic diagnoses have no formal criteria schemes, and there should be a commonsense determination made by the clinician and the vocational rehabilitation specialist. An enumeration of the issues sociologically suffices.

These diagnoses must be made at evaluation, updated throughout the course of treatment, and especially at the end of the formal course of treatment. It is important that follow-up be planned for a patient, and this be discussed as part of the goal structure. Because decreasing health care use and time-limited services are required by the payor, it is important that the follow-up plan be specified. It is equally important that the formal criteria-based diagnoses be updated at each contact if appropriate.

Goal Setting

In addition to educating payors and attorneys, it is essential that the physician constantly communicate the prognosis and expectations to these players, as well as to patients and their families. Communication and negotiation are key, and they must be frequent, realistic, and explicit.

Decreased pain is always a goal in pain management programs. It must be communicated, however, that a "cure" or quick fix is rarely possible. Patients and their families, as well as payors, should understand that in most cases it is unrealistic to pursue freedom from pain as a realistic rehabilitation goal. Everyone should understand that the goal is pain management and the development of rational strategies to minimize the pain. Payors sometimes erroneously assume that a patient's report of ongoing pain after a program signifies lack of success. It is essential that the clinician has a realistic idea of what is achievable, knows what the track record of his or her program is for each diagnosis, and communicates these goals to all involved.

Another goal implicit to interdisciplinary pain management is functional optimization. This may take the pleasant role of therapeutic recreation; however, it also usually must include vocational rehabilitation. Because work is a crucial and intrinsic part our identity as humans, a return to work has great value in terms of a patient's sense of self-esteem. Additionally, there are financial benefits to the patient, and return to work is always a requisite of workers' compensation carriers. Return to work also has value for federal disability systems, and, if it is possible and realistic, a methodical assessment of a patient's work aspirations and capabilities should be undertaken. The process should be laid out for the patients and their families, and begun by a general vocational assessment of skills and strengths. The expectations of the employer and compensation carrier should be included in the decision of the vocational direction. Return to work with the same job for the same employer is always the ultimate goal; however, that is not always feasible. Return to work for the same employer, but a different job, is nearly as valuable. Complicated vocational retraining is expensive, and is a therapeutic path that compensation and disability carriers try to avoid. A comprehensive job description; measurement of the worker's capacities for that work; occupational therapy and work hardening for that job; and, ultimately, work simulation (either in the laboratory or in the workplace) are the idealized processes. It is critically important, forensically and in terms of delivering the goals that have been set, that the clinician carefully document the entire process and unequivocally release the patient to work when it is appropriate. This release to work should never come as a surprise to the patient; the goal of return to work should be discussed in the evaluation phase.

Interdisciplinary pain rehabilitation programs are best able to deliver the standard of care for low back pain diagnoses. All players in the scenario need closure, and it is especially important for patients to believe that they have had everything that medical science can provide for them to get on with their lives. The payor needs closure so that he or she can minimize unnecessary ongoing health care expenditures in the fruitless pursuit of unrealistic goals, and the attorneys need closure so that they can obtain their fee. Once the "standard of care" has been provided, the patient can be declared at maximum medical improvement. This standard of care is a nebulous entity that is variously determined on the basis of the community, the national or the international standard. The standard can be determined through scientific literature and textbooks; however, because pain research is not sufficiently advanced to have definitive answers for many questions, anecdotal evidence and empirical experience often determine the institutional standard of care. The standard, however, should be interdisciplinary because unidisciplinary programs are inadequate here.

Achieving maximum medical improvement should be identified as a goal at the evaluation, and it is essential that the clinician document and declare this when it is appropriate. This has value for the patients and their families because it allows them to understand the residual disability that they have and to begin the process of planning for their long-term future. If the patient believes that the medical community has done everything it can reasonably do to help and that they have all the self-management tools that allow them to do everything they can do themselves to manage their pain, then the process of closure is natural and acceptable to all players.

Impairment and Disability

Impairment is defined as *an alteration of an individual's health status* and is assessed by medical means. It is a deviation of a body part or organ system and its functioning. This can be either temporary or permanent, which is defined as *a static process that is unlikely to change, despite further medical or surgical therapy.* It can also be a loss or abnormality of psychological function.

Disability is defined as *an alteration of an individual's capacity to meet personal, social, or occupational demands because of an impairment.* It implies that the individual is unable to accomplish certain tasks, which can be any activity of daily living, specifically work. These definitions and guidelines for determining impairment can be found in *Guides to the Evaluation of Permanent Impairment* by the American Medical Association.[11] The World Health Organization also defines impairment and disability.[12]

Testimony

The clinician is often called to testify in legal proceedings involving his or her patients. This process should not be considered intimidating, and is an opportunity to clarify and referee issues for the patient to allow closure. The principles of testimony are that the clinicians should be as clear as possible, avoid the use of jargon, and stick to the record. It is an opportunity to portray the facts in a fashion that allows a fair and justifiable compensation to occur, but to prevent the system from continuing to support and maintain pain behaviors. Testimony actually represents an important and valuable milestone. With testimony and case closure, the patient can get on with his or her life without reservation.

KEYS TO REDUCING LEGAL OBSTACLES AND ISSUES

Some broad-based changes have already been outlined elsewhere,[6] which could significantly reduce the influence of legal obstacles and issues in managing low back pain patients. There continues to be need for reform regarding malpractice and liability issues to moderate the sometimes excessive financial rewards for both the patient and attorney. This could come in the form of increasing the requirement for arbitration, as opposed to litigation, and reducing the percentage awarded to attorneys as part of any settlement. In addition, more state and federal statutes dealing with managed health care activities are badly needed. Such legislation is increasing, with more expected.[13]

There is also a need to increase individual awareness and responsibility for avoiding the onset of acute low back pain and the development of chronic disability. In the United States, this idea has been hampered by an increasing view by consumers that state and federal health–related services are entitlements versus benefits. Such a view has a tendency to reduce the individual's willingness to take more responsibility for his or her health problems, fostering expectations that someone else is responsible for fixing the problem, and that the patient is entitled to such care and compensation. Again, the need here is for balance, not either/or.

In the final analysis, regardless of the best efforts from health care providers and legislative mandates, it is the individual patient and his or her willingness to actively participate in the process of low back pain management that is at the core of success. The balance to be achieved is one of offering legislative protection without encouraging excessive dependency on the legal or medical system to fix or be responsible for the low back pain problem.

REFERENCES

1. Agency for Health Care Policy and Research. Clinical Practice Guidelines for Acute Back Pain Management. Rockville, Maryland: U.S. Department of Health and Human Services, 1994.
2. Mendelson G. Compensation and chronic pain. Pain 1992;48:121–123.
3. Dotleib BS. Chronic pain treatment centers and managed care: starting to work toward the same goals? APS Bulletin 1997;7:7–9.
4. Sanders SH, Harden RN, Benson SE, Vicente PJ. Clinical practice guidelines for chronic non-malignant pain syndrome patients II: an evidenced-based approach. J Back Musculoskeletal Rehab 1989;12:1–12.

5. Gemignani J. Business battles managed care mandates. Business and Health 1998;March:9.
6. Sanders SH. Why Do Most Patients with Chronic Pain Not Return to Work? In MJM Cohen, JN Campbell (eds), Pain Treatment Centers at a Crossroads: Practical and Conceptual Reappraisal. Seattle: IASP Press, 1996;193–202.
7. Merskey H, Bogduk N. Classification of Chronic Pain: Descriptions of Chronic Pain Syndromes and Definitions of Pain Terms (2nd ed). Seattle: IASP Press, 1994.
8. Cephalalgia: Classification and Diagnostic Criteria for Headache Disorders, Cranial Neuralgias and Facial Pain. An International Journal of Headache (Vol 8). Headache Classification Committee of the International Headache Society. Oslo: Norwegian University Press, 1988;[Suppl 7].
9. Schumacher HR, Klippel JH, Koopman WJ. Primer on the Rheumatic Diseases (10th ed). Atlanta: Arthritis Foundation, 1993.
10. American Psychiatric Association. Diagnostic and Statistical Manual (4th ed). Washington, DC: American Psychiatric Association, 1994.
11. AMA Guides to the Evaluation of Permanent Impairment (4th ed). Chicago: American Medical Association, 1995.
12. International Classification of Impairments, Disabilities, and Handicaps, World Health Organization, 1980.
13. Olsen GG. Proposals insuring quality medical care while instating federal regulations. Rehab Manage 1998;February:112–113.

Index